INTERFERON
Theory and Applications

INTERFERON
Theory and Applications

V. D. Solov'ev

Director, Department of Virology
Central Postgraduate Medical Institute
Moscow, USSR

and

T. A. Bektemirov

Department of Virology
Central Postgraduate Medical Institute
Moscow, USSR

**Translated from Russian by
Basil Haigh**

**With a Foreword by
George J. Galasso**

Head, Antiviral Substances Program and
Chief, Infectious Disease Branch
National Institute of Allergy and Infectious Diseases
National Institutes of Health
Bethesda, Maryland

PLENUM PRESS • NEW YORK–LONDON

Library of Congress Cataloging in Publication Data

Solov'ev, Valentin Dmitrievich, 1907-
  Interferon; theory and applications.

  Translation of Interferon v teorii i praktike mediŝiny.
  1. Interferons. I. Bektemirov, Tagir Abdullaevich, joint author. II. Title. [DNLM:
1. Interferon. 2. Viral interference. QW160 S689i 1973]
QR187.5.S6413   576'.64   73-79428
ISBN-13: 978-1-4684-2033-3   e-ISBN-13: 978-1-4684-2031-9
DOI: 10.1007/978-1-4684-2031-9

Valentin Dmitrievich Solov'ev, eminent Soviet virologist, Academician of the Academy of Medical Sciences of the USSR, Professor and Doctor of Medical Sciences and State Prizewinner, was born in 1907. In the 1930's he took part in a study of the etiology and epidemiology of tick-borne encephalitis, for which, along with a group of scientists, he was awarded a State Prize. In addition to his comprehensive study of influenza, V. D. Solov'ev has made important contributions to the theory and practice of smallpox vaccination and to the question of rabies control. He has made equally important contributions in other branches of virology: in the development of vaccines against poliomyelitis, in the study of intestinal and respiratory virus infections, and in recent years in the study of the general virology and immunology of virus infections.

Tagir Abdullaevich Bektemirov, Doctor of Medical Sciences, was born in 1929. His principal fields of research are the epidemiology of rickettsioses and, in particular, experimental virology. He has devoted much time to the study of the formation and action of interferon from both the experimental and clinical standpoints and has made a significant contribution to the analysis of this problem. He is actively interested in the training of young virologists and gives a course of lectures at the Department of Virology. At present he is pursuing his research into the problem of interferon at the Department of Virology, Central Postgraduate Medical Institute, Moscow.

The original Russian text, published by Meditsina Press in Moscow in 1970, has been corrected by the authors for the present edition. The translation is published under an agreement with Mezhdunarodnaya Kniga, the Soviet book export agency.

INTERFERON V TEORII I PRAKTIKE MEDITSINY
Интерферон в теории и практике медицины

V. D. Solov'ev and T. A. Bektemirov
СОЛОВЬЕВ ВАЛЕНТИН ДМИТРИЕВИЧ
БЕКТЕМИРОВ ТАГИР АБДУЛЛАЕВИЧ

© 1973 Plenum Press, New York
A Division of Plenum Publishing Corporation
227 West 17th Street, New York, N.Y. 10011

United Kingdom edition published by Plenum Press, London
A Division of Plenum Publishing Company, Ltd.
Davis House (4th Floor), 8 Scrubs Lane, Harlesden, London, NW10 6SE, England

Foreword

Interferon has been and continues to be one of the more fascinating substances produced by apparently all animals in response to particular stimuli. It has led to major revisions in concepts of cellular immunity and theories on the recovery of multicellular systems from viral infection. Since its discovery, interferon has held the interest of the molecular biologist, and definitive answers as to its clinical value are close at hand.

The following treatise is an attempt by the authors to present a complete picture of the many aspects of interferon. Having recently had the privilege of visiting the laboratories of the authors and several others of our Soviet colleagues working in the interferon field, I was most impressed with the amount of research being done in this area. Since a great deal of this work is published in the Russian language, there is unfortunately a time lag until it can be received and translated. We are therefore most grateful to Drs. Solov'ev and Bektemirov for having produced this impressive work which offers the opportunity to review the entire field and, very importantly, some of the work being done by our Soviet counterparts, and also to Plenum Publishing Corporation for providing the English translation.

Work on the mechanism of interferon induction, the relative role of the cellular constituents, and work in cell-free systems and the molecular mechanism of the antiviral action of interferon continues to excite scientists in the field. However, one of the major goals must continue to be the role of interferon in clinical medicine. Our Soviet colleagues are currently using exogenous human leucocyte interferon clinically against a variety of viral diseases. A cooperative effort by American and British scientists has also conclusively demonstrated that exogenous interferon has a prophylactic role in upper respiratory diseases. It is currently under investigation in the United States in double-blind studies against serious viral infection. Although there is still some question as to the proper dosage and whether increased dosage will be therapeutic as well as prophylactic, it does appear that interferon will prove to be of clinical value.

We are most grateful to Drs. Solov'ev and Bektemirov for the preparation of this significant contribution.

George J. Galasso, Ph. D.
Head, Antiviral Substances Program
        and
Chief, Infectious Disease Branch
National Institute of Allergy and
        Infectious Diseases
National Institutes of Health
Bethesda, Maryland 20014, USA

Preface to the American Edition

In the introduction to the book "Interferons" edited by N. B. Finter (North-Holland Publishing Company, Amsterdam), published in 1966, Alick Isaacs stated that "interferon was born 9 years ago, of parents whose family name is viral interference and who are now 30 years old — a very suitable age for parents of a 9-year-old child." Before turning to the question of interferon, it must therefore be remembered that the first account of interference was given in 1935, when Magrassi presented evidence of competition between encephalitogenic and nonencephalitogenic strains of herpes virus in rabbits. Hoskins described experiments in which a neurotropic strain of yellow fever virus had a protective effect in monkeys infected with a viscerotropic strain of the same virus. In 1937, Findlay and MacCallum obtained evidence that the existence of this form of virus interference is a unique phenomenon independent of the specific immune response of the body, and that mutual competition between and inhibition of viruses takes place with both antigenically similar and antigenically different viruses.

Later work by Henle (1943), Huang (1943), and Lennette and Koprovski (1946) extended these observations and obtained evidence that the phenomenon of interference exists in developing chick embryos, in tissue explants, and in cultures *in vitro* . The phenomenon has three chief components: the virus inducing interference, known as the interfering (or inducing) virus, the cell or cell system in which resistance develops, and the virus to be inhibited, known as the challenge virus. The interfering virus need not necessarily reproduce, as is shown by the fact that ultraviolet irradiation, heating, or treating in other ways to deprive the virus of its infectivity leaves intact its properties as an inducing virus.

A criterion of interference is partial or complete loss of the ability of the challenge virus to reproduce. The mechanism of this new and very interesting phenomenon remained unexplained until 1957, when Isaacs, working at the National Institute for Medical Research in London, together with the Swiss virologist Jean Lindenmann, proved the existence of a hitherto unknown special substance of decisive importance in interference. Using heat-inactivated influenza virus for this purpose, and a piece of chorioallantoic membrane as the cell substrate, they obtained interference to the challenge influenza virus when the inducer virus (and later the tissue substrate) was removed from the system, while fresh pieces of tissue again showed resistance to the challenge virus. These workers postulated that this resistance is due to a factor present in the fluid. Subsequent experiments confirmed this hypothesis and the factor was called "interferon."

Sixteen years have elapsed since those days. To continue with Isaacs' metaphor, the 9-year-old child has become a youth. The phenomenon discovered by Isaacs and Lindenmann can now be numbered among the major biological achievements of the mid-twentieth century.

This discovery soon attracted the attention of scientists in many different specialities and since then more than a thousand investigations into various aspects of the study of interferon have been published. The formation and mechanism of action of interferon have been studied and are being studied at the present time at the level of macroorganism and cell and by the methods of molecular biology. It is this last line of research which has revealed which aspects of the virus—cell system influenced these processes and how they do so.

The discovery of interferon has contributed to the development of our knowledge of interaction between viruses and cells. Ability to induce interferon has been shown to be a property not only of viruses, but also of other microorganisms and of their metabolic products and of various chemical compounds and has taken the problem far beyond the limits of experimental virology. Interferon must also be regarded as a chemotherapeutic agent, acting on both infectious and oncogenic viruses, thus paving the way for its therapeutic use.

The prophylactic value of interferon in many virus infections is now established beyond all doubt, and its important role in their pathogenesis and in antiviral immunity is firmly established. The role of the reticuloendothelial system of the host organism in interferon formation has broadened our knowledge of immunity and brought together the concepts of humoral and cellular factors into a single and unified system of immunological reactivity of the host organism.

The authors of the monograph greeted the suggestion made by their American colleagues that the book be translated into English and published in the United States with a feeling of great satisfaction. In the monograph they have attempted to give a systematic account of the existing information on interferon obtained both from the extensive literature and from the authors' own observations made over a period of several years in the laboratories directed by Academician of the Academy of Medical Sciences of the USSR V. D. Solov'ev.

We hope that the publication of this book in the United States will be useful both for the exchange of knowledge between American and Soviet scientists and also because its publication is in the spirit of the intergovernmental agreements signed by the Heads of Government of the United States and the USSR regarding joint efforts toward the solution of current health problems.

V.D.S.
T.A.B.

Preface

It is now 13 years since the late Alick Isaacs, with his assistant Jean Lindenmann, working at the National Institute of Medical Research in London on the study of the mechanism of interference in experimental influenza, found that this phenomenon is due to the action of a special factor which was first obtained from the chorioallantois of developing chick embryos, and later from the cells of many species of animals after exposure to various viruses and virus nucleic acids. The factor responsible for interference proved to be a hitherto unknown low-molecular-weight protein with antiviral action. It was given the name "interferon."

The discovery of interferon aroused great interest in scientific circles and its importance is on a par with many of the leading scientific advances in the field of biology and medicine made in the middle of this century.

Interferon formation and the mechanism of action of interferon have been studied at the level of the organism and cell and also by the methods of molecular biology. Research in this last field has shown which aspects of the virus—cell system are concerned and how they influence these processes. At the same time interferon is used as a criterion for assessment of the behavior of antimetabolites and of agents which inhibit or stimulate the formation of cellular nucleic acids and proteins, and it has thus contributed to the development of knowledge of interaction between viruses and cells. For example, in the first stage of reproduction of the virus of a vaccine new enzymes, including DNA-polymerase and thymidine kinase used for synthesis of virus DNA, are formed in the cells. Interferon inhibits the production of these virus-induced enzymes without affecting the metabolism of the host cell and it thus promotes differentiation of the viral and cellular functions.

The great importance of the lymphoid tissues in interferon formation adds to our knowledge of immunity and welds the concepts of humoral and cellular factors into a single and integral system of immunological reactivity. In addition, the discovery that interferon can be induced not only by viruses but also by other microorganisms and by certain chemical compounds extends the problem of interferon far beyond the confines of experimental virology.

Interferon must also be regarded as a chemotherapeutic substance acting on infectious and oncogenic viruses, so that there are prospects for its therapeutic use. The prophylactic activity of interferon in certain virus infections is already firmly established and is of considerable interest to epidemiologists and to those responsible for organizing the control of epidemics.

More than a thousand papers have been published in these various fields and the many experimental facts obtained as a result require generalization and evaluation.

Soviet investigators have paid considerable attention to the problem of interferon. The monograph now offered to the reader is an attempt to give a systematic account of the factual data described in the literature and of the authors' own observations made during the last few years in the Department of Virology of the Central Postgraduate Medical Institute and the Department of Virology of the N. F. Gamaleya Institute of Epidemiology and Microbiology, Academy of Medical Sciences of the USSR.

V. D. S.
T. A. B.

Contents

PART I

The Properties of Interferon.
The Formation and Action of Interferon Induced in Cell Cultures and Chick Embryos

The Principal Properties of Interferon

Interferon possesses certain characteristic properties which distinguish it from other virus inhibitors. These include:

1. Tissue and species specificity.
2. Insensitivity to the action of virus-neutralizing antibodies [336, 373].
3. Resistance to the action of an acid medium and thermo-stability at 56°C.
4. Sensitivity to proteolytic enzymes.
5. Ability to inhibit reproduction of certain viruses in tissue cultures, i.e., absence of virus specificity.

Besides these properties, interferon also possesses others which characterize it as a protein of low molecular weight with particular physicochemical properties. Details of the various properties of interferon are given below.

1.1. Physicochemical Properties

Interferon is a protein of low molecular weight. Its molecule contains the following components: tyrosine 2.3%, tryptophan 2.6%, arginine 7.2%, lysine 11.1%. It does not contain nucleic acids and only traces of carbohydrate are present [410].

Several types of interferon are believed to exist, i.e., the interferons are a heterogeneous class of proteins [583]. The heterogeneity of interferon is based to some extent on variation in its physical properties, especially its molecular weight.

The molecular weight of interferon induced by viruses in tissue cultures ranges from 26,000 to 38,000 [406, 411, 451, 452, 461, 690]. The sedimentation constant is 2.2-2.3 Svedberg units [406, 410].

The initial results indicated that interferons induced by viruses in tissue cultures and *in vivo* were homogeneous. However, more recently it has been shown that interferons with different molecular weights are formed under the influence of the same inducer. In particular, two components of interferon have been discovered [412] in the sera of mice infected with NDV: component A with a molecular weight of 38,000 and isoelectric point 7.7 and component B with a molecular weight of 23,500 and an isoelectric point of 7.4. Interferon induced by the same virus in a culture of mouse spleen cells and in L cells had molecular weights of 26,000 and 25,000, respectively, and an isoelectric point of 7.0. Inhibitor induced in a tissue culture of rabbit spleen, on the other hand, had a molecular weight of 33,000 and an isoelectric point of 7.4.

Two types of rabbit interferons with molecular weights of 100,000 and 42,000 were found by Ke and co-workers [392]. Since the heavier "early" interferon was found in the blood stream before the lighter, it was postulated that the heavier interferon already exists in the body, evidently in the cells of the reticuloendothelial system and it is quickly liberated after the action of the interferon inducer. However, it has so far proved impossible to disintegrate the "heavy" interferon into the "light."

Recent work has provided evidence that the molecular weight of interferon depends both on the properties of the inducing agent and on the properties of the cells producing the inhibitor. For instance, the molecular weight of interferons induced *in vivo* by nonviral inducers (bacterial endotoxins, polysaccharides) was found to be 89,000-90,000 [329, 459]. Merigan and Hanna [458] obtained two types of interferons (with molecular weights of 53,000 and 77,000) in L cells infected with trachoma-inclusion conjunctivitis virus. It has also been reported that two different types of interferons are formed *in vitro* by rabbit macrophages [540]. One of the interferons, with a molecular weight of 37,000, could also be formed in the absence of the virus, while the other, with a molecular weight of 45,000, was induced by NDV. Differences between interferons formed *in vivo* are also demonstrated by results [908] indicating differences in the sensitivity of inhibitors synthesized in different organs of mice to mercaptoethanol.

The molecular weight of human interferons also was found to be heterogeneous. The inhibitor produced by human leukocytes and cultures of human fibroblasts had a molecular weight of 25,000 [281, 457], while that produced by amnion cells had a molecular weight of 160,000 [279].

Interferon has a slightly acid reaction and contains disulfide bridges [461]. The number of polypeptide chains has not been established. However, the reaction of this protein is alkaline and the isoelectric point is close to pH 6.9-7.1 [411] or 7.2-7.8 [29, 34].

The study of the resistance of interferon to temperature and other factors has yielded inconsistent results. However, the thermostability of interferon has been shown to be largely determined by its origin. In particular, chick interferon is more resistant to heat than mammalian interferon.

The activity of chick interferon is not reduced by heating for 1 h to 75°C. Heating to 80°C for 1 h leads to a fourfold, and heating at 85°C to an eightfold decrease in its activity [351, 372, 577]. Vilček and co-workers [573] found a decrease of 63% in the activity of chick interferon after heating for 1 h at 76°C.

The thermostability of purified preparations has been found to be similar. The activity of chick interferon remained unchanged after heating for 1 h at 66°C [411].

Somewhat different results were obtained by Ermol'eva and co-workers [62]. They found that chick interferon undergoes considerable inactivation when heated for 30 min at 56°C.

Interferons produced by mammalian cells have lower thermostability. Mouse interferon, for instance, loses much (up to 95%) or even all of its activity after heating for 30-60 min at 56-60°C [336, 342, 410, 569]. Similar results after heating to 57-60°C were obtained with purified human interferon [249, 319, 320, 457, 597, 598].

Interferon keeps its activity for long periods at 4°C [239, 302, 461] and also in the frozen state [461]. With further purification of interferon it becomes progressively more sensitive to the action of temperature. If lyophilically dried, interferon remains active for a long time [88, 277].

Interferon is stable over a wide range of pH values [365, 429]. Its preparations are stable at pH 1.0-10.0. Even at pH 12.5, interferon is not completely destroyed but preserves up to 10% of its activity. At pH 1.0, 67% of its activity is lost [578].

Strongly acid pH values are lethal to viruses, but interferon is resistant to them for at least 7 days. The resistance of interferon to acids is therefore used to remove (or inactivate) infective virus in interferon preparations.

Since it is a protein, interferon is inactivated by proteolytic enzymes: trypsin, chymotrypsin, and papain [351, 373, 457, 567, 577]. In the experiments of Lindenmann and co-workers [429] incubation with 0.01% and 0.001% solutions of trypsin at 37°C for 2 h led to a sharp decrease in interferon activity. Later investigations showed that the activity of interferon either disappears completely as a result of treatment with trypsin or it is considerably weakened [312, 410, 411, 567]. The trypsin sensitivity test is widely used to identify interferon and it is of considerable value for its differentiation from the "blocker" which inhibits interferon formation [375].

Interferon is not sedimented at 100,000 g in the course of 2 h, i.e., it is not bound with the virus particle [372, 373, 577].

Conflicting results have been obtained for the resistance of interferon to ether. For instance, interferon obtained by infection of KB cells with parainfluenza virus is resistant to ether [249]. The inhibitor induced by measles virus in HeLa cells has also been shown to be resistant [260]. However, treatment of mouse interferon with ether at 4°C for 2 h destroyed up to 90% of its activity [312, 410].

Total inactivation by ether also was described in one of the earliest studies of interferon [429]. This work also showed that interferon: a) is resistant to $6M$ urea; b) undergoes no change in its activity if treated at room temperature for 1 h with $NaIO_4$ in final concentrations of 0.001, 0.0001, and 0.00001M; c) is resistant to 0.001% ribonuclease, deoxyribonuclease, and RDE; d) is filterable through Gradocol membranes with a pore diameter of 1-8 μ and loses some of its activity if the pore diameter is 1μ; e) is resistant to ultrasound; f) is precipitated by ammonium sulfate and retains its activity after redissolving; g) does not dialyze.

The resistance of interferon to ultraviolet irradiation has received little study. According to Lampson and co-workers [411], native and relatively unpurified preparations of chick interferon are highly resistant whereas purified preparations have marked sensitivity to this agent. Exposure for up to 10 min to x-rays does not reduce the biological activity of interferon [12].

Interferon can be purified and concentrated by precipitation with ethanol, acetone [599], zinc acetate [461], or ammonium sulfate [141, 180, 429, 497].

Filtration through Sephadex gel is at present used to purify and concentrate interferon [34, 122, 406].

We have studied the properties of interferon preparations experimentally. The resistance of interferon was determined during keeping in a cold room (4-10°C), during heating, and during repeated freezing and thawing. Chick, mouse, rabbit, and human interferons, induced by NDV, strain N, were used in these experiments. The interferon preparations were kept at 4°C in 5-ml tubes and samples were taken after an interval of 2 months. Tubes containing 1 ml of the preparation were heated on a water bath for 1 h or longer, and in the other experiments the material was frozen to −40°C and thawed at 4-10°C.

As Table 1 shows, titers of interferons kept for 8 months at 4°C were virtually unchanged except in the case of mouse (serum) interferon, the activity of which was reduced fourfold during this period. Chick interferon was most resistant, for its activity was reduced by only half after keeping for 15 months. The other interferons tested were more labile, but their activity was reduced by only 4-8 times after keeping for 15 months in a cold room. The resistance of serum interferons to heating at different temperatures is shown in Table 2.

These experiments gave further confirmation of the thermostability of chick interferon. With these facts in mind, the combinations of temperature and time necessary to inactivate this preparation were determined (Table 3).

TABLE 1. Stability of Interferons at 4°C

Interferon preparation	Interferon titer after keeping for							
	0 months	2 months	4 months	6 months	8 months	10 months	12 months	15 months
Chick	64	64	64	64	64	64	32	32
Human (leukocytic)	256	256	256	256	256	128	64	64
Human (diploid)	32	32	32	32	32	n.i.	n.i.	n.i.
Mouse (serum)	1024	1024	1024	512	256	256	128	128

Note: n.i., not investigated.

TABLE 2. Resistance of Serum Interferons to Heating for 1 Hour

Interferon preparation	Interferon titer			
	unheated	after heating to		
		56°	60°	70°
Chick	64	64	64	64
Mouse	2048	256	256	<4
Rabbit	1024	256	256	<4
Human	32	4	4	<4

TABLE 3. Thermostability of Chick Interferon

Temperature of heating	Duration of heating, h	Interferon titer
Unheated	0	64
60°	1	64
70°	1	64
80°	1	16
80°	2	4
80°	3	<4
90°	1	4
100°	10 min	<4

The preparation of chick interferon thus obtained was thermostable and did not lose any of its inhibitory activity even after heating to 90°C for 1 h. Freezing and thawing human and chick interferons three times caused no decrease in their activity.

The interferon titer likewise was not reduced after lyophilic drying of preparations of human leukocytic interferon and chick cultural interferon. Subsequent storage of the dried interferon for 18 months at 4°C likewise was not accompanied by any decrease in the biological activity of the interferon.

The lyophilic drying method was tested as a means of increasing the interferon concentration. Chick interferon was dried in a volume of 3 ml. The dry residue was diluted in 0.5 ml distilled water. Theoretically this should have resulted in a preparation which was six times more active. However, the interferon titer was increased by only four times, from 1 : 32 to 1 : 128 when diluted to 0.5 ml.

The sensitivity of interferon to trypsin in a final concentration of 1% was tested. The mixture of interferon and trypsin was incubated at 37°C for 1 h. The trypsin was then inactivated by heating to 56°C for 30 min and the interferon activity was determined. There was a fourfold decrease in its titer after treatment with the proteolytic enzyme.

The activity of interferon preparations remained practically unchanged after centrifugation at 180,000 g for 2 h and filtration through a Seitz EKS-2 filter. The results of a study of some properties of an interferon preparation obtained from cultures of chick fibroblasts are given in Table 4.

1.2. Species Specificity

One of the most important properties of interferon is its well-marked species specificity. This property of interferon was first described by Tyrrell [559]. In his experiments the inhibitors obtained in the chorioallantoic membranes of the chick embryo and in cultures of calf kidney cells possessed antiviral activity only in homologous cells. Isaacs and Westwood [377] also showed that vaccinal lesions in the rabbit's skin were actively inhibited by inter-

TABLE 4. Effect of Different Methods of
Treatment on Activity of Chick Interferon

Method of treatment	Material	Interferon titer
Centrifugation at 180,000 g for 2 h	Original	16
	Supernatant	8
	Residue	<2
Treatment with 0.1% trypsin	Original	16
	Treated	4
Ultrafiltration	Original	24
	Filtrate	12

feron produced in cultures of rabbit cells, whereas chick interferon gave a very weak effect in such cases. The opposite effect
was obtained in experiments on chick embryos, i.e., only chick and
not rabbit interferon was active. Later the marked species specificity of interferon was confirmed by most investigations [31, 32,
34, 188, 207, 303, 315, 328, 410, 411, 451, 461, 493, 529, 535, 554].

Meanwhile workers who studied the species specificity of
interferon reported that this property is not absolute and that
antiviral activity may be exhibited in heterologous tissues obtained
from closely related species [207, 231].

In some investigations, antiviral activity was also discovered
in heterologous tissues. Sutton and Tyrrell [554] found inhibitory
activity of a preparation obtained from monkey kidneys in heterologous cells. Ermol'eva and co-workers [62] discovered antiviral
activity in interferon obtained on the chorioallantoic membrane of
a chick embryo in both homologous and heterologous cells. In
particular, chick interferon inhibited the development of vaccinia
virus in a culture of transplanted human HEp-2 cells. Other workers
also found inhibitory activity in cells of heterologous species [8,
118, 123, 130, 177, 196]. In the experiments of Priimyagi and
Fadeeva [131], for instance, interferons obtained in primary cultures of chick fibroblasts and also in transplanted lines HeLa and
HEp-2 possessed equal inhibitory activity in both homologous and
heterologous cells.

However, it must be emphasized that in most investigations
interferon activity in heterologous cultures was much lower than
in homologous. Buckler and Baron [231] determined the level of
activity in heterologous tissue and found that it varied from 1 to
10% of the interferon activity in homologous tissue. It must be
remembered that activity in heterologous systems was demonstrated
for unpurified interferon preparations. For this reason some workers [143, 220, 231, 451, 583] consider that activity in heterologous
tissues is due to the presence of other inhibitors or of interferon-
inducing activity of residual virus in the interferon preparations.
That this hypothesis is correct is confirmed by the high species
specificity of purified interferon preparations and by the demon-
stration of other inhibitors besides interferon.

Merigan [451] found that a highly purified preparation of
mouse interferon with a titer of 1:20,000 in homologous cells

showed no antiviral activity in chick cells even in a dilution of 1 : 30.
Chick interferon with a titer of 1 : 4000 in chick fibroblasts likewise was inactive in mouse cells in the same dilution.

A study of the action of interferon on RNA-synthetase activity
in homologous and heterologous cells confirmed its species specificity [315].

Evidence that interferon-like substances are present was
obtained by the work of Paucker [480] and also of Buckler and Baron
[231]. Paucker found an inhibitor with antiviral activity which was
not interferon in the native preparation obtained in mouse line L.
A feature distinguishing the inhibitor found by Buckler and Baron
was that the resistance of the cells disappeared when they were
washed before infection with the virus. The resistance of cells
treated with interferon, however, still remained even if the cells
were washed before addition of the indicator virus.

We also carried out an investigation to determine the species
specificity of chick and human interferon preparations. Some of
these experiments were carried out with the collaboration of A. E.
Gumennik.

A strain of vaccinia virus passed more than 20 times through
chick embryos was used to obtain the chick interferon. Since active
vaccinia virus does not induce interferon formation by chick fibroblasts, the interferon was obtained by treatment of these cells with
inactivated vaccinia virus. The test viruses used for interferon
assay were smallpox and WEE viruses. Interferon was produced
in diploid cells by treatment with vaccine strain V1 of Newcastle
disease virus.

In the experiments to assay inhibitory activity these preparations were diluted in medium 199. Each twofold dilution of interferon was tested in three tube cultures to which 0.9 ml of the corresponding dilution was added at once and 0.1 ml of smallpox or
WEE virus, containing 100-1000 TCD_{50}, 24 h later. The results
were read after 4-5 days, when degeneration of the control cultures infected with virus alone was about to take place. Primary
monolayer cultures obtained from a trypsinized cell suspension
were used. The cultures were grown in 0.5% lactalbumin hydrolysate solution containing 2-10% of bovine serum depending on the
type of cell. Transplanted cell lines were grown on medium 199

with 10% serum and diploid cells on Eagle's medium with 10% bovine serum and 30% of 0.5% lactalbumin hydrolysate.

In the initial experiments the inhibitory action of the native interferon obtained in chick fibroblasts was determined. To study its species specificity primary tissue cultures, diploid cells, and transplanted cell lines of different origin were used. Chick, mouse, rabbit, pig, and calf embryonic tissues, adult monkey kidney tissue, L-44 (human) diploid cells, and transplanted lines A-1, J-96, D-6, Liv, and Ph (of human origin), SOTs, PAO, MIO, and PO (of monkey origin), and mouse cells were tested.

The species specificity of purified and concentrated interferon prepared at the Institute of Poliomyelitis and Virus Encephalitis, Academy of Medical Sciences of the USSR, was tested on the same tissue cultures. The results are given in Table 5.

The results in Table 5 show that despite their well-marked activity in homologous tissues, neither the native nor the purified

TABLE 5. Results of the Study of Species Specificity of Interferon from Tissues of Different Origin

Origin of tissue			Interferon titer		
species from which tissue was obtained	type of cells	name of strain	native chick	purified and concentrated chick	human (diploid)
Man	Diploid	L-44	<2	<2	32
	Transplanted	J-96	<2	<2	—
Man	Transplanted	A-1	<2	<2	—
		Liv	<2	<2	—
		D-6	<2	<2	—
Monkey	Primary (kidney)		<2	<2	4
	Transplanted	SOTs	<2	<2	—
		PAO	<2	<2	—
		MIO	<2	<2	—
		PO	<2	<2	—
Chick	Primary, embryonic		32	1000	<2
Mouse	Primary, embryonic		<2	<2	<2
	Transplanted		<2	<2	—
Rabbit	Primary, embryonic		<2	<2	—
Pig	Primary, embryonic		<2	<2	—
Cow	Primary, embryonic		<2	<2	—

Note. A minus sign indicates no test.

and concentrated chick interferon exhibited any antiviral action
in tissue cultures of heterologous origin. Only interferon obtained
in human diploid cells also exhibited some of its activity in monkey
cells.

Besides its species specificity, the tissue specificity of the
interferon also was determined. Little attempt had previously
been made to study this problem and all that was known was that
different tissues of the same species of animal under the influence
of the same inducer can produce different interferons [459]. According to another report [408] interferons from different organs
of the same animal differ in their sensitivity to mercaptoethanol.
These results are evidence of differences between the interferons
induced *in vivo*. Presumably these differences are also reflected
in the sensitivity of the tissues to the interferon produced by them
or by other organs.

Experiments were carried out on 16-day chick embryos from
which the kidneys, spleen, and lungs were removed after exsanguination. Monolayer cultures were obtained in 100-ml Pavitskaya
flasks from each type of organ from several embryos by tryp-
sinization, and after growth for 6 days in an incubator they were
infected with Chikungunya virus at the rate of 1 TCD_{50} per cell.
The virus was inactivated in the usual way 24 h later and the inhibitory activity was then determined in cells of the homologous
and heterologous organs. The results are given in Table 6.

Analysis of the results in Table 6 shows that interferon titers
determined in cells of the homologous organ were appreciably
higher than in cells of the heterologous organ. The only exception
was found on titration of "kidney" interferon in spleen cells. In
this case, however, the fact that the spleen cells are more sensitive to interferon than cells of the lung and, in particular, the
kidney evidently played a role. This probably also reduced the
differences in tissue specificity of the kidney interferon.

The role of the inducer virus in the virus specificity of interferon also was studied. For this purpose chick fibroblasts were
infected with NDV (strain N), Chikungunya virus, and inactivated
vaccinia virus. The interferon preparations obtained were assayed
with 100 TCD_{50} of Chikungunya, vesicular stomatitis, and WEE
viruses.

TABLE 6. Determination of
Tissue Specificity of Interferon

Organ in whose cells interferon was obtained	Cells in which interferon was assayed	Interferon titer*
Lung	Lung	26
	Spleen	21
	Kidney	7
Spleen	Spleen	43
	Lung	12
	Kidney	11
Kidney	Kidney	13
	Spleen	16
	Lung	8

*Mean results for 3 flasks.

TABLE 7. Effect of Inducer Virus on
Specificity of Interferon

Virus inducing interferon formation	Titer of interferon with		
	Chikungunya virus	vesicular stomatitis virus	WEE virus
Chikungunya	128	32	32
Vaccinia	128	32	32
Newcastle disease	64	16	16

The results in Table 7 show that the viruses exhibit identical sensitivity to the inhibitory action of interferon regardless of whethe the homologous or a heterologous agent was used to induce it.

The results so far obtained thus indicate marked species specificity of interferon. The antiviral activity of interferon discovered in the tissues of widely different species of animals must be reexamined in order to clarify the nature of the action of the inhibitors in native preparations.

1.3.   Antigenic Properties

Studies of the antigenic properties of interferon have given conflicting results. The attempts of Burke and Isaacs [237] to induc antibody formation in rabbits by immunization with concentrated chick interferon, with or without adjuvant, were unsuccessful.

However, other workers have obtained antibodies against rabbit [466, 467, 469] and mouse interferons [482]. Paucker [480] repeatedly obtained specific antiserum against chick and mouse interferons. It has been found that interferons of different species of animals differ in their antigenic properties. Differences in the antigenic structure of interferon and of the cells producing it also have been observed. Although the investigations cited above are evidence that interferon has antigenic properties, it must be remembered that antibodies against it have been discovered, and in low titers, only after prolonged and repeated immunization (in the experiments of Paucker and Cantell [482] 13 injections were given in the course of 5 months).

The weakness of the antigenic properties of interferon is confirmed by the results obtained by Falcoff and co-workers [277], who found that repeated intravenous injections of human leukocytic interferon into adults and children were not accompanied by the formation of any detectable quantities of antibodies. No antibodies could be detected even in a child aged 6 years who received 3620 ml of leukocytic interferon intravenously over a period of 400 days.

We also attempted to obtain a specific anti-interferon serum. Rabbits weighing 2.5-3 kg were immunized intramuscularly. Besides a native preparation of mouse serum interferon, a mixture of interferon with methylated bovine serum albumin, obtained from Braun as the dry substance, also was used for immunization. According to Braun, this substance stimulates antibody production *in vivo* and its action is more marked if it is combined with Freund's adjuvant. As recommended by Braun, the dose of methylated albumin given in each course of immunization was 2 mg.

The technique of preparing the mixture of albumin and interferon was as follows. Initially a 1% solution of albumin was made up in distilled water. This was then added drop by drop to the native preparation of interferon until turbidity appeared. Equal volumes of Freund's adjuvant and of the mixture of interferon with albumin were then mixed.

Four rabbits were used in the experiments, two of which received 2 ml of native mouse serum interferon (titer 1 : 4096) intramuscularly at each immunization, while the other two each received 2 ml of the above mixture with Freund's adjuvant.

In the course of 4 months and 10 days 8 injections of interferon with and without the adjuvants were given. One of the rabbits receiving interferon only died, evidently from serum anaphylactic shock. Thereafter immunization was carried out only by Besredka's method. The schemes and dates of immunization are given below.

Blood was taken from the rabbits 10 days after the 4th and 8th immunizations and the anti-interferon activity of the resulting rabbit serum was determined in tests on cells. It must be stated at once that no antibodies against mouse interferon could be found in the serum of the rabbits. To detect anti-interferon activity tests were carried out in two modifications. In the first, contact between antigen and hypothetical antibody was carried out *in vitro*. For this purpose two series of twofold dilutions of each test serum, from 1 : 10 to 1 : 320, were prepared. To each dilution of the serum in the first series four units of interferon in an equal volume was added, while two units of interferon was added to the second row of tubes. The mixture was incubated (37°C) for 3 h and the inhibitory activity of the mixtures was then tested on mouse cells. If anti-interferon antibodies had been present, the biological activity of the interferon would have been depressed and the mixture would not have induced resistance in the cells. However, after incubation of the mixture with the cells for 18 h at 37°C and subsequent addition of 100 TCD_{50} of vesicular stomatitis virus all cultures except the control proved to be resistant to the virus. Neither 4 nor 2 units of interferon activity neutralized any of the dilutions of the sera obtained.

In the second modification of the test different dilutions of serum were added initially to tubes containing the tissue culture and incubated (37°C) for 18 h, after which 2 or 4 units of interferon, in a volume of 0.5 ml, was added to each tube, followed after 18–20 h by 100 TCD_{50} of the indicator virus. Just as in the first case, no neutralization of the inhibitory activity of the interferon was found.

Immunization with interferon eight times in the course of 4 months and 10 days, whether with the native preparation or with the addition of adjuvants, thus failed to demonstrate any antigenic properties of the interferon.

To sum up, the properties of interferon are independent of the properties of the virus inducing it but are determined by the genetic features of the producing tissue.

1.4. Conclusion

Determination of the species specificity of interferon has played the decisive role in the study of its possible use in the prevention and treatment of virus infections. We used native (titer 1 : 32) and purified and concentrated chick interferons (titer 1 : 1000) in our experiments. They were tested on a wide variety of primary, diploid, and transplanted cell cultures of different origin. Both types of preparations proved to be strictly species-specific. Consequently, purification and concentration of chick interferon do not enable it to be used with success in heterologous tissues. Investigations by other workers, who have found inhibitory activity in heterologous cells, showed that during purification of interferon its species specificity becomes increasingly more marked [31, 282].

Our investigations have confirmed the partial activity of interferon in cells of closely related species of animals. In particular, interferon obtained in human diploid cells was found to be active in monkey cells. These results are in agreement with those obtained by other workers [231].

We have shown for the first time that interferon possesses not only species, but also a certain degree of tissue specificity. Interferon prepared in homologous tissues proved to be more active than that prepared in heterologous tissues of the same species of animal.

A study of the thermostability of interferons of different origin showed that the preparation of chick origin is most resistant to heating at 56–60°C. The thermostability of human, rabbit, and mouse interferons was similar.

Preparations of interferon obtained by us and used in our experiments possessed the properties of the classical interferon [373, 429].

An attempt to obtain an anti-interferon serum by immunization of rabbits proved unsuccessful. Addition of Freund's adjuvant and methylated bovine serum albumin to the interferon likewise failed to achieve success.

The absence of antibodies in the serum of immunized rabbits, a result which conflicts with the findings of other workers [466, 467, 469, 480, 482], may be due to inadequate immunization because where success was achieved 13 immunizations had been given over a period of 5 months. Nevertheless the results do confirm the low antigenic activity of interferon.

The Formation of Interferon in Cell Cultures and Chick Embryos

2.1. The Interferon-Inducing Activity of Viruses

By interacting with the cells of tissue cultures or of chick embryos, viruses may induce the formation of interferon in them. Interferonogenic properties are found in viruses belonging to different families.

2.1.1. The Interferon-Inducing Activity of Poxviruses

Ability to induce interferon formation has been studied in only a few of the poxviruses. The first investigation in this direction was published by Nagano and Kojima [464]. These workers described the appearance of a virus inhibitor in the skin of a rabbit injected with vaccinia virus. This inhibitor was later identified [463, 465] as interferon. A study of the interferon-inducing activity of vaccinia virus *in vitro* showed [312] that virus inactivated by ultraviolet rays is less able than infectious virus to induce interferon production by both primary and transplanted mouse embryonic cells. Interferon production takes place more intensively in one of the two transplanted lines tested (*M*-21) than in primary cells. Peterson and Li Yü [118] found that heat-inactivated vaccinia virus induced interferon formation in cultures of chick fibroblasts and monkey kidneys but they found no interferonogenic activity in transplanted lines HeLa, HEp-2, and SOTs (Cynomolgus heart). Induction of interferon by infectious viruses of vaccinia [40, 120], ectromelia, and fowlpox [120] was described later.

19

However, results of an opposite kind have been obtained. No
interferon could be detected by Sellers and Fitzpatrick [536] in
cultures of dog kidney cells or by Lindenmann and Gifford [431]
in cultures of chick fibroblasts infected with vaccinia virus.

Relatively little information is thus available on the interferon-inducing activity of viruses of the smallpox—vaccinia subgroup
and the results obtained with vaccinia virus are contradictory.
These contradictions can be partly explained by the observations
of Litvinov [108]. The same strain of vaccinia virus (the dermal
variant) showed unequal inferferon-inducing activity in cultures
of chick fibroblasts. Litvinov studied the causes of the variability of the results and found that the freshly obtained vaccinia virus
cannot induce interferon formation, but becomes capable of doing
so if stored at 4°C. Litvinov explained his results by the appearance of inactivated virions in the virus-containing suspension.

Because of the insufficient attention paid to the study of the
interferon-inducing activity of the poxviruses and the conflicting
nature of the results obtained we undertook a comparative investigation of the ability of several viruses belonging to the smallpox—vaccinia subgroup to induce interferon formation. Because
of the heterogeneity of strains of vaccinia virus, a comparative
study within this series also was required. Some of the work
described in this section was carried out jointly with A. E. Gumennik and S. S. Marennikova.

The following viruses were used in the experiments: a) natural smallpox, strains Sh and T, isolated during an outbreak of
smallpox in Moscow in 1960 and subsequently passed more than 20
times through chick embryos, and strain Sokolov, after 3 successive
passages through chick embryos; b) alastrim virus, strains Nos. 1
and 2; c) ectromelia virus, strains K and G, adapted to chick embryos; d) rabbit smallpox; e) cowpox, strain Brighton; and f) variants of vaccinia virus. The latter group included the following
strains: 1) Lister; 2) MNIIVP, used previously at the Institute of
Virus Preparations for the production of smallpox vaccine; 3)
Tashkent; 4) EM-63; 5) a neurovaccine adapted by Yu. N. Mastyukova by intracerebral passage through rabbits; 6) ovovaccines
also adapted by Mastyukova and subjected to more than 400 passages through chick embryos; 7) a white variant, consisting of
a clone isolated by Marennikova from a production strain of der-

movaccine of the Tashkent strain. Besides the latter, strains Lister, MNIIVP, Tashkent, and EM-63 also were dermal variants. The interferon-inducing activity of the viruses was first studied in cultures of chick fibroblasts. All the above viruses were added to the cultures in an infective state at the rate of 1 TCD_{50} per cell. The culture fluids were investigated for their interferon content for 3 days, but no inhibitory activity against the virus of Western equine encephalomyelitis (WEE) could be found in any of the samples tested, even in a dilution of 1 : 2.

The interferon-inducing action of smallpox and vaccinia viruses also was studied in experiments on 12-day chick embryos which were infected in the chorioallantoic membrane in doses of 10^5, 10^3, and 10^1 TCD_{50} per embryo. At intervals of 24 h for 4 days groups of five embryos infected with different doses of active virus were examined. The allantoic fluid and the chorioallantoic membranes were collected separately. A 10% suspension was made from the membranes. The suspension and the allantoic fluid were treated with hydrochloric acid to inactivate the virus, the pH was adjusted to 7.4, and the materials were then tested for inhibitory activity. The results showed that the allantoic fluid and suspension of chorioallantoic membranes of the chick embryos infected by different doses of smallpox virus and obtained after incubation for various periods showed no inhibitory properties.

Consequently, both in cultures of chick fibroblasts *in vitro* and in chick embryos *in vivo* the viruses tested showed no interferon-inducing activity. No inhibitory properties could be detected in the materials studied whether by the use of inhibition of cytopathogenic action as the method of indication or by testing by Dulbecco's method of plaque inhibition.

Having demonstrated the absence of interferon-inducing activity of infectious vaccinia virus in cultures of chick fibroblasts it was decided to study this property of the virus in other types of tissue cultures, also using heat-inactivated virus for comparison.

Monolayer cultures of chick and mouse fibroblasts, of monkey kidney cells and chick embryonic cells, and also cultures of rat, guinea pig, and rabbit embryonic fibroblasts were used in comparative experiments. Side by side with primary cultures, transplanted lines MIO, PAO, HEp-2, SPEV, and J-96 were tested.

TABLE 8. Interferon Formation in Cell Cultures Inoculated
with Vaccinia Virus

Type of culture	Source of tissue	Titer of interferon after addition of vaccinia virus	
		native	heated
Fibroblasts	Chick embryo	<2	16-128
	Mouse embryo	4-32*	<2
	Rat embryo	<2	8
	Guinea pig embryo	<2	4
	Rabbit embryo	<2	<2
Epithelial	Monkey kidney	<2	16
	Pig embryonic kidney	<2	<2
Transplanted lines	J-96, HEp-2, SPEV, MIO, PAO	<2	<2

*Here and in subsequent tables reciprocals of the interferon titer are given.

The virus was added to the cultures at the rate of 1 TCD_{50} per
cell and incubation continued for 4-5 days.

The results of the experiments with strain MNIIVP are shown
in Table 8. Similar results were obtained with natural smallpox
virus.

As Table 8 shows, heated vaccinia virus induced interferon
formation in primary monolayer cultures of chick, rat, and guinea
pig embryos and in monkey kidney cells without inducing its production in pig and rabbit embryonic cells or in any of the transplanted
cultures used. Active vaccinia virus did not induce interferon synthesis in any of the cultures tested except the primary mouse embryonic culture. Ability to stimulate interferon formation, incidentally, was also characteristic of other strains of vaccinia
virus taken in the active form (Table 9).

The results described above show that vaccinia and smallpox
vaccines in principle can induce interferon formation both in the
infectious and in the inactivated state. However, heating the viruses
to certain temperatures potentiates their interferon-inducing
properties.

2.1.2. The Interferon-Inducing Activity of Myxoviruses

Of all the myxoviruses, interferon-inducing properties have
been most fully studied in influenza virus and Newcastle disease

TABLE 9. Interferon-
Inducing Activity of Strains
of Vaccinia Virus in
Mouse Embryonic Cells

Name of strain	Interferon titer
Ovovaccines	8
Lister	16
EM-63	8
White clone	4-8

virus (NDV). Ability to induce interferon formation was found
originally in the inactivated [376], and later in active influenza virus
[559, 578]. Subsequently the influenza viruses, both infectious and
inactivated by ultraviolet rays, have been repeatedly investigated
as inducers of interferon in cultures of fragments of chorioallantoic
membrane and chick embryos [13, 14, 62, 63]. It has been shown
that interferon formation can also be stimulated by incomplete
virus containing nucleoprotein, whereas virus hemagglutinin, without nucleic acid, does not possess this property [235]. After influenza virus, interferon-inducing activity was discovered in fowl
plague virus and NDV [236], mumps virus [238, 336], Sendai virus
[244, 336], and measles virus [259, 260]. The interferon-inducing
activity of the above viruses differed with the experimental conditions and depended both on the species of virus and its infectivity
and also on various other factors. In particular, active influenza
virus induced the formation of the largest quantities of interferon
during reproduction in chick embryos [13, 14, 80, 82, 244, 578].
In tissue cultures infected with influenza virus small quantities
of interferon were usually found. Its titer was increased if virus
inactivated by ultraviolet rays was used [235, 372, 429].

Similar relationships are found if cultures of chick fibroblasts are infected with NDV. In particular, a comparative study
of this virus with four other (Chikungunya, Semliki forest, vaccinia,
and pseudorabies viruses) revealed its weak interferonogenic activity [40]. NDV treated by various methods was also found to be
capable of inducing interferon synthesis [602]. The experiments
were carried out in two cell systems: chick embryonic fibroblasts
and transplanted L cells. In the latter large quantities of inter-

feron were synthesized if both infectious and inactivated viruses were treated with ultraviolet rays. In chick fibroblasts, on the other hand, the active virus did not induce interferon while virus inactivated by ultraviolet rays induced the formation of large quantities of interferon.

Investigations [143, 517, 236, 350] have shown that NDV induces little interferon in chick fibroblasts. At the same time, this virus gave a high yield of interferon in thyroid cells [137, 517], in diploid [40, 45, 132] and primary human fibroblasts [132], and also in mouse embryonic cells [517].

Active and ultraviolet-inactivated NDV induced interferon in transplanted cells [240, 241, 485]. Under the same conditions influenza virus had no interferon-inducing action. A study of the effect of γ-rays on the interferon-inducing activity of the myxoviruses showed that this activity is exhibited only if the virus is still capable of reproducing in sensitive cell systems [12].

To this must be added the fact that myxoviruses and, in particular, NDV and Sendai viruses have proved to be the most active interferon inducers in suspensions of human leukocytes [277, 549], followed by influenza B and A viruses.

Comparative studies have been made of the interferon-inducing activity of NDV and other myxoviruses in chick embryos. Comparison of eight strains of NDV differing in virulence showed [206] that all are weak inducers of interferon. Strains with low (lentogenic) and with high (velogenic) virulence induced the smallest amounts of interferon. Strains with moderate virulence (mesogenic) induced larger amounts of interferon.

Tests of several myxoviruses in the allantois of chick embryos have shown that of influenza viruses A, B, and C, parotitis and Sendai viruses, and NDV, influenza virus B is the best inducer and Sendai the worst [244].

In some experiments [13, 106, 108, 190, 532] NDV induced the formation of interferon in comparatively high titers.

Swine influenza virus has also been used as inducer to obtain allantois interferon [34, 82, 176-179].

These various investigations can be summarized by stating that influenza viruses were best able to induce interferon in chick embryos. In mammalian tissue cultures the largest quantities of interferon are induced by active NDV, and in chick fibroblast cultures by the same virus when inactivated by ultraviolet rays.

2.1.3. The Interferon-Inducing Activity of Rhabdoviruses

In the family of the rhabdoviruses, interferon-inducing activity has been studied in the viruses of vesicular stomatitis and rabies.

Comparative-studies have shown that vesicular stomatitis virus possesses weak interferon-inducing activity both in cell cultures and in chick embryos [243, 244]. This virus induced significant quantities of interferon only in leukocyte suspensions [277].

In the study of the ability of rabies virus to induce interferon formation in cell cultures conflicting results have been obtained.

Kaplan et al. [655], for instance, when studying the ability of street rabies virus to interfere with western equine encephalomyelitis virus, found that this interference is due to interferon. Joshing et al. [664] found that autointerference of rabies virus of strain Hep Flury in cultures of chick fibroblasts also induced interferon. Interferon was found in the nutrient fluid of cultures infected with a multiplicity of 0.1-0.5 LD_{50} per cell in titers of 1:4-1:16.

Similar results were obtained by Vorob'ev et al. [611], who infected cultures of chick fibroblasts with strain Flury LEP of fixed rabies virus. The interferon titer in samples of culture fluid 3 days after infection was 1:16, and by the 6th-7th day it reached 1:64 to 1:128.

Meanwhile American workers [694] found no interferon in WY-38 diploid cultures infected with fixed rabies virus adapted to them. On the basis of these results, Depoux [640] postulated that rabies virus cannot induce interferon formation.

Bektemirova [608] observed that the interferon-inducing activity of fixed rabies virus in cell cultures is directly dependent on the ability of the virus to reproduce in the given type of cell culture.

Reflecting the weak reproduction of fixed rabies virus or its complete absence, no interferon could be found in the culture fluid of transplanted L, BHK, and WY-38 cells, while in a strain of human myodermal cells and in a monolayer culture of chick fibroblasts it was found only in a titer of 1 : 4. At the same time, strains "Moskva" and "CVS" of fixed rabies virus, replicating in monolayer cultures of Syrian hamster kidneys and of Japanese quail embryonic fibroblasts, induced considerable quantities of interferon in them (titers 1 : 16 to 1 : 64). The dynamics of interferon production in these cell cultures correlated with replication of the virus.

Suspensions of mouse and rabbit leukocytes, when treated *in vitro* with fixed rabies virus, produced moderate amounts of interferon.

2.1.4. The Interferon-Inducing Activity of Herpes Viruses

The study of the interferon-inducing activity of herpes virus in cell cultures has yielded conflicting results. Lampson et al. [411] observed moderate interferon-inducing activity of herpes virus in a culture of chick embryonic fibroblasts. However, Germanov [613] found interferon in comparatively high titers (1 : 320 to 1 : 640) in the culture fluid of chick fibroblasts infected with strain K of herpes virus. Weak interferon production was observed in dog kidney cells infected with herpes virus [199, 200]. It was also found that if the cell culture was infected with a replicating mutant of herpes virus, no interferon could be detected in the culture fluid. Conversely, a mutant not replicating in the particular cell culture induced interferon in a titer of 1 : 4 to 1 : 8. The inability of the replicating mutant to induce interferon in a culture of dog kidney cells is attributed to inhibition of the synthesis of cell RNA, which was not observed in the case of infection with a nonreplicating mutant. The weak interferon-inducing activity of herpes virus in cultures of chick fibroblasts has also been described by Smorodintsev et al. [145] and by Vaczi et al. [560, 691].

Induction of interferon in 10-day chick embryos infected with herpes virus was observed by Fruitstone et al. [302].

In experiments carried out by us jointly with S. A. Moisiadi, the interferon-inducing activity of six strains (L2, K, US, OSh, KUB, GUL) of herpes virus, belonging to six antigenic groups in accordance with the classification of Shubladze and Maevskaya [625], was studied.

The experiments were carried out in cell cultures of two types: chick (CEF) and human embryonic fibroblasts (HEF).

The intensity of interferon formation in the cell cultures was found to depend primarily on the infecting dose of virus. With a multiplicity of 1 LD_{50} per cell, for instance, from 2 to 4 times more interferon was formed than with a multiplicity of 0.1 LD_{50}. With a multiplicity of 0.01 LD_{50} per cell, no interferon was found in the CEF and HEF tissue cultures.

A study of the ability of herpes virus, incubated at 60°C for 30 min, or 1 and 2 h, to induce interferon showed that under these conditions none of the strains of virus tested could induce interferon formation. After heating for 30 min, nearly all the strains (except US) retained a residual infectivity.

In view of these results, experiments were then carried out to determine the interferon-inducing activity of herpes virus in tissue culture by infection with active virus in an infecting dose of 1 LD_{50} per cell.

The highest interferon titers in a culture of human embryonic fibroblasts were induced by strains L2, K, and US. Its titers were 1 : 223, 1 : 160, and 1 : 170, respectively. Strains OSh, KUB, and GUL induced the formation of smaller amounts of interferon (1 : 120, 1 : 56, 1 : 56). The time taken for the interferon titer to reach its maximum differed for the various strains tested. Strains L2, K, and OSh, for instance, induced maximal interferon titers 24 h after infection, and strains US, KUB, and GUL 72 h after infection.

Similar results were obtained by determination of the interferon-inducing activity of different antigenic variants in cultures of chick fibroblasts. However, all strains induced interferon more slowly and in smaller amounts in chick embryonic fibroblasts. Consequently, the interferon-inducing activity of herpes virus depended not only on strain differences, but also on the properties of the cell cultures in which their inducing activity was tested.

The interferon-inducing activity of other members of the herpes group of viruses (cytomegalovirus, the viruses of chickenpox, herpes zoster, and pseudorabies) has so far received comparatively little study.

Glasgow (cited in [652]), for instance, stated that human cytomegalovirus does not induce interferon formation in cell cultures. Similar results were obtained by Osborn and Medearis [477], who found that no interferon is produced in cultures of mouse cells. However, Henson and Smith [652] observed interferon formation in mouse embryonic cells infected with cytomegalovirus. A direct correlation was found between the titer of virus and the interferon production. Interferon production in cultures of human embryonic fibroblasts was observed by Vaczi et al. [560, 691], and in strain WY-38 of diploid cells and in human preputial fibroblasts by Vaczi et al. [314]. These workers showed that cytomegalovirus induced small quantities of interferon in these cultures.

Vaczi et al. [560, 691] found marked interferon production in cultures of human embryonic fibroblasts induced by chickenpox virus.

In a study of the interferon-inducing activity of pseudorabies virus, Belady and Bakny [632] found no interferon in cultures of calf kidney cells. However, in the experiments of Litvinov [106] this virus induced interferon formation in chick embryonic fibroblast cultures and in transplanted lines of hog kidney and BHK cells. Interferon with a varied level of activity was obtained by intraallantoic infection of chick embryos.

2.1.5. The Interferon-Inducing Activity of Arboviruses

The first investigations to determine the ability of arboviruses to induce interferon formation were carried out by Vilcek [567]. The results showed that interferon is produced in a culture of chick fibroblasts during reproduction of tick-borne encephalitis virus but is not formed under the influence of the same virus when inactivated by ultraviolet radiation or by heating to 56°C [570]. This work was confirmed by Vil'ner et al. [38] and by Andzhaparidze et al. [5, 6].

Subsequently other arboviruses also were found to possess interferon-inducing activity. Many of them are active interferon inducers in tissue cultures of various types and, in particular, in chick fibroblasts. Ability to induce interferon synthesis was originally discovered only in infectious arboviruses. For instance, interferon formation was observed only in culture of cells infected by Sindbis virus [490]. If this virus was inactivated by heat, however, it did not induce interferon in cultures of chick fibroblasts. Large quantities of interferon were formed on infection of L cells and chick fibroblasts by Eastern equine encephalomyelitis virus [578, 579]. However, in the inactivated state this same virus did not induce interferon formation [44].

According to some observations [434, 436] the virus of Western equine encephalomyelitis lost its interferonogenic activity in L cells after heating to 37°C.

Detailed investigations of the ability of Western, Eastern, and Venezuelan equine encephalomyelitis viruses to induce interferon formation in chick fibroblasts were carried out by Ershov and Zhdanov [75].

Interferonogenic properties have been found in Mayaro [335], Chikungunya [40, 306, 307, 427, 516], and Japanese encephalitis viruses [91, 92, 143, 146, 149, 442].

An investigation [536] has shown that Bunyamwera virus reproduces in dog kidney cell cultures but does not induce interferon formation whereas Semliki forest virus, which reproduces poorly in these cells, induces interferon synthesis.

Several workers later showed that under certain conditions inactivated arboviruses can nevertheless induce interferon formation. In particular, interferon formation has been observed under the influence of Chikungunya virus inactivated by heating to 65°C for 30 min or to 35°C for 23 h [305, 306]. The heat-inactivated virus proved to be a better stimulator of interferon formation than the infectious virus.

Similar results were obtained with Western equine encephalomyelitis and Sindbis viruses [416]. These viruses, completely inactivated by heating to 37°C for 10-14 days, induced interferon production in chick embryonic fibroblasts in larger quantities than the infectious virus. However, in L cells, in which the infectious virus was a good inducer of interferon, inactivated viruses did not stimulate interferon formation.

Eastern equine encephalomyelitis virus, if gently inactivated by ultraviolet rays, likewise preserved its interferonogenic activity [75, 76].

Certain arboviruses, if special methods of inactivation are chosen, thus not only do not lose their ability to induce interferon formation but may actually become more active inducers.

Inactivated viruses with no interferon-inducing activity were found to have the distinctive property of stimulating interferon induction by active viruses. In particular, heat-inactivated Sindbis virus stimulates interferon production induced by the homologous infectious virus [349]. Similar results were obtained with other arboviruses [75]. On the basis of these results [75, 305] it is recommended that partially inactivated viruses be used as interferon inducers, for they give a better effect than completely inactivated arboviruses.

In the experiments of Ershov and Zhdanov [75] the maximum yield of interferon was observed when a method of double infection was used. Chick fibroblast cells were treated first with virus inactivated by ultraviolet rays and later with infectious virus. The optimal interval between the two infections was 3 h. It is interesting to note that interferon production in cell cultures contaminated by mycoplasmas was higher than in cultures freed from these organisms [74]. This applies also to transplanted cell lines HeLa, A-1, L, KB, and KEM, in which interferon production was negligible under ordinary conditions under the influence of EEE and WEE viruses.

2.1.6. The Interferon-Inducing Activity of Other Viruses

The interferon-inducing activity of the enteroviruses has received comparatively little study. Several workers failed to find interferon in the nutrient fluid of cultures infected with enteroviruses [114, 417, 552]. Other workers found interferon but consider that the enteroviruses have low interferon-inducing activity [50, 333, 352].

Gendon (1966) observed that strains Mahoney (type I) and Saukkett (type III) of poliovirus did not induce interferon in HeLa cells. Meanwhile the mutant ML/15 obtained by Gendon from the first strain induced interferon formation in this cell culture in titers of 1:16 to 1:64.

It is claimed [352] that the onset and continuation of chronic poliovirus infection in transplanted human amniotic cells depends to some extent on interferon production. In these experiments the inactivated virus was unable to induce interferon formation.

However, the interferon-inducing activity of poliovirus, both active and inactivated by ultraviolet rays, was discovered by Priimyagi et al. [125, 132]. Bovine enterovirus M_6 did not induce interferon in cultures of dog kidney cells (535, 536); nor did Coxsackie B viruses in chick fibroblasts [552] and in cultures of strains of human diploid cells [129]. Parkman et al. (1965) detected interferon in primary cultures of green guenon kidney cells infected with rubella virus.

Herpes [143, 242, 411, 560] virus, adenoviruses [239, 355], and cytomegalovirus [314] possess weak or, according to some observations, moderate interferon-inducing activity in cell culture.

Interferon is also induced in tissue culture by oncogenic viruses: the viruses of polyoma [193], Rous sarcoma [201], SV 40 [271], etc. This property is found not only in active, but also in inactivated viruses [201].

2.2. Nonviral Induction of Interferon in Cell Cultures

In the first stage of the study of interferon-induction it was held that only viruses and their nucleic acids can induce its formation. In 1963, Isaacs et al. [370] showed that viruses are not the only inducers and that "foreign" cell nucleic acids possess similar powers. In particular, cultures of chick fibroblasts synthesized an inhibitor when treated with RNA obtained from mouse cells. Under the influence of isologous RNA no interferon was formed. If, however, the purine and pyrimidine bases were denatured by treatment with sulfuric acid, the nucleic acid of homologous cells became foreign and exhibited interferon-inducing properties. Later the ability of foreign cell nucleic acids to induce interferon formation *in vitro* and *in vivo* was confirmed by a number of investigators [107, 173, 381, 471, 555].

Interferon-inducing properties *in vivo* have also been found for Rickettsia tsutsugamushi [359] and for the trachoma-inclusion conjunctivitis (TRIC) viruses [458].

Bacterial polysaccharides, unlike viruses, cannot stimulate interferon synthesis in growing tissues. *In vitro*, bacterial endotoxins and lipopolysaccharides exhibit interferon-inducing activity only by their action on human and animal macrophages and leukocytes [409, 551].

Of the other nonviral agents which induce interferon formation only in suspensions of leukocytes and macrophages *in vitro*, mention must be made of mannan, isolated from <u>Candida</u> <u>albicans</u> [228], phytohemagglutinin [592] and other mitogenic agents [297], and also pyran, a copolymer of the divinyl ester of formic acid [677].

Statolon and helenine, obtained during fermentation of the respective fungi <u>Penicillium</u> <u>stoloniferum</u> and <u>Penicillium</u> <u>funiculosum</u> [399, 522], have been found to be active interferon inducers in cell cultures. It was first considered that the active principle of statolon is a complex anionic polysaccharide with a high content of galacturonic acid. However, it has recently been shown that the active components of both statolon and helenine are double-stranded RNAs, which are evidently the replicative form of viruses parasitizing the mycelium of these fungi [627, 668]. It was later shown that, as well as natural double-stranded RNAs from viral sources, interferon synthesis can also be induced *in vitro* by synthetic double-stranded polyribonucleotide self-polymers [644-646]. A comparative study of the antiviral activity of RNA and DNA copolymers on tissue cultures showed that an RNA-RNA complex has the highest activity. Mixed RNA-DNA complexes have much lower activity and DNA-DNA complexes none whatever. The inhibitory activity of RNA-RNA and RNA-DNA complexes can be enhanced by preliminary treatment of the cells with DEAE-dextran, whereas DNA-DNA complexes still remain inactive as before [641]. Single-stranded RNAs also acquire the ability to inhibit viruses in the presence of DEAE-dextran. For these reasons it has been suggested that the interferon-inducing activity of polynucleotide complexes is dependent on the stability of their secondary structure. To determine antiviral activity, direct protection of tissue culture cells is a more sensitive test than measurements of the interferon concentration. Minimal amounts of the double-stranded poly I:C complex for interferon production in different cell cultures vary from 0.001 to 5.6 $\mu g/ml$ [655, 656]. At the same time, to induce interferon formation with equal intensity, from 100 to 1000 times more of the single-stranded self-polymer (poly I or poly C) than of the double-stranded is required.

Buckler et al. [633] suggest two explanations for the inter-feron-inducing activity of single-stranded structures when tested in high concentrations: either the preparations are contaminated with double-helical material or poly I and poly C in high concentrations can form double-stranded secondary structures. The formation of a double-helical structure in the first case is facilitated by the presence of magnesium ions and in the second case by the presence of an excess of magnesium and a low pH.

2.3. Factors Influencing the Intensity of Interferon Production

Interferon can be produced both by stationary monolayer cultures and in cultures of suspended cells. Cells in the suspended state are considered to produce more interferon [125, 241, 447]. In a comparative study of the interferon yield in stationary and suspended cultures, L. S. Priimyagi showed that interferon can be obtained in higher concentration and in a shorter time by the second method.

Both primary, diploid, and transplanted lines of fibroblastic and epithelial types are capable of synthesizing interferon. White blood cells of man and animals are also active interferon producers.

In the first stages of the study of the ability of various types of tissue cultures to form interferon it was found that transplanted cell lines are weaker producers of interferon than primary cultures [352, 374, 444]. It was later shown, however, that some transplanted lines can synthesize interferon more actively than primary cultures of homologous origin. In particular, transplanted amniotic cells were found to produce more interferon than primary cultures under the influence of Chikungunya virus [325]. A similar relationship in interferon production was found between transplanted cells (M-29 and L) and primary mouse fibroblasts [287, 321, 545, 546].

It must also be remembered that differences in interferon productivity are found not only between primary and transplanted cultures, or between different transplanted cell lines, but also between different variants of the same transplanted line. In a comparison of two variants of HeLa cells [240] fiftyfold differences in interferon production were obtained. In experiments with three lines of L cells, quantitative differences also were detected [435]. Interferon production in one line was much greater than in the other two.

The intensity of interferon production is also influenced by the age of the chick embryo and the duration of incubation of the culture cells *in vitro* before infection with virus. For example, 11-day chick embryos produced ten times more interferon than 6-day embryos [368]. Stimulation of interferon synthesis with an increase in the period of incubation before infection has also been described in the case of primary cultures of human amnion [351], green guenon kidneys, and chick embryonic fibroblasts, and also human diploid cells and L cells [40, 45, 188]. In some experiments, however, the intensity of interferon production in mouse [517], hamster [514], and human [383] cells was independent of the time of incubation of the cultures before infection with virus. These differences evidently indicate that not all cell cultures can stimulate interferon production if the duration of their incubation before infection is increased.

The quantity of interferon formed in cell cultures is determined by the species and strain of the viruses, the activity of the viruses in the given cell culture, and the multiplicity of infection. The same virus can induce interferon synthesis in one cell system but not exhibit this property in another [434, 517, 518].

According to Wagner [577], the highest production of interferon is observed when there is competition between reproduction of the virus and interferon formation, i.e., when reproduction of the virus in the given culture is slow. Smorodintsev [143] and other authors [286, 534, 554, 559] found that the largest quantities of interferon are induced as a rule by viruses with a latent type of infection for the particular type of cell culture concerned. If a virus causes rapid and complete destruction of the cells, little or no interferon will be formed. As a result of observations on a chronic type of virus infection of cell cultures it was concluded that it is due to interferon formation [103, 221, 312, 336, 352]. Some workers found no definite correlation between the cytopathogenicity and the quantity of interferon formed. For example, Sindbis virus, which causes complete and rapid destruction of the cells of a chick fibroblast culture, induced the formation of interferon in them in considerable quantities [349]. Chikungunya virus adapted to the same culture is one of the most active interferon inducers despite the rapidity and completeness of its cytopathogenic action [40, 45, 307].

Interferon is also formed in large amounts after infection of
L cells and cultures of chick fibroblasts by Eastern equine encephalomyelitis virus, which produces rapid degeneration of cultures
if added in high concentration [75, 76, 579].

The intensity of interferon production also was independent
of the intensity of the cytopathogenic action of the virus of tick-
borne encephalitis on cultures of chick fibroblasts in Grokhovskaya's
experiments [54]. A study of the correlation between the time of
appearance of cytopathogenic changes in the cells and the presence
of maximal amounts of interferon showed that these are found in
the culture fluid after most cells in the culture have degenerated
[260]. There is thus no strict correlation between the interferon-
inducing ability of viruses and their cytopathogenic activity.

It was shown previously that induction of interferon is a
property of both infectious and inactivated viruses. However, the
ability of inactivated viruses to induce interferon is largely dependent
on the method of inactivation. Optimal conditions are created where
gentle methods of treatment are used, such as ultraviolet irradiation
and heating. Other methods, especially inactivation with acid and
formalin, have proved to be unsuitable. During inactivation it is
evident that the site in the nucleic acid which is responsible for
inducing interferon must not be damaged during inactivation. When
virus-containing material is treated with an excessive dose of ultraviolet rays or by prolonged heating the interferon-inducing activity
of the viruses is lost. Irradiation of influenza virus for 1-4 min,
for instance, gave a high yield of interferon, but irradiation for
8 min almost completely deprived it of its interferon-inducing
properties [429]. Data showing the importance of the method of
inactivation are given in the same paper. In particular, cells of
the chorioallantoic membrane produced eight times more interferon when treated with irradiated virus than with virus heated
to 56°C. Virus inactivated at 60°C did not induce interferon synthesis at all. It has been shown [310, 602] that NDV irradiated
by ultraviolet rays for 30-60 sec is the best inducer of interferon.
If the virus was irradiated for a longer or shorter period, it induced
the formation of little or no interferon. In addition, NDV inactivated by heating at 56°C did not induce interferon formation either
in chick fibroblasts or in L cells.

The importance of the method and conditions of inactivation for the induction of interferon by viruses has already been mentioned. To this it must be added that in some virus—cell systems ability to induce interferon synthesis is exhibited by both active and inactivated virus, while in other systems only the infectious or the inactivated virus can induce interferon. Different mechanisms are evidently at the basis of these differences. An essential element of the interacting systems is the tissue culture. The quantity of interferon produced by the cells in some cases depends on the multiplicity of infection. This factor is particularly important during induction of interferon by inactivated viruses. Lindenmann and co-workers [429] showed that interferon production was maximal when about 800 a.u. of inactivated influenza virus was used to 1 chorioallantoic membrane. Diluting the virus by 100 times led to an appreciable decrease in the interferon yield. Interferon likewise was not produced or only small quantities were obtained in chick fibroblasts after addition to 10^6 p.f.u. (plaque-forming units) of virus or less to the culture [516, 517].

The effect of multiplicity of infection on interferon formation in cell cultures has been described with respect to the following systems: Chikungunya virus and chick fibroblasts [305], Eastern equine encephalomyelitis, Sindbis, and vesicular stomatitis viruses and chick fibroblasts [40], Eastern and Venezuelan equine encephalomyelitis viruses and chick fibroblasts [75], and Scottish encephalomyelitis virus and chick fibroblasts and L cells [149].

However, in the case of infection with infective viruses some investigators found no relationship between the dose of virus inocculated and the yield of interferon. For instance, in experiments with Newcastle disease virus added to suspended cultures, identical interferon production was obtained regardless of whether the dose added was 0.5 or 500 ID_{50} per cell [241]. Nor was any such dependence found if chick fibroblasts were infected with the viruses of Japanese encephalitis [91, 92] or of tick-borne encephalitis [6]. However, a high multiplicity of infection led to the earlier appearance of maximal amounts of interferon in the culture. The titers of interferon in chick fibroblasts infected with Chikungunya virus in doses of 12 and 0.12 p.f.u. per cell were 1 : 2 and 1 : 23, respectively. Some workers [40], attaching importance to the multiplicity of infection, conclude from these findings that the optimal interferon-inducing dose is not necessarily the largest dose. There are evidently certain optimal virus–cell ratios which lead to the most marked interferon production [40, 130, 131].

The intensity of interferon formation is also influenced by the incubation temperature, the pH, and other factors.

An investigation [516] has shown that supraoptimal temperatures of cultivation of viruses in chick embryos provide more favorable conditions for interferon formation. In particular, Chikungunya, O'nyong-nyong, and Kumba viruses with an optimal propagation temperature of 35°C induced more interferon at temperatures of (for Chikungunya virus) 39 and 42°C. Newcastle disease virus induced more interferon at 42°C than at 37 and 39°C. The optimal temperature for induction of interferon by the virus of tick-borne encephalitis in chick fibroblasts cultures is 36-39°C, and for Chikungunya and Semliki forest viruses it is 40°C. At 30°C no interferon was produced [188]. Dubov [56] and Henslova and Libikova [337] found the highest interferon titers in a system of fibroblasts and tick-borne encephalitis virus at 37°C. At 39°C more interferon was produced by virulent strains than by avirulent strains, which possessed weak interferon-inducing activity at this temperature. In chronically infected cells interferon production depended on the incubation temperature. At 39°C the interferon titers were higher than at 36°C, while at 32°C they were lower [543, 544]. Solov'ev and co-workers [168] found no significant difference in interferon production by chick fibroblast cultures infected with influenza virus within the temperature range from 36.5 to 39.5°C. However, interferon was formed most rapidly at 39.5°C. No interferon could be detected at 30°C.

Interferon formation was also studied in chick embryos in relation to the virulence of the virus and the incubation temperature. No definite correlation could be detected between these properties of the virus [206].

In a series of investigations the effect of hydrogen ion concentration was studied. Between 2 and 4 times more interferon was induced by Sindbis virus in a nutrient medium at pH 6.8 (bicarbonate concentration 0.1%) than in a medium at pH 7.2 (concentration 0.3%) [265]. The opposite relationships were obtained if interferon was induced by Semliki forest virus in mouse embryonic tissue. Less interferon was formed in a weakly acid medium than in a neutral or alkaline medium [563].

No changes were observed in the quantity of interferon inducers by influenza virus in a chick fibroblast culture [234] by a change in pH from 6.8 to 8.1. In the experiments of Smorodintsev and co-workers [149] most interferon was formed in tissue cultures incubated in a medium at pH 6.5 to 7.1.

We also studied the effect of certain factors on the production of interferon by vaccinia and natural smallpox viruses in chick embryonic tissue cultures. Let it be stated at once that no appreciable difference was obtained between them. Accordingly, only results obtained with strain MNIIVP of vaccinia virus will be discussed below.

It has already been stated that the conditions of inactivation of viruses so that they can be used to induce interferon are of considerable importance.

Since this problem has not been studied with respect to vaccinia virus, experiments were carried out to test different conditions of inactivation in order to determine the optimal temperature and duration of heating the virus. The virus was inactivated in a volume of 1 ml in sealed ampules completely immersed in a water bath under different conditions. A volume of virus suspension sufficient to contain 1 TCD_{50} per cell of the culture, calculated as active virus, was then added to each flask. Subsequently every 24 h samples of culture fluid were taken from the flasks and its inhibitory activity determined. The largest quantity of interferon was found in samples obtained 72 h after addition of the virus to the chick fibroblast cultures. However, the intensity of interferon production by the cells was absolutely dependent on the conditions of inactivation of the virus. The results of these experiments are given in Table 10.

The most stable results were obtained with virus heated to 55°C for 30-60 min (Table 10). Inconstant results obtained at lower temperatures or after shorter periods of heating were evidently dependent on the completeness of inactivation of the virus. Negative results were due to the presence of residual activity of the virus in the heated materials. Tests of these samples by passing them twice or three times through chick embryos showed that even very slight residual activity of the virus completely inhibited interferon production by the cells. To confirm this fact either inactivated

TABLE 10. Effect of Conditions of
Inactivation of Vaccinia Virus on Its
Ability to Induce Interferon
Production by Cells

Temperature of heating	Duration of heating, min	Interferon titer
50°	60	0-32
55°	15	0-32
	30-60	32
60°	10	2-16
	20	0-2
	40-60	0
70°	5	2
80-100°	5 and over	0

virus alone or a mixture of completely inactivated virus with active vaccinia virus was added to flasks containing chick fibroblasts.
In the second variant of the experiment interferon production by
the cells was completely inhibited whereas it was found in sufficiently high titer in the culture fluid in the flasks to which only inactivated vaccinia virus was added (Table 11).

The use of higher temperatures to inactivate the virus led to
partial or complete loss of its ability to induce interferon production by the cells. The negative results of these experiments can
evidently by explained by destruction of certain substances of the
vaccinia virus responsible for the ability of the heated vaccinia
virus to induce interferon production by chick fibroblast cells. In

TABLE 11. Interferon For-
mation after Addition of Active and Noninfective Vaccinia Viruses Separately
and Together

Material added	Interferon titer
Active virus	<4
Heated to 55°C	
for 60 min	32
Active + heated	<4

TABLE 12. Interferon Formation in Monolayer Cultures of Chick Fibroblasts Inoculated with Vaccinia Virus Heated to 55°C

Dose (in TCD_{50}) of vaccinia virus calculated per cell	Interferon titer
1-10	128
0.1	64
0.01	16
0.001	4
0.0001	0

TABLE 13. Effect of Age of Culture on Interferon Formation

Age of culture	Interferon titer
24 h	0
48-72 h	4
6-7 days	32

all subsequent experiments to study the conditions of interferon production, vaccinia virus inactivated by heating to 55°C for 1 h was therefore used.

The level of interferon production by cells as a function of the dose of added virus was studied in a series of experiments. The results given in Table 12 show that interferon production by cells infected with inactivated vaccinia virus is directly dependent on the dose of virus added. The maximal quantity of interferon was produced by a dose of 1 CPD_{50} per cell. A further increase in the dose caused no increase in interferon production by the cells. Interferon production by the cells was virtually absent with a dose of 0.0001 TCD_{50} per cell; intermediate doses gave a smaller yield of interferon.

Interesting experiments were carried out to determine the effect of age of the culture and dose of the cells on the intensity of interferon formation. In the experiments with cultures of different ages inactivated virus was added after various times to cultures with a continuous monolayer (Table 13).

In these experiments the most intensive interferon production was observed in cultures incubated at 37°C for 6-7 days before addition of the virus-containing material.

To determine the effect of the number of cells in the culture, 1000-ml Pavitskaya flasks were used and were seeded with between 6 million and 100 million cells. A standard dose of heated virus (10^7 TCD_{50}) was added to the flasks on the 6th day after seeding.

TABLE 14. Effect of Dose of Cells on
Intensity of Interferon Formation

Dose of cells, millions	Time of taking sample, h	Interferon titer
6	24	4
	72	4
20	24	16
	72	64
30	24	32
	72	64
50	24	64
	72	128
100	24	64
	72	64

Samples of culture fluids were titrated after 24 and 72 h. The results are given in Table 14.

It is clear from Table 14 that addition of a larger dose of cells leads to a higher intensity of interferon production by the cells. However, this rule is observed only within certain limits, after which no further increase in interferon production takes place under these experimental conditions. The highest interferon titer (1:128) was obtained in flasks containing 50 million cells. The interferon titers were lower by only one dilution when the standard seeding dose adopted for cells of this type in the production laboratory of the Moscow Research Institute of Virus Preparations was used.

The effect of hydrogen ion concentration and incubation temperature of the cultures on interferon production and the effect of composition of the medium on the intensity of interferon formation also were studied (Tables 15 and 16).

The results in Tables 15 and 16 show that optimal conditions for interferon production by chick fibroblasts are a temperature of 37°C and a pH between 7.0 and 7.4.

Hormones, carcinogens, and other substances have been shown to exert some action on interferon production by the cells of tissue cultures. In particular, the substances "Dianabol" (a derivative of methyltestosterone) and cortisol inhibited interferon formation induced by Sindbis virus [258]. The inhibitory effect of

TABLE 15. Effect of Incubation Temperature on Interferon Formation by Cultures of Chick Embryonic Cells

Incubation temperature	Time of taking samples, h	Interferon titer
4°	24	0
	48	0
	72	0
22°	24	0
	48	4
	72	16
37°	24	16
	48	16
	72	32
42°	24	0
	48	0
	72	0

TABLE 16. Effect of Hydrogen Ion Concentration on Interferon Formation

pH	Interferon titer
6.6	32
7.0	64
7.4	64
7.8	32

cortisol on interferon synthesis was also observed in cultures of chick fibroblasts and of cells of transplanted line 3B infected with Chikungunya virus and vaccinia virus [450]. Suppression of interferon formation under the influence of cortisol also took place after treatment with inactivated viruses. A decrease in interferon formation results from the treatment of cultures of chick fibroblasts infected with influenza A virus by steroid hormones [508-510].

In experiments by Solov'ev and co-workers [167] colchicine inhibited interferon formation. These workers consider that the inhibitory action is based on a disturbance of the synthesis of RNA which is essential for interferon formation.

Interferon synthesis was suppressed in rat embryonic cultures infected with Sindbis virus by treatment with the carcinogens 3-methylcholanthrene, benzpyrene, and 7,12-dimethylbenzanthracene [261, 262, 264], in cultures of chick fibroblasts infected with the same virus by the action of adenine, adenosine, deoxyadenosine, and 6-mercaptopurine [448], and in cultures infected with Kumba virus by the action of triethylenimine.

Interferon formation is also suppressed by ultraviolet irradiation of cell cultures [54, 255, 263]. The reason for this effect may be that interferon synthesis is coded at a certain site of the cell DNA. Destruction of this region by UV-irradiation also affects the ability of the cells to produce interferon.

Interferon production may also be affected by preliminary treatment of the tissue cultures with interferon. It was discovered initially that cells first treated with interferon synthesize more interferon during subsequent action of the virus [369]. A later report [574] described the opposite effect of preliminary treatment of the cells with interferon. However, these contradictory results were explained after experiments [295, 434] which showed that treatment of the cells with small doses of interferon in fact potentiates the ability of the cells to produce interferon, while high concentrations depress this ability. It was also shown [426] that RNA appears sooner and interferon is formed more rapidly in cells treated with low concentrations of interferon. In an attempt to explain the results of these experiments to study the effect of different doses of interferon on its production, Friedman [295] postulated that the mechanism controlling the inhibition of subsequent interferon synthesis is an excess of the end product, i.e., interferon itself. This hypothesis was confirmed by the discovery of the fact that an effect similar to that observed after addition of a large dose of exogenous interferon was also observed as the result of the subsequent treatment of the cultures with a small dose of interferon and a small dose of virus.

It may be pointed out in conclusion that interferon production can be influenced by antibiotics which inhibit the synthesis of RNA, DNA, and cell proteins (see "Mechanism of Formation and Action of Interferon," p. 263) and also by certain viruses, especially NDV, parainfluenza and vaccinia viruses, and polioviruses [49-51, 339, 365, 477].

2.4. Comparative Study of Induction of Interferon by Viruses in Different Cell Cultures

The study of the interferon-inducing activity of viruses is of interest in two ways. First, it can give some idea of the role of interferon in the pathogenesis of virus infections and, second, it can help to discover the most active interferon inducers. The

TABLE 17. Interferon-Inducing Activity of Viruses in Cultures of Chick Fibroblasts and Monkeys' Kidneys

Virus	Interferon titer after treatment with virus					
	chick fibroblasts			monkey's kidneys		
	native	heated to		native	heated to	
		37°	56°		37°	56°
Western equine encephalomyelitis	0	0	0	0	0	0
Sindbis	16	0	0	n.i.	n.i.	n.i.
Chikungunya	16	0	0	0	0	0
Vesicular stomatitis	0	0	0	2	4	4
Newcastle disease (strain H)	16	2	0	0	0	0
Influenza A (PR-8)	2	2	0	0	0	0
Coxsackie B3	0	0	2	0	0	0
Poliovirus type I	0	2	4	0	0	0
ECHO 11	0	0	2	0	0	0

second of these aspects is particularly important because of reports of the desirability of using viruses which stimulate endogenous interferon in the prevention and treatment of virus infections [39, 41, 82, 83, 144, 186].

Accordingly the ability of a series of viruses to induce interferon production in primary cultures, strains of diploid cells, and transplanted lines of different origins was compared. Some of these experiments were carried out jointly with A. E. Gumennik.

The results of these experiments are given in Table 17.

The results in Table 17 show that after heating to 56°C for 30 min only poliomyelitis, Coxsackie, and ECHO viruses induced interferon production, poliomyelitis virus did so after heating to 37°C for 14 days, whereas Newcastle disease, Sindbis, and Chikungunya viruses induced interferon production only in the active state. Under these experimental conditions, the viruses of Western equine encephalomyelitis and vesicular stomatitis induced no interferon production whatever by chick fibroblasts. Influenza A viruses, whether active or inactivated at 37°C, induced weak interferon synthesis.

Only vesicular stomatitis virus, both active and inactivated, induced interferon production in monkeys' kidney cells. The other viruses used in these experiments did not induce interferon production.

Comparison of the results given in Table 17 shows that the same virus exhibits different interferon-inducing activity in different tissue cultures. The manifestation of this ability is affected also by the conditions of inactivation of the viruses. At the same time the results of these experiments show that to determine whether a particular virus is suitable as an interferon inducer, it must be investigated under homologous conditions. The results of the study of this ability in a heterologous system cannot serve as a reliable basis for the use of a virus to induce interferon.

In the search for accessible sources of human interferon, we carried out research to determine the ability of strains of diploid cells to produce interferon. As inducers, viruses possessing different degrees of cytopathogenic activity were tested.

As a first step the interferon-producing ability of a strain of human diploid cells, obtained by R. I. Rapoport from a fetal lung and generously provided by him, was determined. The results are given in Table 18.

Of the myxoviruses, enteroviruses, and arboviruses tested, as Table 18 shows only poliovirus type I and Sendai and Newcastle disease viruses possessed interferon-inducing activity in a culture of a strain of human diploid cells of pulmonary origin, and in the last two of these viruses this property was more strongly

TABLE 18. Interferon-Producing Activity of Viruses
in Strain L-44 of Diploid Cells

Virus	Cytopathogenicity	Interferon titer
Influenza A	−	0
Western equine enceph- alomyelitis	−	0
Vesicular stomatitis	+	0
Chikungunya	−	0
Foot and mouth disease	−	0
Poliovirus type I	+	0
ECHO 11	+	2
Sendai	−	8
Newcastle disease	+	8-16

Note. + Degeneration complete; − no degeneration present.

TABLE 19. Interferon Formation in Monolayer Cultures
Inoculated with Newcastle Disease Virus

Composition of cells	Source of tissue	Titer of interferon induced by	
		native virus	heated virus
Fibroblasts	Chick embryos	8	0
	Mouse embryos	32	0
	Rat embryos	16	0
	Guinea pig embryos	0	0
	Rabbit embryos	32	0
Renal epithelium	Monkeys	0	0
	Pig embryos	0	0

marked. It was therefore interesting to determine whether this
activity of NDV extends to tissue cultures from other species of
animals. Experiments were accordingly carried out in which primary trypsinized cultures of fibroblasts and epithelial cells were
treated with infective virus which had been heated to 56°C for 30
min, in the proportion of 1 TCD_{50} per cell (Table 19).

Interferon production in the test cultures was induced only
by infective NDV and this induction, moreover, was observed only
in cultures of fibroblast type. Heat-inactivated virus did not induce
interferon formation in any of the test cultures.

These results show that NDV induces interferon formation in
tissue cultures of different species, but in the experiments described
it exhibited this activity only in cultures of fibroblasts. However,
this does not mean that NDV is in general incapable of inducing inter
feron formation in cultures of epithelial type. From information in
the literature it is known that NDV induces large quantities of interferon in cultures of amnion cells [277, 279].

Later the ability of NDV to induce interferon production was
demonstrated in various strains of diploid cells obtained from the
myodermal tissue of 8- to 12-week embryos and from the lung of
a 5- to 6-month human fetus after 4-5, 10-12, and 25 subcultures.
No significant difference in interferon production by the same strain
of cells could be discovered after this number of subcultures. However, appreciable differences in interferon production were found
between strains of cells obtained from the lungs and myodermal
tissue and between strains of the same origin (Table 20).

TABLE 20. Interferon Production by Strains
of Diploid Cells of Different Origin

Source of cell strain	Name of strain	Interferon titer
Human fetal lung	L-44	16
	L-45	4
	L-46	8
Myodermal tissue of human embryo	KM-1	32
	KM-2	64
	KM-3	64
	KM-4	32
	KM-5	16

It will be noted in Table 20 that strains from the fetal lung produced different quantities of interferon but this quantity in most cases was less than the amount of interferon formed by cells derived from myodermal tissue. These differences can be attributed either to the genetic features of the donors from whose tissues the strains were obtained or to the unequal ability of lung and myodermal tissues to produce interferon. The importance of the donor's genetic characteristics is shown by the different titers of interferon obtained with different strains from the fetal lung or from myodermal tissues.

However, the role of the type of tissues for interferon production could be demonstrated only if the different types of tissue cultures were obtained from the same embryos. To investigate the role of organ or tissue specificity of the cells, tissue cultures were therefore prepared from the organs and tissues of the same chick embryos at the age of 16 days. Cultures of myodermal tissue, spleen, lung, and kidney were obtained from the embryo and their ability to produce interferon was tested under identical experimental conditions. Chikungunya virus was used as the inducer.

The technique of preparation of the cultures was as follows. The organs of ten embryos exsanguinated by decapitation were pooled and trypsinized in the usual way. The cell suspensions were added in equal amounts (5 million cells) to not less than three 100-ml Pavitskaya flasks. After 5 days of growth Chikungunya virus was added to the flasks at the rate of 1 TCD_{50} per cell. The virus was inactivated after 18-20 h in the usual way (pH 2.4) and the material was titrated on primary cultures of chick fibroblasts.

TABLE 21. Ability of Various Tissues of 16-Day Chick Embryo to Produce Interferon

Source of tissue	Interferon titer
Spleen	128
Myodermal tissue	128
Lung	64
Kidney	48

The results (Table 21) demonstrate that different tissues of the body differ in their ability to produce interferon. The most active interferon producers in the experiments described were cultures from the spleen and myodermal tissue, followed by the culture from the lung, and the smallest quantity of interferon was produced by kidney tissue cultures.

The interferon-inducing activity of viruses was compared with their cytopathogenic activity in experiments on chick fibroblasts. In these experiments cultures were infected at the rate of 1 TCD_{50} per cell and the culture fluid was collected 48 h after infection. The results (Table 22) showed no correlation between ability to induce interferon formation and cytopathogenic activity.

TABLE 22. Comparison of Interferon Inducers and Cytopathogenic Activities of Viruses

Virus	Rate of onset of degeneration, days	Interferon titer
Newcastle disease	3-4	16
Chikungunya	1-2	64
Sindbis	1-2	16
Vesicular stomatitis	1-2	<2
Western equine encephalomyelitis	1-2	<2
Vaccinia	3-4	<2
Smallpox	5-6	<2

Western equine encephalomyelitis and vesicular stomatitis viruses caused rapid destruction of the cells without inducing interferon synthesis, whereas Chikungunya and Sindbis viruses, with similar cytopathogenic activity to the above-mentioned viruses, were active stimulators of interferon formation.

2.5. Dynamics of Formation and Liberation of Interferon in Cell Cultures

The dynamics of formation and liberation of interferon in cell cultures was also compared experimentally in our laboratory. Investigation of these processes is of considerable practical as well as theoretical importance because it can be used to establish the optimal times for "harvesting" interferon.

According to reports in the literature interferon is formed at different rates in different virus—cell systems. In most cultures tested maximal interferon production occurred within the first 24 h [34, 543]. Wagner [58] found interferon 4 h after infection of chick fibroblasts with Chikungunya virus. In suspensions of human leukocytes, interferon appeared under the influence of Sendai virus 2-3 h after infection [277].

In the experiments of Ershov and Zhdanov [75] the first appearance of interferon in the culture fluid was observed 6-8 h after infection, coinciding with the time of ending of the replication cycle of the viruses used. Later the interferon titer rose gradually to reach a maximum at 24 h. The curve of interferon formation resembled the curve of replication of Eastern and Venezuelan encephalitis viruses and Semliki forest virus which were used in these experiments.

In some virus—cell systems, however, interferon was found relatively late. For instance, the quantity of interferon in cultures of chick fibroblasts infected with herpes simplex virus reached its maximum on the 4th day after infection [411]. In cultures of monkeys' kidneys infected with SV_{40} virus, on the other hand, interferon did not begin to appear until the 4th day and its content increased until the 12th day [271]. Interferon was found later still (on the 11th day) in cultures of human amnion cells infected with measles virus [260].

The rate of interferon formation also depends on the method of cultivating the cells. In cultures of suspended cells interferon synthesis takes place twice as fast as in monolayer cultures of the same cells [125, 447].

In practice the formation of interferon in tissue cultures infected with active viruses takes place simultaneously with or immediately after reproduction of the virus [6, 91, 193, 273, 349].

Several investigations have shown that interferon diffuses into the surrounding nutrient medium continuously as it is formed in the cells [149, 344, 582]. Ho and Wagner consider that this leads to the development of equilibrium between the interferon formed in the cells and the interferon liberated into the surrounding medium. By cultivation in inverted flasks, so that the cells were not in contact with the liquid, Smorodintsev and co-workers [149] obtained a sharp increase in the content of intracellular interferon.

It follows from the investigations cited above that the rate of interferon formation has now been studied in tissue cultures of different types and under the influence of different viruses. However, it is not yet clear which element of the interacting virus—cell system determines the rate of formation of interferon. This

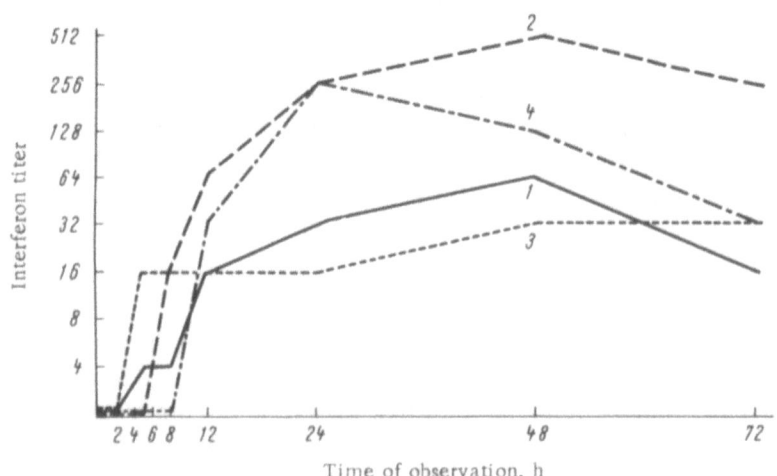

Fig. 1. Dynamics of interferon production induced by Newcastle disease virus in various tissue cultures: 1) chick fibroblasts; 2) rabbit fibroblasts; 3) strain of human diploid cells; 4) transplanted line L mouse cells.

problem can be solved only by experiments in which the same interferon inducer is used with different types of tissue cultures. For this purpose the writer infected primary monolayer cultures of chick and rabbit fibroblasts, a strain of human diploid cells, and transplanted cells of mouse line L (clone 929) with NDV. The cells were grown in Roux flasks and virus was added at the rate of 10 TCD_{50} per cell. Samples were taken at once and 2, 5, 8, 12, 24, 48, and 72 h after addition of NDV. The virus was inactivated in the usual way and the inhibitory activity of the samples was determined by titration in homologous cells with vesicular stomatitis virus. The results are given in Fig. 1.

Although in all these experiments the same virus was used as inducer, the dynamics of interferon formation in cultures of different types varied (Fig. 1). Interferon production was most rapid in the strain of human diploid cells. In this case interferon synthesis actually ended 5 h after infection and its content remained at the same level until 48 h. Interferon formation in the transplanted mouse cell line occurred at the slowest rate of all. It was not until 12 h had elapsed that the inhibitor was first found in these cultures, but its synthesis ceased completely during the next 12 h, i.e., interferon formation in these cultures ended 24 h after infection. A different picture was observed in primary cultures of chick and rabbit embryonic fibroblasts. Although interferon was liberated into the medium by them sooner and could be detected after 5-8 h, its concentration in the culture medium reached its maximum after 48 h. Usually between 24 and 48 h the titer of the inhibitor was doubled. The decrease in titer after this period was evidently due to the destructive action of cellular enzymes or other factors on the interferon.

The results show that the properties of the cell culture have a marked influence on the rate of interferon formation. Presumably the rate of interferon production depends on the rate of formation of interferon-specific mRNA transmitting information to the ribosomes. This hypothesis is supported by the results of experiments on rabbit macrophages [732]. It has been shown, in particular, that mRNA for interferon synthesis is formed later in rabbit kidney cells than in macrophages.

The importance of the properties of the cells as a factor determining the dynamics of interferon formation is also confirmed by

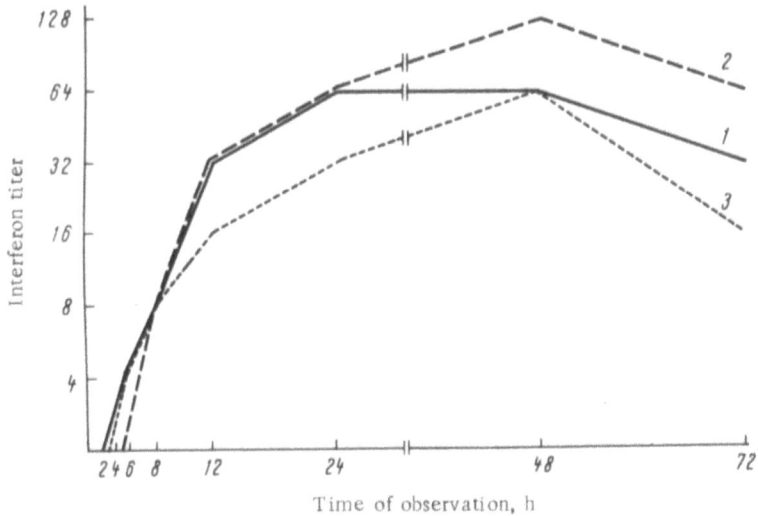

Fig. 2. Dynamics of interferon production by chick fibroblasts induced by different viruses: 1) Chikungunya virus; 2) Sindbis virus;
3) Newcastle disease virus.

the results of our experiments on chick fibroblasts with infective
Chikungunya, Sindbis, and Newcastle disease viruses (Fig. 2) and
with heat-inactivated vaccinia virus (Table 23). They show that
different viruses induce a similar dynamics of interferon formation
in the same culture.

TABLE 23. Dynamics of In-
terferon Formation Induced
by Inactivated Vaccinia Virus

Duration of incubation	Interferon titer
0	<4
1	<4
2	<4
5	8
8	16
12	64
24	64
48	64

The results given in Fig. 2 and Table 23 show that the four viruses tested on chick fibroblasts induced interferon formation at the same rate. Given an equal multiplicity of infection, the properties of the cell culture are thus decisively important for the rate of interferon formation.

A fact which will be clear from these results is that NDV was an active inducer of interferon production not only in mammalian cells, but also in cultures of chick fibroblasts. These results are in conflict with those obtained by other workers who found that the ability of NDV to induce interferon formation in chick embryonic cells is weak. These differences could be due to differences in the properties of the NDV strains used by us and those used by other workers. In particular, there are statements to the effect that virulent strains of measles virus [174, 351] induce less interferon than avirulent strains and are less sensitive to its action.

In the experiments described earlier the writer used a vaccine strain (N) of NDV, which is nonpathogenic to chickens. It was therefore important to study the effect of virulence of NDV strains on their ability to induce interferon formation.

These investigations revealed a connection between virulence, interferon-inducing activity, and other properties of NDV in cultures of chick fibroblasts and of certain other cells. In particular, the correlation between virulence and intensity of interferon formation, on the one hand, and such features as the level of virus replication and of hemagglutinin formation, the intensity of the cytopathogenic action, and the effect of temperature on the manifestation of these properties was studied.

Five strains of NDV with three different levels of virulence were used in the experiments: strains K and Tomilino, virulent toward chick embryos, chickens, and hens; strains N and GNKI, virulent to chick embroys and chickens under the age of 15 days, and strain V1, virulent to chick embryos only. The last three strains are used in vaccine production.

In the first stage of these investigations the character of the cytopathogenic action and the level of inteferon formation and replication of the viruses used in the experiments at 37°C were studied (Table 24).

TABLE 24. Comparison of Interferon-Inducing and Other Properties
of Strains of Newcastle Disease Virus

Strain	Virulence[*]	Cytopath-ogenic activity	Intensity of reproduction of virus TCD_{50}	Intensity of hemagglutinin formation	Interferon titer
K	Velogenic	Marked	$10^{6.5}$-10^8	1:40-1:160	2-4
Tomilino	Velogenic	Marked		1:40-1:160	2-4
N	Mesogenic	Marked	10^5-$10^{6.5}$	1:5-1:10	16-32
GNKI	Mesogenic	Marked		1:5-1:10	16-32
V1	Lentogenic	Weak	10^4-10^5	1:4	2-4

[*]Velogenic: pathogenic to chickens and chick embryos; lentogenic means pathogenic
to chick embryos only.

The experiments showed that the cytopathogenic action of
Tomilino, K, N, and GNKI viruses is well defined and appears rapidly if small doses of virus (10-100 CPD_{50}) are used. The corresponding action of strain V1 is weak and total degeneration of
the culture is not observed even after infection with 10^4-10^5 TCD_{50}
of virus.

Titration in chick embryos after the most severe degeneration of the cell culture showed that the level of reproduction of the
viruses in the embryos is also correlated with virulence. After
infection of the cultures with 100-1000 TCD_{50} of each virus strains
K and Tomilino reproduced up to a titer of $10^{6.5}$-10^8, strains N and
GNKI up to 10^5-$10^{6.5}$, and strain V1 up to 10^4-10^5.

Meanwhile appreciable differences also were found in the
hemagglutinin titers in the culture fluid in experiments with 1%
hens' erythrocytes. The hemagglutination test was positive with
the virulent strains in a dilution of 1:40 and 1:160 and with strains
N and GNKI in dilutions of 1:5 to 1:10; with strain V1 it was
negative.

Comparison of the interferon inducing activity and the properties described above showed definite correlation between the intensity of interferon formation and the intensity of reproduction.
In particular, the velogenic strains K and Tomilino, which induced
interferon formation weakly, reproduced more intensively (up to
higher titers) in chick fibroblasts. These differences are presumabl
based on the unequal interferon-inducing activity of strains of NDV
with different virulence. However, different relationships were

TABLE 25. Interferon-Inducing
Activity of Various Strains
of NDV

| Strain | Interferon titer | |
	in human dip-loid cultures	in primary mouse fibroblasts
K	2-4	8
N	6-32	128
V1	2-4	8-16

TABLE 26. Sensitivity of Different Strains of NDV
to Interferon

| Method of determining sensitivity to interferon | Strain | | | | |
	K	Tomilino	N	GNKI	V1
Number of TCD_{50} inhibited by 8 units of interferon	1	1	10	10	100
Interferon titer using a constant dose of virus (100 TCD_{50})	2	2	4	4	8

found for the least virulent strain V1. Strain V1 reproduced with least intensity in chick fibroblasts but, at the same time, it induced interferon in the same amounts as the virulent, epizootic strains K and Tomilino.

Taking into consideration these features of the five strains in cell cultures from a naturally susceptible host, it was decided to investigate their interferon-inducing activity in cell cultures of less susceptible or resistant organisms. As Table 25 shows, the same principles as those indicated above were found with cultures of human and mouse origin.

The most and least virulent strains induced less interferon in these cultures than strains of moderate virulence. Consequently, mechanisms other than the intensity of interferon induction are responsible for the fact that V1 virus reproduces less intensively in chick fibroblasts. In particular, one factor responsible could be the higher sensitivity of strain V1 to interferon. Experiments were carried out with all five strains of NDV and they showed that the

TABLE 27. Effect of Incubation Temperature on Induction of Interferon
by NDV Strains

Strain	Interferon titer			
	at 34°	at 37°	at 40°	at 42°
K	0	2	4	0
T	0	2	2	0
N	16	16	64	4
GNKI	4	16	4	2
V1	2	8	0	0

least virulent strain V1 is the most sensitive to interferon. Velogenic
strains K and Tomilino were more resistant to the inhibitory action of interferon. The mesogenic strains N and GNKI occupied an
intermediate position in their sensitivity to interferon (Table 26).

Consequently, one of the factors determining the lower
virulence of strain V1 was its higher sensitivity to interferon.

Since our experiments [27] had shown a definite relationship
between virulence and ability of Newcastle disease viruses to form
plaques at higher temperatures, interferon formation was studied
at different temperatures.

Chick fibroblasts in 100-ml Pavitskaya flasks were infected
at the rate of 1 TCD_{50} per cell and their interferon titer was investigated 24 h after addition of the virus. The results are shown
in Table 27.

Raising the incubation temperature of the cultures did not
increase but decreased the intensity of interferon production (Table
27). However, a more important aspect of these results would
appear to be that although the absolute quantities of interferon
induced by each strain were lower at 40 and 42°C, the relative
abilities of the different strains to induce interferon remained the
same as at 37°C. Consequently, the assumptions made at the beginning of this chapter apply also to the results of experiments at higher
temperatures.

These results show that strains which differ in their virulence
also differ in their intensity of reproduction in chick fibroblast

cultures. More virulent strains, which are weak inducers of interferon and less sensitive to it, reproduced to the highest titer ($10^{6.5}$–10^8). Moderately virulent vaccine strains, which induced more interferon and were more sensitive to it, reproduced up to titers of 10^5–$10^{6.5}$. The least virulent strain induced little interferon but was most sensitive to it and reached titers of 10^4–10^5.

The intensity of reproduction of the different strains of NDV in chick fibroblasts thus depended both on their activity as inducers of interferon and on their sensitivity to it.

It will be noted that the interferon-inducing activity of NDV strains was independent of the character of their destructive action on the cells.

2.6. Blocking of the Formation and Action of Interferon by Viruses

In 1960 Lindenmann [428] described a phenomenon which he called inverse interference. He found that infective influenza virus (strain MEL) inhibited interferon production induced by inactivated virus of the same strain.

Ability to inhibit interferon formation induced by other viruses was later discovered in Newcastle disease and fowl plaque viruses [365] and in parainfluenza virus 3 [338]. Isaacs showed that virulent myxoviruses (NDV and fowl plague) inhibit interferon formation induced by Chikungunya virus in chick fibroblasts. Hermodsson used Newcastle disease virus with a low intensity of reproduction in bovine kidney cells but which induced large quantities of interferon in them. Parainfluenza virus 3, which reproduced readily in the same cultures, did not induce interferon formation. However, the behavior of NDV in the cultures changed if they were additionally infected with parainfluenza virus. If cells chronically infected with NDV were infected with parainfluenza virus, the NDV ceased to induce interferon but began to reproduce more actively.

Another example of the stimulation of NDV by parainfluenza virus was described by Maeno et al. [674], who showed that NDV reproduced to much higher titers in a culture of HeLa cells which was a latent carrier of type I parainfluenza virus (HVY) than in HeLa cells not infected with HVY, and induced a marked cytopathogenic action. When comparing interferon induction by NDV in HeLa and HeLa–HVY cells, these workers found that interferon

was present in the first culture but absent in the culture chronically infected with HVY. Furthermore, culture fluid from HeLa cells
containing interferon did not reduce the number of plaques of test
poliovirus in the HeLa-HVY culture. It is clear from these experiments that HeLa-HVY cells, unlike normal HeLa cells, cannot
produce interferon on infection with NDV and are insensitive to its
antiviral action.

Interferon formation induced by NDV was also found to be
inhibited by bovine diarrhea virus [272], vesicular stomatitis virus
[384], and cytomegalovirus [314].

A similar phenomenon has been described in the case of
poliomyelitis virus [50]. Yurov [190] observed inhibition of interferon formation in chick embryos infected successively with the
viruses of Newcastle disease and infectious bronchitis or laryngotracheitis.

The potentiating action of Sendai virus on reproduction of
vesicular stomatitis virus has also been described [243, 565]. In
particular, preliminary infection of cell cultures with parainfluenza
virus led to the formation of vesicular stomatitis virus in 2-8 times
as many plaques. These workers postulated that their results are
due to the blocking action of the virus on the antiviral activity of the
interferon.

It was stated in the publication cited above that the phenomena
of inverse interference were due to the direct action of the virus.

Meanwhile there are other reports in the literature of nonviral factors which can potentiate the reproduction of a virus. A
factor called a "stimulon" has been described [230, 250, 251]. It
is found when rat embryonic cells are infected with adenovirus
type 12 and it potentiates reproduction of viruses. Its nature and
mechanism of action have not yet been established. However, it
is known that the stimulon does not affect interferon production
but blocks its action. The formation of a factor potentiating reproduction of viruses in the allantoic fluid of chick embryos infected with parainfluenza type I and influenza A (PR-8) viruses has
been reported by Katoi and co-workers [387-389]. Gendon and co-
workers [48-51] have described an inhibitor which blocks the action
of interferon. In their opinion this factor, like interferon itself,

is formed during reproduction of certain viruses in tissue culture and does not possess strict virus specificity.

In 1966, Isaacs and co-workers [375] described an inhibitor of interferon production which they called a "blocker." In their opinion, in some of its properties this blocker is similar to interferon but differs from it in its relationship to proteolytic enzymes. Interferon is partially sensitive to trypsin and highly sensitive to pepsin, whereas the blocker is resistant to both these enzymes. They suggest from these results that the blocker is nonprotein in nature. Since the blocker is more easily found when chick embryos are infected by more virulent viruses (NDV and fowl plaque), it may possibly play a role in virus virulence.

In 1967, Ota (cited in [675]) described a substance which he called an "interferon depressor." It was produced in a culture of chick embryonic cells infected with NDV or in the allantoic fluid of chick embryos infected with HVY parainfluenza virus. The depressor inhibited interferon production by NDV or by Sindbis virus in cultures of chick embryonic cells and in some of its properties it resembled the blocker: it was not sedimented during ultracentrifugation, not neutralized by virus antiserum, not dialyzed, and was stable on heating (90°C for 1 h). Truden et al. [689] published a report on a substance which they called an interferon antagonist. This substance was produced by mouse cells infected with NDV and it stimulated reproduction of Mengo virus in Ehrlich's ascites cells. The semipurified antagonist could be isolated from interferon by filtration through CM-Sephadex, and it was found in two zones of the chromatographic column. One of these peaks was identified as a protein. The purified preparation was inactivated by trypsin, while the unpurified was resistant to the action of the enzyme. Sheaff and Stewart [688] also observed the formation of an interferon antagonist in the supernatant of cultures of BHK-21 and chick fibroblasts infected with Sindbis virus. This substance stimulated replication of the homologous virus and was sensitive to trypsin but resistant to the action of ribo- and deoxyribonucleases.

At this stage, therefore, a number of papers have been published on the ability of certain viruses to induce special inhibitors in infected tissues which inhibit the formation or action of interferon. It must be emphasized that these properties described were possessed as a rule by only certain strains of viruses and there is some evidence to suggest that they are exhibited only in certain types of cultures [565].

In our investigations of vaccinia virus a phenomenon similar to that of inverse interference was encountered and an attempt was made to study some of its aspects.

It was pointed out on page 38 that a strain of vaccinia virus previously used at the Moscow Institute of Virus Preparations for the production of smallpox vaccine does not induce interferon formation in cultures of chick fibroblasts. If, however, it was inactivated at 55°C for 50 min it exhibited this property distinctly.

The combined addition of active and inactivated viruses to a culture likewise does not induce interferon formation. It was postulated that active vaccinia virus induces the formation of an inhibitor which blocks the ability of the cells to produce interferon. The technique used to detect the inhibitor was a modification of the method described previously by Gendon [49] to detect an inhibitor blocking the action of interferon.

In our experiments chick fibroblasts were infected, 48 h after seeding in Roux flasks, with vaccinia virus in a multiplicity of 2–3 TCD_{50} per cell and incubated at 37°C. One hour later the cells were washed 3 times with Hanks's solution, 100 ml of medium 199 was added to each flask, and the contents were again incubated for 2 h. The medium was then removed and the cells were collected mechanically and suspended in 15 ml of medium 199. The contents of three flasks were pooled and the cell suspension treated with ultrasound (800 kHz, 10 W/cm², 10 min). The material was centrifuged for 10 min at 1000 rpm. The supernatant was centrifuged at 180,000 g twice for 2 h. The supernatant from this procedure was tested for the presence of an inhibitor blocking the formation and action of interferon.

These experiments were carried out on chick fibroblasts grown for 5–6 days in 100-ml Pavitskaya flasks. The total number of flasks was divided into 6 groups, to which the following were added, respectively:

1) 5 ml supernatant and 3 ml Chikungunya virus (titer 10^6 TCD_{50});

2) 3 ml Chikungunya virus;

3) 5 ml supernatant;

4) 5 ml supernatant, 4 ml interferon (titer $1:128$), and 1000 TCD_{50} WEE virus;

5) 1000 TCD WEE virus;

6) 4 ml interferon and 1000 TCD_{50} WEE virus.

Instead of WEE virus, 100 TCD_{50} vaccinia virus was added to the flasks of groups 4-6 in some experiments.

The flasks of the first 3 groups with tissue culture served to demonstrate the ability of the inhibitor to block interferon formation, while the purpose of the flasks of groups 4-6 was that of a system to detect the ability of the inhibitor to inhibit the action of interferon.

The volume of fluid in all the flasks was adjusted to 15 ml with medium 199. All the ingredients were added on the day that the supernatant was obtained, and the WEE virus was added 24 h later. The supernatant was tested for the presence of residual virus, which was absent in all the experiments.

A supernatant of uninfected chick fibroblasts, treated in the same way, was used as the control.

All the flasks were incubated at 37°C until the beginning of degeneration of the cells of the chick fibroblast cultures infected with virus only. The contents of the flasks of groups 1-3 were then treated with hydrochloric acid to pH 2.4, and 48 h later the pH was adjusted to 7.4 with alkali and the interferon content was determined. Flasks with cultures of groups 4-6 were repeatedly frozen and thawed, after which the virus contained in them was assayed by titration in chick fibroblasts.

The results of the first series of experiments are given in Table 28. They show that the supernatant had a blocking action on interferon formation. Interferon was found in a titer of $1:16$ only in cultures infected with Chikungunya virus alone; in cultures to which both virus and supernatant were added no interferon was present.

The blocking effect of the inhibitor on the action of interferon also was studied. However, when WEE virus was used as the test virus no blocking action on interferon could be demonstrated.

TABLE 28. Blocking of Interferon Formation
by Vaccinia Virus

Group of culture	Material added to cells	Interferon titer
1	Supernatant of infected cells	0
2	Chikungunya virus	16
3	Supernatant + Chikungunya virus	0
Control	Supernatant of normal cells	0

In the presence of the supernatant, interferon completely suppressed reproduction of WEE virus, which is known to be highly sensitive to interferon. Presumably even if some of the activity of the interferon were suppressed, the action of the inhibitor would not become manifest because of the high sensitivity of the test virus to interferon. This could be established either by the use of limiting dilutions of interferon or by the use of viruses only moderately sensitive to the inhibitory action of interferon. A strain of vaccinia virus, obtained by cloning from the Mastyukova strain of vaccinia virus, which possesses all these properties, was chosen for the purpose.

The results of the second series of experiments are given in Table 29.

As Table 29 shows, the action of interferon was blocked only when vaccinia virus was used as the test virus. If the supernatant was added to the virus—interferon mixture, 100 times more virus

TABLE 29. Blocking of the Action of Interferon by
Inhibitor Induced by Vaccinia Virus

Material added to cells	Titer of virus, CTD_{50}/ml
Supernatant, vaccinia virus, and interferon	10^4
Vaccinia virus and interferon	10^2
Vaccinia virus	10^5
Supernatant, WEE virus, and interferon	0
WEE virus and interferon	0
WEE virus	10^7

was reproduced than in the cultures inoculated with virus and interferon only. It should be noted, however, that the blocking action of the inhibitor in these experiments was only partial. The titer of virus was ten times less than in cultures infected with vaccinia virus alone, despite the presence of inhibitor in the medium. Consequently, the inhibitor formed in chick fibroblasts through the action of the vaccinia virus is capable of blocking not only the formation, but also the action of interferon.

The effect of the time of addition of the inhibitor on interferon formation when Chikungunya virus was used as the inducer was studied in the next experiments. The inducing virus and supernatant were added in these experiments at different intervals and the interferon was assayed after complete degeneration of the cultures. The blocking action of the inhibitor on interferon formation was revealed only when the supernatant was added to the culture not later than 6 h after infection of the chick fibroblasts with the interferon-inducing virus. Total suppression of interferon formation was observed in the cultures to which virus and supernatant were added successively at an interval not exceeding 1 h. If the intervals were from 1 to 6 interferon production gradually increased, and if the interval exceeded 6 h it was at the control level (Table 30).

2.7. Conclusion

The study of interferon formation in tissue cultures has shown that it is determined by the properties both of the virus and

TABLE 30. Effect of Interval between Addition of Virus and Inhibitor on Interferon Formation

Material added to cells	Interval between addition of virus and supernatant, h	Interferon titer
Supernatant + Chikungunya virus	0	0
The same	1	0
The same	3	4
The same	6	16
The same	8	32
The same	24	32
Chikungunya virus	–	32

of the producing tissue. The cell systems used responded differently to the action of the same viruses. For instance, native vaccinia virus did not induce interferon production in chick embryonic and other cells. It did induce interferon production, however, in these cells after inactivation by heating to 55°C for 30-60 min. Meanwhile, active vaccinia virus induced interferon production in mouse embryonic cells.

The quantity of interferon produced by the cells depends on the age of the culture, the dose of added virus, the incubation temperature, the number of cells, and the hydrogen ion concentration. In chick embryonic cells the largest quantity of interferon was produced at 37°C, pH 7.4, and with a dose of virus of 1-10 TCD_{50} per cell. The maximal interferon concentration under these conditions was observed in cultures incubated for 6-7 days before addition of the inducer virus.

The conditions of inactivation are of great importance to the induction of interferon by vaccinia and natural smallpox viruses.

Having regard to the species specificity of interferon, it is interesting to study the ability of strains of human diploid cells to produce interferon. In the event of success they could be used as a readily available source of interferon. However, most viruses tested under these conditions induced interferon only weakly, the virus of Newcastle disease (NDV) exhibiting the greatest activity. It was active in strains of cells obtained from the fetal lung and from the myodermal tissue of the human embryo. Although all these strains are fibroblastic, cells of myodermal origin produced more interferon under identical conditions. These differences are evidently due to the fact that the tissues are derived from different embryonic layers. We regard the discovery of this fact to be of fundamental importance. As will be shown later, myodermal tissue is also highly sensitive to interferon. These facts, when considered together, may play an important role in the pathogenesis of virus infections and, in particular, of those whose agents penetrate through the skin.

It is also important to note that strains of diploid cells of identical (myodermal or lung) origin produced different quantities of interferon, evidently because of genetic differences between the cells from which the strain originated. These results suggest that different individuals may differ in their ability to produce interferon. This hypothesis was later confirmed by us in a study of the capacity of leukocytes from different donors to produce interferon.

Results obtained with cell cultures prepared from different organs are also noteworthy. First, they are additional evidence of the importance of lymphoid tissue in interferon formation. In particular, spleen cells produced more interferon *in vitro* than kidney and lung cells. Another interesting fact is that cultures of myodermal cells possessed equal interferon-forming ability. There are thus, it seems, three principal tissues in the body which produce interferon. Although some workers assert that the intensity of interferon formation depends on the intensity of the cytopathogenic action of the virus on the particular type of cell culture, we were unable to demonstrate such a relationship. In our experiments NDV proved to be an active inducer of interferon not only in mammalian cells, but also in cultures of chick fibroblasts, a result which contradicts the findings of other investigators. These differences were shown to be due to differences in the properties of the strains used.

A study of the dynamics of interferon formation has confirmed the results obtained by other workers who found that interferon is produced in maximum quantities during the first 24-48 h after infection. Experiments on tissues of different origin and on different types of cell cultures have shown significant differences between the duration of the incubation period, i.e., the time required for interferon to be liberated into the culture medium after infection with the virus. These differences are evidently based on the rate of formation of the messenger RNA transmitting information to the trigger mechanisms of interferon synthesis. This hypothesis is supported by the results obtained by Smith and Wagner [539], who showed that mRNA is synthesized much more rapidly in rabbit macrophages than in kidney cells, with the consequent more rapid formation of interferon. The predominant role of the properties of the cells in the dynamics of interferon formation is also demonstrated by the results of our experiments to study its induction by different viruses in cultures of chick fibroblasts. Irrespective of the properties of the inducing virus, interferon was formed at the same rate.

Several workers have described the inhibition of the formation and action of interferon by viruses or by substances induced by them in cells. Gendon [49] was unable to find an inhibitor blocking interferon formation. In our experiments using a modified Gendon's technique such an inhibitor was found, probably because different strains of viruses were used. It is interesting to note that the action of the inhibitor was exhibited only for the first 6 h after addition of the interferon inducer. The inhibitor thus obtained acts in the early stage of the cycle of interferon formation. It is evidently a repressor of interferon synthesis. Further research is undoubtedly necessary to enable the mechanism of action of the inhibitor to be finally established, but the inhibitor we discovered most probably differs from the blocker described by Isaacs and co-workers [375], for the blocker was found only in the late stage of the process. However, considering that our experiments were carried out on tissue cultures and not in chick embryos, and also with other viruses, differences in the experimental techniques may be a significant factor. So far as the suppression of activity of exogenous interferon by the inhibitor is concerned, it is not yet possible to state whether this action is brought about by the same mechanism as that which blocks interferon formation. It can be assumed that in chick fibroblasts the formation of two inhibitors of different nature is stimulated by the action of vaccinia virus. In the time of its appearance the inhibitor discovered by the writer is similar to the "stimulon" and the potentiator. The blocking action of our inhibitor was exhibited if it was added not later than 6 h after infection of the cultures with the inducing virus, which indicates that it exerts its effect in the early stages of interferon formation.

Chapter 3

The Action of Interferon in Cell Cultures

3.1. The Sensitivity of Viruses and Cells to Interferon*

One of the chief properties of interferon is its ability to inhibit reproduction of viruses *in vitro* and *in vivo* . Detection and titration of the biological activity of interferon are based on this property.

Interferon has no selective antiviral activity and it acts on virtually all viruses. In the width of its spectrum of action on viruses interferon can be compared with the antibiotics of the tetracycline series, which are active against most species of bacteria.

However, it must be remembered that the intensity of action of interferon on different viruses varies: some viruses are more susceptible, others less, to its action.

Many of the RNA viruses, which are usually used as indicators of interferon, are highly sensitive to its inhibitory action.

The virus most sensitive to the action of interferon is evidently Chikungunya virus [85, 234, 307].

Other highly sensitive viruses are those of vesicular stomatitis, of Eastern and Western equine encephalomyelitis, Semliki forest,

---

*"Sensitivity of cells to interferon" is taken to mean the effect of the cells on the antiviral activity of interferon. These differences between the cell cultures are evidently due to differences in the ability of the cells to produce antiviral protein under the influence of interferon (see "Mechanism of Formation and Action of Interferon," p. 263).

Sindbis, and O'nyong-nyong viruses [75, 76, 85, 108, 266, 286, 294, 574], and encephalomyocarditis virus [527, 561]. All these viruses have been widely used as indicators for the detection and assay of interferon activity.

Influenza A and A1 viruses are moderately sensitive to interferon [58, 62, 235].

According to Cantell and co-workers [238, 239] vaccinia virus is less sensitive than poliovirus but more sensitive than herpes simplex virus to interferon. Vaccinia virus has been shown [535] to be less sensitive to interferon than bovine enterovirus, and according to other investigations [511, 512] vaccinia virus is 5.5 times more sensitive than vesicular stomatitis virus and 1.4 times more sensitive than Semliki forest virus to interferon.

In Litvinov's experiments [109] vaccinia virus was 4 times less sensitive to interferon than vesicular stomatitis virus.

Glasgow and Habel [312] arrange the viruses which they studied in the following order of decreasing sensitivity: vaccinia, Sindbis, mouse encephalomyocarditis, herpes simplex, Eastern equine encephalomyelitis, and vesicular stomatitis. Their data for the last virus differ significantly from those obtained by other workers.

Most authors consider that Newcastle disease virus, adenoviruses, and herpes virus are least sensitive to interferon [79, 85, 108, 109, 130, 143, 239, 242, 328, 516, 574, 577].

According to Wagner [577], NDV is a thousand times less sensitive than WEE virus. Zhdanov and co-workers [79] consider that ECHO 2, 6, 13, and 24 and Coxsackie B2 viruses are insensitive to interferon. The resistance of certain enteroviruses to interferon has also been reported by Priimyagi [132].

An important factor in the selection of an indicator virus for interferon titration is its cytopathogenic activity in different types of tissue cultures. Among the viruses listed above as most susceptible to the action of interferon, vesicular stomatitis virus occupies a special place. It has a destructive action on most cell cultures of widely different origin. Because of the combination of these two properties, vesicular stomatitis virus is widely used as an indicator.

Differences in sensitivity to interferon have been found not only between viruses of different species, but also between different strains of the same species. In particular, an avirulent small-plaque variant of vesicular stomatitis virus was 4–8 times more sensitive than virulent variants [580]. Similar relationships have been observed for foot and mouth disease [533], Semliki forest [286], Newcastle disease and influenza [171, 244], and herpes simplex viruses [200]. Differences in the sensitivity of strains of polyoma virus have also been described [298].

There is no definite connection between interferon-inducing activity and the sensitivity of a virus to interferon. Some viruses induce interferon synthesis rapidly, but at the same time they possess low sensitivity to its action.

It must also be remembered that the results of assay of interferon activity depend not only on the sensitivity of the virus, but also on the sensitivity of the tissues to interferon. Some cells in tissue cultures are known to be good interferon producers but to be insensitive to its action. In particular, the action of interferon induced by tick-borne encephalitis virus in HeLa cells cannot be demonstrated in the homologous cells, although it is demonstrable in primary human amnion or monkey kidney cells [444, 569].

However, this rule cannot be applied to all transplantable cell lines. For instance, when interferon from mouse brain was titrated in primary embryonic fibroblasts and L cells [436, 575], much higher titers of inhibitor were obtained in the latter. The interferon titer in primary cells was regularly 16 times lower than in L cells.

Various factors have been shown to affect the sensitivity of cells to the action of interferon. In particular, higher interferon activity is found with an increase in the age of the cell system [45, 240]. These differences were particularly important in primary chick fibroblasts and monkey kidney cells [45]. The titer of chick interferon was 1:40 in a 1-day and 1:128 in a 6-day culture. However, some investigators [244, 337] found no difference in anti-

viral activity of interferon when assayed on chick fibroblasts and
a transplanted line (FL) of human amnion cells incubated for different periods.

An investigation [265] showed that the activity of interferon
induced by Sindbis virus in a transplanted line of rat tumor cells
was higher at pH 6.8 than at pH 7.2. However, in Gifford's experiments [304] interferon activity was unchanged between pH 6.8
and 7.6. No significant differences were found during titration of
interferon at 35 and 39°C [516]. Addition of methyltestosterone
derivatives or cortisol before or together with the interferon
potentiated its activity; this has been explained [263] by a change
in the permeability of the cell membranes, facilitating penetration
of the interferon into the cells. However, in Reinicke's experiments
[508-510] neither steroid hormones nor growth hormone affected
interferon activity in chick fibroblasts. The antiviral action of
interferon can be inhibited by viruses or by substances induced by
viruses in the cells [49, 250, 251, 338, 365, 375, 428, 477, 478].

3.2. Methods of Indication and Assay of Interferon

Several methods are used to determine the biological activity of interferon. The first method of assay, suggested by Isaacs
and Lindemann [372], was to determine the inhibitory activity of
interferon against influenza virus in a culture of fragments of the
chorioallantoic membrane of a chick embryo. An original method
was suggested by Porterfield [496]: interferon activity was assayed
by counting the plaques of virus reproduction under an agar over-
lay through which the interferon could diffuse. Dulbecco's plaque
technique was later used by Wagner [578] for interferon assay.

Most investigators [336, 351, 567] have used a tube method
to assay interferon activity based on inhibition of the cytopathogenic action of a virus by interferon. Other methods of interferon assay in vitro have also been suggested but they have not
yet been widely used [105, 283, 430, 564].

It must be remembered that the methods suggested differ
in their sensitivity. For instance, Dulbecco's plaque method is
16-32 times more sensitive than the method of assay based on inhibition of cytopathogenic action in tube cultures, and the method

of inhibition of hemadsorption suggested by Finter [283] is 8 times less sensitive than Dulbecco's method.

The most sensitive method of titrating interferon is by determining its action on the intensity of reproduction of the virus in cells. This can be obtained either from the decrease in the content of virus hemagglutinins, as in the method of Isaacs and Lindenmann cited above [372], or from the decrease in the "yield" of infective virus [209, 535]. This method has not been used extensively because of its laboriousness and because of the long time required to titrate the biological activity of each sample of virus.

The Dulbecco plaque method and the method based on inhibition of viral cytopathogenic effects (the CPE-inhibition method) are both used at the present time for determining the biological activity of interferon. The interferon preparation for testing is usually added to the culture 18-20 h before its infection by the indicator virus. Some workers remove the interferon before adding the virus, while others do not.

It must be remembered that the cells treated with interferon did not develop their maximal resistance in under 7-8 h after addition of the preparation [214]. If interferon from the cell cultures was removed by washing after the resistance had reached its maximum, the cells remained resistant to the virus for some time. However, prolonged incubation of the cells after removal of the interferon led to gradual loss of resistance.

As an alternative to the assay of interferon activity *in vitro*, a method based on inhibition of intradermal multiplication of vaccinia virus in rabbits has been recommended [464]. However, this method gives inconsistent results and has not been widely used.

It must also be borne in mind that a certain, and sometimes considerable, variability of the results is also observed in the tests carried out *in vitro*, when it depends on the indicator virus used, the sensitivity of the tissue culture, and so on.

Factors which cannot at present be fully taken into consideration may also influence the manifestation of the inhibitory properties even of the same interferon preparations. For this reason, on the basis of their analysis of an extensive material, Zeitlenok and co-workers [88] concluded that each test must incorporate a

well-studied standard of interferon activity and determination of
the activity of the test material in units of this standard. Until
an international standard has been adopted, in their opinion there
should be a national standard preparation which could be used for
both practical and pure scientific purposes at the present time.

3.3. Studies of the Sensitivity of Some Virus—Cell Systems to Interferon

It has already been said that the evidence on the sensitivity
of viruses to interferon is conflicting, and that the sensitivity of
some viruses of the smallpox—vaccinia subgroup has not yet been
studied. The results obtained by interferon assay in different virus-
cell systems have been found to differ significantly. It must also
be pointed out that the sensitivity of virus—cell systems to preparations of human interferon has been inadequately studied.

Experiments with mouse interferon [436, 575] showed that if
vesicular stomatitis virus was used as indicator, clone L-929 of
transplanted mouse cells was more sensitive to interferon than a
primary culture of mouse fibroblasts. Consequently, the results
of determination of the sensitivity of viruses to interferon and of
interferon assay depend both on the properties of the virus and
on the properties of the cell culture. To investigate these problems
the writer therefore used particular cell systems on which comparative investigations were carried out.

In particular, the sensitivity of different viruses to interferon, the intensity of the inhibitory action as a function of the
time after infection of the culture, the role of the type of cell culture,
and other related problems were studied experimentally.

Some experiments described in this chapter were carried
out jointly with Gumenik and Rapoport. In experiments to
determine the sensitivity of viruses to interferon, cultures of chick
fibroblasts and a strain of human diploid cells (L-42) obtained by
Rapoport from fetal lungs were used. One batch of interferon was
prepared for the cells of each type and the sensitivity of the
different viruses was tested with it on homologous cells.

The technique of these experiments was as follows. Tube
cultures were treated with 1 ml of twofold dilutions of interferon
and, after incubation for 18-20 h at 37°C, 100 TCD_{50} of each virus

TABLE 31. Sensitivity of Viruses
to Chick Interferon

Virus	Interferon titer
Western equine encephalomyelitis	32
Vesicular stomatitis	32
Sindbis	32
Chikungunya	128
Vaccinia	8
NDV, strain N	4
Ectromelia	16

in a volume of 0.1 ml was added. The results were read after complete degeneration of the control cultures infected with virus only (Tables 31 and 32).

It will be clear from Tables 31 and 32 that the highest dilution of interferon inhibiting Chikungunya virus was 1:128, vesicular stomatitis and Sindbis viruses 1:32, ectromelia virus 1:16, vaccinia virus 1:8, strain N of Newcastle disease virus 1:4, and poliovirus 1:4.

Since there is no discussion in the literature on the sensitivity of natural smallpox virus to inteferon and since information on vaccinia virus is contradictory, comparative experiments were carried out with these and other viruses of the same subgroup, paying particular attention to different strains of vaccinia virus. It was essential to study this problem because, despite a number of common properties, the viruses of vaccinia and natural smallpox differ in the character of the pathological process produced by them in

TABLE 32. Sensitivity of Viruses
to Human Interferon

Virus	Interferon titer
Vesicular stomatitis	32
Poliomyelitis	4

the body and in the character of the cytopathogenic changes observed
in the cells in vitro. The possibility cannot be ruled out that these
differences may be due to a certain difference between the sensitivity
of these viruses to interferon. The interferon used in the experiments was obtained by treating a monolayer culture of chick fibroblasts with heated vaccinia virus.

The inhibitory action of interferon was assayed on a monolayer culture of chick embryonic cells by a tube method based on
cytopathogenic action. The dose of smallpox virus added 24 h after
addition of the interferon was 100-10000 TCD_{50} in all experiments.

The results (Table 33) show that the sensitivity of smallpox
virus to the inhibitory action of interferon is commensurate with
that of the highly sensitive viruses of vesicular stomatitis and
Western equine encephalomyelitis. This property of smallpox virus
is appreciably more marked than in vaccinia virus and the difference between the sensitivities of vaccinia and natural smallpox
viruses to interferon is not a strain-specific feature of the latter
but was characteristic of several different strains tested.

The sensitivity of different numbers of the smallpox subgroup of viruses was compared by titration in the presence of 8
units of activity of the same interferon preparation.

The method of titration in the presence of interferon was
as follows. Interferon, in a volume of 1 ml, was added to one
group of tubes containing chick fibroblasts, while the same volume
of medium 199 was added to another group. The test virus, in a
volume of 0.1 ml, was titrated 18-20 h later on the tubes treated and
untreated with interferon. Each tenfold dilution of virus in medium
199 was tested in four experimental and four control tubes. The
results were read 6 days after addition of the virus and the number

TABLE 33. Comparative Sensitivity of Viruses to Interferon

Virus	Interferon titer
Smallpox	32
Vesicular stomatitis	32
WEE	32
Vaccinia	8

TABLE 34. Number of TCD_{50} Inhibited by the Same Interferon Preparation

| Virus | Strain | Titer of virus in medium | | Number of TCD_{50} inhibited by interferon |
		with interferon	199	
Vaccinia	Lister	10^2	10^5	10^3
	MNIIVP	10^6	10^7	10^1
	WR	10^6	10^6	$<10^1$
	EM-63	10^2	10^5	10^3
	Neurovaccine	10^5	10^6	10^1
	Ovovaccine	10^5	10^6	10^1
	Tashkent	10^6	10^7	10^1
	Grey clone	10^2	10^7	10^5
	White clone	10^6	10^6	$<10^1$
Natural smallpox	T	10^2	10^5	10^3
	Sh	$<10^2$	10^4	$>10^2$
	Sokolov	$<10^2$	10^4	$>10^2$
Ectromelia	G	10^2	10^7	10^5
	K	$<10^2$	10^4	$>10^2$
Cowpox	Brighton	10^4	10^4	$<10^1$
Rabbit pox	Utrecht	10^6	10^6	$<10^1$
Alastrim	1	$<10^2$	10^4	$>10^2$
	2	10^2	10^6	10^4

of TCD_{50} of each virus or strain, inhibited by interferon, was determined. The results are given in Table 34.

It will be clear from the results in Table 34 that the same
preparation of chick interferon inhibited multiplication of different
members of the subgroup of smallpox viruses to different degrees.
Viruses of natural smallpox, alastrim, and ectromelia were most
sensitive to interferon. The preparation of interferon used inhibited
not less than 10^3 TCD_{50} of these viruses. The viruses of cowpox
and rabbit pox were generally insensitive to the inhibitory action
of interferon. A wide range of differences in sensitivity to interferon was found in the various strains of vaccinia virus tested.
The number of cytopathogenic doses inhibited by the same propagation of interferon varied from 10^1 to 10^5 for different strains. The
grey clone (inhibition of 10^5 TCD_{50}) and strains EM-63 and Lister
(10^3 TCD_{50}) were most sensitive to interferon. The other strains
tested possessed comparatively low sensitivity. For instance,

TABLE 35. Sensitivity of Different Strains of
Herpes Virus in Cultures of Human Fibroblasts

Strain	Antigenic group	Titer of virus (in LD_{50}) in	
		control	experiment
L2	I	6.1 ± 0.1	4.8 ± 0.4
K	II	2.4 ± 0.6	1.9 ± 0.1
US	III	1.55 ± 0.05	1.25 ± 0.05
KUB	V	1.8 ± 0.2	1.6 ± 0.2

strains WR and the white clone were insensitive under the experimental conditions used, and inhibition of reproduction by strains
MNIIVP, neurovaccine, ovovaccine, and Tashkent was observed only
in the case of infection with not more than 10 TCD_{50}.

In experiments conducted jointly with Moisiadi on cultures of human embryonic fibroblasts the sensitivity of four strains
of herpes virus, belonging to different antigenic groups, to interferon was tested. The degree of sensitivity was judged from the
intensity of inhibition of reproduction of herpes virus in the presence
of 30 units/ml of homologous interferon. The cell culture was
infected at the rate of 1 LD_{50} per cell.

As Table 35 shows, the strains of herpes virus tested are only
slightly sensitive to interferon. Strains L2 and US were most susceptible to its inhibitory action. The other two strains, tested *in
vitro,* showed no statistically significant inhibition of their replicative activity in the presence of interferon (p > 0.05).

TABLE 36. Inhibitory Action of Interferon in
Relation to Time of Addition of Smallpox Virus

Order of addition of interferon and virus	Interferon titer
Interferon, virus 48 h later	32
Interferon, virus 24 h later	32
Interferon at same time as virus	32
Virus, interferon 3 h later	32
Virus, interferon 24 h later	2
Virus, interferon 48 h later	<2

TABLE 37. Intensity of Action of Interferon in Relation to Time of Infection of Tissue Cultures with WEE Virus

Order of addition of interferon and virus	Interferon titer
Interferon, virus 48 h later	64
Interferon, virus 24 h later	64
Interferon, virus 4 h later	64
Interferon and virus simultaneously	32
Virus, interferon 3 h later	32
Virus, interferon 6 h later	16
Virus, interferon 24 h later	<2

In some experiments the importance of the time of addition of smallpox virus (strain T) to the manifestation of the inhibitory action of interferon also was determined. It is clear from Table 36 that the maximal interferon titer can be demonstrated even if smallpox virus is added several hours after the interferon.

Since smallpox virus exhibits its cytopathogenic action slowly in cultures of chick fibroblasts, experiments similar to those described above were carried out with WEE virus. A cytopathic effect of rapid onset is characteristic of this virus. As Table 37 shows, the interferon was added before or after infection with the virus in the different experiments.

Examination of the results in Table 37 shows that interferon has a predominantly prophylactic action and is ineffective in the case of a developed infection. Addition of interferon 24 h after infection of the cells with WEE virus did not prevent their destruction.

The effect of dose of the test virus on titers of inhibitory activity of interferon also was studied experimentally. Addition of WEE, vesicular stomatitis, or smallpox viruses in doses of between 1 and 1000 TCD_{50} to tube cultures 18-20 h after interferon showed no difference in the titers of inhibition.

The influence of the composition of the medium on sensitivity of the cell system to interferon was examined in experiments on cultures of chick and mouse fibroblasts. Medium 199, medium 199 with 2% serum, and 0.5% lactalbumin hydrolysate were tested.

TABLE 38. Effect of In-
cubation Temperature on
Inhibitory Activity
of Interferon

Incubation temperature	Interferon titer
4°	8
22°	16
37°	32
42°	16

TABLE 39. Effect of Re-
moval of Interferon on
Its Titer

Change in medium	Interferon titer
Changed	32
Not changed	64

The interferon titers determined in the presence of the synthetic and semisynthetic media showed no appreciable difference.

The next series of experiments was aimed at discovering the optimal temperature for interferon action. Different dilutions (twofold) of interferon were added to four groups of tubes containing chick fibroblasts and these were then incubated overnight at 4, 22, 37, and 42°C, respectively. At the end of incubation, 100 TCD_{50} of WEE virus in a volume of 0.1 ml was added to the tubes and incubation continued at 37°C. The results were read three days later (Table 38).

The weakest inhibitory action was found in the group of cultures incubated at 4°C and the strongest in cultures incubated at 37°C. Some differences were found in the inhibitory activity of the interferon depending on whether it was kept in or taken from the tubes before addition of the indicator virus (Table 39).

The effect of age of the culture of chick fibroblasts and of the duration of incubation of the chick embryos before preparation of the cell cultures on the interferon titer also was studied. The importance of age of the cell culture was demonstrated by titrating the interferon on 1-day and 6-day tube cultures of chick fibroblasts. The effect of age of the chick embryo was tested by interferon assay in tissue cultures prepared from the spleens of 10- and 16-day embryos and day-old chicks. The results of these experiments are given in Tables 40 and 41.

They show that the age of the cell system had no significant effect on the sensitivity of the cells to interferon. We found more marked differences in our experiments to titrate interferon in cell

TABLE 40. Effect of Age of Cell
System Used to Determine
Interferon Titer

Age of culture	Interferon titer
1 day	16-32
6 days	32-64

TABLE 41. Interferon Titers
in Relation to Age of Embryo
Used for Preparation of
Cell Culture

Age of embryo or chick	Interferon titer
10-day embryo	4-8
16-day embryo	4-16
Day-old chick	8-32

cultures prepared from chick embryos and day-old chicks. They were most clearly seen on comparing the results of interferon assay in cells of 10-day embryos and day-old chicks. Fourfold differences in interferon titer were observed. Intermediate results were obtained during interferon assay in cultures of 16-day embryos.

Various factors can thus influence the intensity of the inhibitory action of interferon and these must be taken into account when its antiviral activity is estimated.

Because interferon shows promise for practical use in the prevention and treatment of human virus diseases and because of its species specificity, a comparative study of the sensitivity of certain virus—cell systems to interferon produced by human cells, notably leukocytes, is an essential task. Some workers have used a number of different virus—cell systems for the assay of human interferon material [277, 457, 549]. However, it is not yet known which, if any, of these systems provides optimal conditions for detection of minimal quantities of interferon.

To study this problem we used vesicular stomatitis virus and strain K of smallpox virus for testing purposes. Both viruses are highly sensitive to interferon and have a cytopathic effect on a wide spectrum of tissue cultures.

Primary trypsinized cultures, strains of diploid cells, and transplanted lines from human tissues were used to detect and assay the interferon preparations. Primary trypsinized human cells were obtained by the usual method and grown before use in the experiment on 0.5% lactalbumin hydrolysate solution with 10% bovine

TABLE 42. Comparative Interferon
Assay by Inhibition of Plaque Formation and by Cytopathic Effect

| Material | Interferon titer[*] based on inhibition | |
	plaque for- mation	cytopathic effect
Interferon from hens	1024	32
Human interferon	512	32

[*]Titration carried out on homologus cells with virus
added 18-20 h after interferon.

serum. Strains of diploid cells were obtained by Hayflick's method
and cultivated on Eagle's medium containing 30% of 0.5% lactalbumin hydrolysate and 10% of bovine serum. The transplanted cell
lines were grown on medium 199 with 10% bovine serum. For the
interferon assay experiments 100 TCD_{50} of virus was used; its
concentration was determined on the corresponding type of cells.

To obtain comparable results, a single batch of interferon
was prepared and tested in the different systems. The interferon
preparation was obtained in a suspension of human leukocytes,
using Newcastle disease virus, strain N, as the inducer.

Comparative assay of the preparations of human and chicken
interferon by Dulbecco's plaque inhibition method and by the
cytopathic effect method in tubes confirmed that the former is more
sensitive, in agreement with results obtained by other workers
(Table 42).

Although the plaque inhibition method is more sensitive and
gives interferon titers 16-32 times higher than the inhibition of
cytopathic effect method, there are difficulties associated with its
use, especially for titration on human cells. Efforts were therefore made to choose a system which would be conveniently available
and would exhibit comparable sensitivity during titration on the
basis of inhibition of cytopathic effect. Having regard to the species
specificity of interferon, experiments were carried out on various
types of human tissue cultures. The results of comparative assay
on the same preparation of leukocytic interferon in different cell
systems are given in Table 43.

It will be clear from Table 43 that diploid cells from human embryonic myodermal tissue are most sensitive to interferon. The interferon titers obtained in cells of this type were from 4 to 256 times higher than the titers in other cell systems. The highest indices were obtained in the system of diploid cells of myodermal tissue and smallpox virus. It will be noted that the results in Table 43 were obtained with strains of diploid cells which had gone through at least 15 subcultures in Eagle's medium with 10% serum. It was therefore interesting to determine the effect of the number of subcultures *in vitro* on the sensitivity of strains of diploid cells to interferon. For this purpose, titers of the same batch of interferon were determined with smallpox virus in primary cultures and in a diploid strain of myodermal tissue obtained from them during subculture (Table 44).

As Table 44 shows, during subculture *in vitro* the sensitivity of the strain of diploid cells to interferon increases gradually, to reach a maximum between the 12th and 30th subcultures.

The next stage was to determine the sensitivity of different strains of diploid cells obtained from myodermal tissue of different

TABLE 43. Comparative Assay of Interferon in Different Types of Human Cells

Type of cell culture	Interferon titer with virus of	
	vesicular stomatitis	smallpox
Primary myodermal tissue of 8-week embryo	16	32
Primary myodermal tissue of 12-week embryo	16-32	32
Primary lung tissue of 6-month fetus	4	8
Primary kidney tissue of 6-month fetus	8	8
Strain of diploid cells of myodermal tissue of 8-week embryo (18-28 subcultures)	128	512
Strain WI-38 of diploid cells from fetal lung (20-22 subcultures)	8	n.i.
Strains L-44 and L-49 of diploid cells from fetal lung (12-22 subcultures)	128	n.i.
Transplantable lines:		
A-1 (amniotic)	2	n.i.
D-6	2	n.i.
HeLa	2	n.i.
HEp-2	4	n.i.

Note: n.i., not investigated.

TABLE 44. Titers of Interferon in Relation to Number of Subcultures of Strain of Diploid Cells from Myodermal Tissue

Number of subcultures	Interferon titer
Primary tissue	32
The same culture after 5 subcultures	32
The same culture after 8 subcultures	64
The same culture after 12-30 subcultures	128

TABLE 45. Sensitivity of Different Strains of Diploid Cells to Interferon

Strain	Interferon titer
KM-1	256
KM-2	32
KM-3	16
KM-4	256
KM-5	8
KM-6	32

human embryos to interferon. Pieces of myodermal tissue obtained on different days were used. They were trypsinized and subcultured in a parallel series on medium described above. After 12 subcultures the sensitivity of the strains to the same batch of interferon was tested with vesicular stomatitis virus. Altogether six strains of diploid cells were tested. The results in Table 45 show that the titers of the same batch of human interferon varied, when assayed on different strains of diploid cells, from 1 : 8 to 1 : 256.

With these results in mind, in the subsequent investigation the most sensitive strains of diploid cells were specially selected for the detection and assay of human interferon, so that minimal quantities of interferon in test materials could be identified.

TABLE 46. Sensitivity of Cultures of Mouse Cells to Interferon

Type of cell culture	Variant	Interferon titer
Primary fibroblasts		64
Transplantable line L	Noncloned	4
	Clone 929 on Eagle's medium	256
	Clone 929 on medium 199	8192

Since the inhibitory activity of preparations of mouse interferon had to be determined frequently in our experiments, in order to choose the most sensitive cells a comparative study was made of a series of mouse cultures with the same batch of mouse interferon and with vesicular stomatitis virus. In particular, primary embryonic fibroblasts and variants of a transplanted line of mouse cells, including a noncloned L line and clone 929 adapted to medium 199 and to Eagle's medium with 10% serum, were investigated. The results are given in Table 46.

The results in Table 46 reveal extreme variation between primary and transplanted mouse cells in their sensitivity to interferon. Particularly marked variations (from 1:4 to 1:8192) in the titers of the same interferon preparation were obtained on different variants of transplanted mouse line L.

3.4. Conclusion

The results of our experiments confirmed the high sensitivity of Chikungunya, WEE, vesicular stomatitis, and Sindbis viruses to interferon and the low sensitivity of poliovirus and NDV.

The sensitivity of smallpox virus had not previously been studied. The sensitivity of ectromelia virus to interferon likewise was not definitely known. Ruiz-Gomez and Isaacs [516], who used this virus in their experiments, did not obtain clear results. Natural smallpox virus was shown by us to be at least equal to vesicular stomatitis and WEE viruses in its sensitivity to interferon. It was much more sensitive than the related vaccinia virus.

Differences in sensitivity to interferon were found not only among different species of poxviruses, but also among different strains of vaccinia virus. This may account for the contradictions between results obtained by different workers who have studied the sensitivity of vaccinia virus to interferon.

To understand the pathogenesis of the process of immunization by vaccination against natural smallpox, it is pertinent to compare the virulence of vaccine strains with their sensitivity to interferon. Vaccinia viruses (EM-63, Lister, grey clone), producing benign lesions on intradermal and intracerebral inoculation of rabbits and chick embryos, were much more sensitive to interferon when. inoculated on the chorioallantoic membrane than more virulent strains (MNIIVP, neurovaccine, WR, etc).

Resistance of the virus of rabbit pox to interferon is particularly interesting. Of all the poxviruses tested, it was the most pathogenic for rabbits.

These experiments confirmed the predominantly prophylactic action of interferon in tissue cultures; however, at the same time they showed that interferon can exert a marked action even when it is added immediately after the virus. In particular, addition of smallpox virus to cultures a few hours after interferon was not too late to demonstrate its antiviral activity.

Our investigations show that fibroblasts are more sensitive than epithelial cells to the inhibitory action of interferon *in vitro*. It can be assumed that differences in the susceptibility of epithelial and fibroblastic cells to a number of viruses are due precisely to this fact.

The sensitivity of human cells to interferon is also affected by the conditions and duration of their cultivation *in vitro* and by the genetic characters of the cell. Whereas transplanted lines of human cells showed minimal resistance, the sensitivity of strains of diploid cells increased with an increase in the number of subcultures *in vitro*. During the first 12 subcultures the sensitivity of this culture to interferon was increased by four times. It is interesting to note that the change in sensitivity of a strain of diploid cells to interferon begins after four subcultures, i.e., at a time when the formation of a homogeneous cell population, consisting entirely of fibroblast-like cells, is complete. During the first four or five subcultures, the culture consists of a mixed population. The unequal sensitivity of different strains of diploid cells obtained from different sources to interferon must also be noted. This fact can evidently be attributed to genetic differences between the organisms from which the cells were obtained, as is confirmed by differences in their susceptibility to viruses.

Consequently, the interferon titer, even if determined in the same virus-cell system, may differ significantly with the duration of existence of the cells *in vitro*. To standardize methods of assay of human interferon preparations it is therefore essential to use a sensitive system which gives reproducible results in different experiments. Other important conditions which must be satisfied are the availability of the culture and the simplicity of its preparation.

In our experiments the system of smallpox virus and diploid cells from the myodermal tissue of a human embryo after 12-28 subcultures possessed the highest sensitivity. The same cells in conjunction with vesicular stomatitis virus also were highly sensitive, and if there are good grounds for supposing that the interferon content in the test material is low, it is better to use this system. Its disadvantage is the variability of the results depending on the origin of the cells and the duration of their subculture *in vitro*. Each strain of diploid cells must therefore be tested beforehand for its sensitivity to interferon and only then should it be used in experiments. An incubation temperature of 37°C without removal of the material to be titrated gave optimal conditions for interferon assay. Under these conditions the age of the cell system and the dose of indicator virus added (between 1 and 1000 TCD_{50}) were of no significant importance.

Chapter 4

Interferon Production by Human and Animal Leukocytes

The ability of the blood leukocytes to produce interferon was first described by Gresser [319]. Human leukocytes were used in these experiments, and after infection with Sendai or measles virus they produced an inhibitor which was shown to be identical with interferon. When the liquid part of a suspension of infected leukocytes from two healthy donors and 18 patients with different diseases, including three patients with congenital agammaglobulinemia, was tested, different concentrations of interferon were found. The quantity of interferon produced was directly proportional to the concentration of leukocytes in the suspension.

It was later found that mouse leukocytes also produced interferon [309, 313, 409, 449]. Peritoneal leukocytes, treated *in vitro* with infective and UV-inactivated vaccinia, Newcastle disease, influenza, and Chikungunya viruses, were used in these experiments. Ability to produce interferon *in vitro* by white blood cells of chickens [166], rabbits [539], monkeys [418], and cattle [403] was discovered.

The optimal conditions for interferon production by chick leukocytes were studied by Solov'ev and co-workers [166]. Of the Chikungunya, Newcastle disease, influenza, vesicular stomatitis, and Coxsackie B3 viruses which were studied as inducer, the first showed the highest activity. With a multiplicity of infection of 10 TCD_{50} per cell, interferon was produced in largest amounts by leukocytes in an initial concentration of 1 million/ml and by incubation at 37°C. Similar titers of interferon were found if leukocytes in whole blood were used or if they were freed from plasma by centrifugation.

Detailed studies of the production of virus-induced interferon
by rabbit macrophages were carried out by Smith and Wagner [539].
These workers compared the rate of formation and the quantity of
interferon synthesized by different rabbit cells. Cultures of kidney
cells and of polymorphonuclear and mononuclear leukocytes produced interferon at the same rate. The interferon appeared 2 h after adsorption of the virus and synthesis reached a maximum between 2 and 16 h. The kinetics of interferon formation was similar
for all types of cells.

Macrophages produced more interferon than somatic (kidney)
cells or polymorphs.

Investigations with actinomycin D showed that the transcription of mRNA for interferon is complete in macrophages between
30 and 60 min, whereas in kidney cells this process begins later
and requires 120 min for its completion. Consequently, interferon
synthesis takes place more rapidly in macrophages than in somatic
cells.

The rapid production of interferon by rabbit macrophages has
also been described by Nagano [463]. In his experiments interferon
appeared after 1 h and its maximum level was reached after 4 h.
Kono [403] compared the rate of formation and quantity of interferons synthesized in cultures of bovine blood leukocytes and kidney cells to NDV. The content of interferon produced by the leukocytes reached a maximum after 4-6 h, whereas in the kidney cells
a significant level was attained only after 20 h. An increase in
production of the inhibitor in cultures of leukocytes was observed
after longer periods of incubation. These workers attribute this
result to transformation of monocytes into macrophages.

Finally, interferon production was found to take place much
more rapidly than reproduction of the virus in leukocytes but not
in kidney cells. In Kono's opinion this may be of great importance
in the pathogenesis of infection. Although the virus multiplies in
leukocytes which disseminate throughout the body, because interferon is formed more rapidly than the virus reproduces, the arrival of infected leukocytes in sensitive organs provides them with
an earlier protection on account of the interferon produced by the
leukocytes. Consequently, regardless of the ability of the virus to
multiply in the leukocytes, induction of leukocytic interferon provides
a rapid protection for the susceptible cells against infection.

Consequently, the considerable ability of human and animal leukocytes to produce interferon by interaction with viruses is now firmly established. Meanwhile, by contrast with cells growing *in vitro*, leukocytes have been shown to be capable of producing interferon after treatment with nonviral agents: phytohemagglutinin and other mitogens, endotoxins, and certain other substances of bacterial origin. The discovery of interferon production by uninfecte rabbit macrophages [468, 539] must also be mentioned. A study of the properties of this inhibitor revealed its similarity with the interferon induced by endotoxin. It should be noted that in order to obtain a peritoneal exudate some workers [468] used liquid paraffin, while others [539] used glycogen. The possibility therefore cannot be ruled out that these substances or other contaminants may have had an interferon-inducing action. The production of interferon by uninduced human leukocytes, macrophages, and bone marrow cells, and also by mouse peritoneal leukocytes has been described by other workers [191, 257, 313, 529] who detected an interferon-like substance in leukocyte suspensions. Consequently, the discovery of interferon in uninduced leukocytes is not just an isolated fact and its origin in "normal" uninfected suspensions of leukocytes requires study. Wheelock [592] gave the first account of the ability of human leukocytes to produce interferon under the influence of a nonviral agent, viz., phytohemagglutinin, an extract of the leguminous plant Phaseolus vulgaris. In these experiments phytohemagglutinin was added to a suspension of leukocytes (2 × 10^6 cells/ml) at the rate of 0.1 ml to 2 ml of suspension. The inhibitor was found after 2 h and reached its maximum after 5 h. In its properties the inhibitor was found to be similar to virus-induced interferon, the only difference being its slightly lower resistance to acids and heat. In particular, at pH 2.0 and 10.0 and during heating for 60 min at 56°C, interferon induced by phytohemagglutinin showed some decrease in activity. However, at pH values between 3.0 and 9.0 it showed similar resistance to virus interferon and there was no decrease in its activity during 24 h. Consequently, the interferon induced by phytohemagglutinin showed great similarity to the inhibitor produced *in vivo* after administration of endotoxins.

These results were subsequently confirmed and extended [297, 549]. In particular, it was shown that besides phytohemagglutinin, other mitogens such as streptolysin O, etc., can induce interferon production [297]. Removal of phytohemagglutinin from the medium interrupted interferon synthesis, to be resumed when a fresh batch of phytohemagglutinin was added. However, the results cited above are not confirmed by another report [274]. Besides phytohemagglutinin, interferon production by leukocytes *in vitro* is also induced by endotoxins [226, 404, 539, 549] and by mannan, obtained by Berkhout [228] from Candida albicans. These workers showed that the addition of endotoxin in a dose of 50-100 μg/ml suspension is followed by liberation of an interferon-like substance with antiviral activity by the leukocytes into the surrounding medium.

In the experiments of Smith and Wagner [539] rabbit macrophages *in vitro* produced interferon under the influence of endotoxin from Escherichia coli added at the rate of 10-100 μg/ml. At 4°C no production of interferon was observed under the influence of the endotoxin.

Borecky and Lackovic [226, 228] showed that mouse peritoneal leukocytes can liberate interferon *in vitro* after stimulation by extracts containing the O antigen of E. coli 0111, E. coli 086, and Salmonella typhi 0901, and also by highly purified mannan from Candida albicans. The largest quantities of interferon in these experiments were found after incubation of leukocytes at between 22 and 26°C. Higher and lower temperatures reduced the yield of interferon. Under the same conditions interferon formation stimulated by NDV followed a course parallel to the rise in temperature up to 40°C. Consequently, the temperature optima for the production of virus- and endotoxin-induced interferons were different. Similar results were obtained in experiments with mannan. It must be pointed out that, in principle, viral inducers are regarded as more active than nonviral inducers of interferon production in leukocytes [539, 549].

These observations evidently support the view that interferon production by leukocytes under the influence of viral and nonviral inducers is based on different mechanisms.

To sum up the results described above, leukocytes have been found to be more active producers of interferon *in vitro* than other types of cells. To obtain large quantities of human inter-

feron the optimal conditions for intensive interferon production
by leukocytes during induction by viruses have been studied. The
most important work in this direction has been undertaken by
Falcoff and co-workers [277, 281] who described a technique for
the large-scale production of human interferon. They showed that
Sendai virus and NDV are the most active inducers of interferon.
The optimal conditions for interferon formation were as follows:
1) concentration of leukocytes in the suspension 5×10^6/ml; 2)
multiplicity of infection 100; 3) incubation temperature 37°C; 4)
duration of the cycle of interferon production 22 h; 5) concentration of human serum in the medium 5%; 6) pH of medium 7.4-7.5.
Serum was of great importance to interferon production. In its
absence no interferon was formed.

Similar results were obtained by Strander and Cantell [549-
551]. However, Falcoff and co-workers prefer to use Sendai virus
as the interferon inducer, while Strander and co-workers prefer
NDV, although these two viruses were found to have identical activity in the investigations cited. In the experiments of Strander
and Cantell the amount of interferon produced reached a maximum
6-7 h after infection, a result which differed from that found by
Falcoff and co-workers.

The question of the relative importance of the different types
of white blood cells in interferon production has not yet been settled
Gresser [319] showed that monocytes are competent producers of
interferon, but he reached no definite conclusions regarding the
role of polymorphs in this respect. Lee and Ozere [449] presented
evidence of interferon formation by polymorphs. The ability of
rabbit polymorphs to produce interferon is shown by the results
obtained by Smith and Wagner [539]. However, the most important
role among the white blood cells in interferon production is ascribed
to mononuclear cells — lymphocytes and macrophages [227, 313, 539
593]. In particular, in Wheelock's experiments [593] human blood
polymorphs did not actively form interferon, although it was actively produced by lymphocytes. Mouse peritoneal leukocytes, predominantly macrophages, also produced interferon in response
to virus infection [309, 313, 409] and to the action of nonviral agents
[409]. Smith and Wagner [539] consider that macrophages are the
main, if not the only, cells producing interferon in rabbit peritoneal
exudate. However, they emphasize that the reticuloendothelial

cells of the spleen are more likely than circulating monocytes to
be the chief source of the interferon appearing in the serum after
intravenous infection of a virus.

Finally, the amount of interferon produced by leukocytes
in vitro depended on the length of time they were kept at 37°C
before infection with the virus [539]. In particular, incubation of
leukocytes at 37°C even for only 4 h led to a sharp decrease in
their interferon production. Care must therefore be taken when
phenomena taking place *in vivo* are interpreted on the basis of
results obtained *in vitro*.

According to Borecky and Lackovic [227], the maturity of
the mononuclear cells is of great significance to interferon production. They postulate that young cells do not significantly affect
interferon formation until they reach maturity, when they are
converted into fully interferon-competent cells.

The intensity of interferon production by leukocytes *in vitro*
is thus influenced by many factors.

At the beginning of our investigations only the first reports
of interferon production by human blood leukocytes and mouse
peritoneal leukocytes had been published. Regarding leukocytes
as one of the most convenient sources of interferon, we [157,
162], simultaneously with Falcoff and co-workers [277] and Strander
and Cantell [549-551], developed a technique for producing human
leukocytic interferon. At the same time, the principles governing
interferon formation by monkey, rabbit, and mouse leukocytes were
studied.

For these experiments packed human leukocytes were obtained from the Institute of Hematology and Blood Transfusion, where
they were prepared as follows. Blood from a donor was added to
preservative solution 7b and kept at 4°C for 18-20 h. During this
period the red cells sank to the bottom of the vessel, the leukocytes
formed a film above them, and the top layer consisted of plasma.
The film of leukocytes was removed and placed in a separate vessel, unavoidably together with a small quantity of red cells and
plasma. Usually 50 ml of packed leukocytes was obtained from
500 ml donor's blood, and it contained from 5-6 to 20 million leu-

kocytes per milliliter (Solov'ev). On arrival at the laboratory
the packed leukocytes were stored at 4°C until required.

In some cases a modified technique of Strander and Cantell
[549] was used, in which the blood was mixed with 5% versene
solution in the ratio of 10 : 1. Eight volumes of 0.83% ammonium
chloride was then added and the mixture allowed to stand for 10
min at 4°C. It was then centrifuged for 10 min at 1000 rpm. The
sedimented leukocytes were resuspended in medium 199 with 10%
bovine serum and heparin (10 units/ml) and used for subsequent
experiments. Versene is used as an anticoagulant, while ammonium
chloride causes lysis of erythrocytes.

Blood from monkeys (Macaca rhesus) was obtained from the
heart and mixed with heparin at the rate of 10 units/ml. From each
monkey weighing 2.5-3 kg it was possible to obtain 40-50 ml blood,
which was kept at 4°C for 18-20 h. After this period the film of
leukocytes was separated and added to medium 199 with 10% serum,
after which the leukocytes were counted.

In all experiments the monkey leukocytes were used not more
than 24 h after the time of taking blood from the donor. Blood from
other animals was obtained and treated in the same way. In most
experiments with rabbit and mouse leukocytes, however, the modified technique of Strander and Cantell was used.

Rabbits weighing 3 kg and mice weighing 25-40 g were chosen.
To irritate the peritoneum the rabbits and mice received an intraperitoneal injection of sodium thioglycollate in doses of 150 and 1.5
ml, respectively. After 24 or 72 h the peritoneal cavity was irrigated with medium 199 with 10% bovine serum and heparin (10
units/ml). The rabbits were treated with 100-150 ml and the mice
with 5 ml of medium. In all experiments, unless for special purposes, the above medium containing 5-10% serum was used. The
leukocyte suspension was diluted in medium 199 with 5-10% bovine
serum to a specified concentration (in most experiments 1 million
cells/ml) and infected with the inducer virus. The mixture was
incubated at 37°C and the inhibitory activity of the culture fluid
tested at various time intervals after inactivation of the virus at
pH 2.0.

4.1. Interferon Production by Rabbit and Mouse Blood Leukocytes

We determined the ability of circulating blood and peritoneal leukocytes of rabbits and mice to produce interferon. Newcastle disease virus was used as the inducer and was added with a multiplicity of 10. A suspension of leukocytes infected with virus was incubated at 37°C, and samples taken from it after various time intervals were acidified to pH 2.0 and kept for 4 days. The hydrogen ion concentration was then adjusted to 7.4 and the inhibitory activity determined in cultures of myodermal tissue from a rabbit embryo subcultured more than ten times *in vitro*, or on cultures of L cells of mouse origin (depending on the material to be titrated). Vesicular stomatitis virus was used as the test virus.

Peritoneal leukocytes were obtained 24 and 72 h after intraperitoneal injection of sodium thioglycollate. The peritoneal cavity of the rabbits and mice was irrigated with medium 199 with 10% serum and heparin (10 units/ml) and the cells were counted. The cell concentration was adjusted to 10^6/ml and the virus was added. The mixture was incubated at 37°C and samples were taken immediately after addition of the virus and at intervals of 2, 5, 8, 12, 24, and 48 h thereafter.

The principles governing interferon production by peritoneal and circulating blood leukocytes of rabbits were found to be completely identical with those governing interferon formation by the mouse leukocytes. Even the quantities of interferons produced by leukocytes of the different species of animals were found to be similar.

The experiments showed that the dynamics of interferon formation by peritoneal leukocytes obtained 24 and 72 h after irritation of the peritoneum was identical (Fig. 3). The quantities of interferon produced, when calculated per million leukocytes, also were identical. The high rate of interferon formation by the leukocytes will be noted. The interferon level had almost reached its maximum 5 h after its induction by the virus. The increase in interferon titers during the first 4–5 h was linear in character.

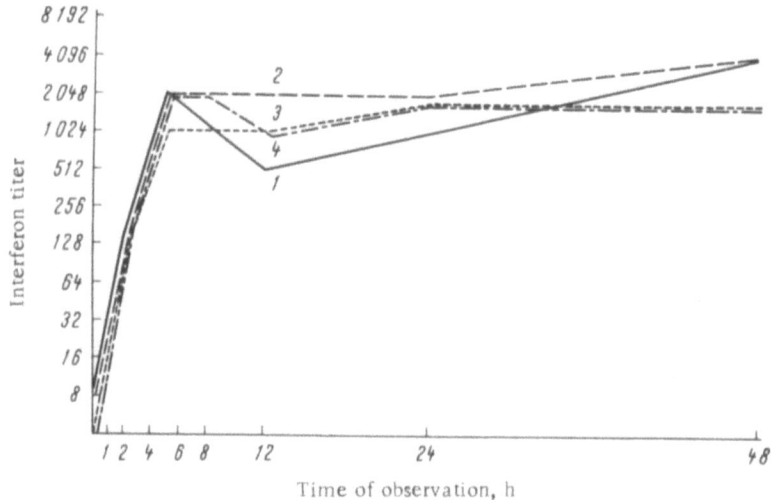

Fig. 3. Dynamics of interferon production by peritoneal leukocytes
of rabbits (1, 2) and mice (3, 4) obtained 24 (1, 3) and 72 (2, 4) h after injection of thioglycollate.

During each 2 hours the quantity of interferon increased by 16
times. Later, the titers of interferon were only doubled.

The distribution of cells producing interferon and obtained
from the peritoneal cavity was compared. In the exudate after
24 h most cells (up to 70%) were polymorphs,. The remaining 30%
were monocytes. After 72 h the peritoneal exudate contained up
to 90% of monocytes and only 10% of polymorphs.

Since peritoneal macrophages differ from the circulating
monocytes [576], it was important to compare interferon production
by blood leukocytes and peritoneal leukocytes obtained from the
same animals. For this purpose, 5-10 ml blood was taken from
a rabbit and thyoglycollate injected intraperitoneally at the same
time. Leukocytes of the peritoneal exudate were removed for
investigation 72 h later. In an analogous experiment with mice,
suspensions of blood leukocytes and exudate were obtained from
different groups of mice with 10 animals in each group. The results
given in Table 47 show that leukocytes in a focus of inflammation
are more active producers of interferon than blood leukocytes.
Moreover, leukocytes of the inflammatory exudate not only pro-

TABLE 47. Dynamics of Interferon Production by
Leukocytes from Blood and Peritoneal Exudate of
Rabbits and Mice

Materials	Time of investigation, h	Interferon titer with leukocytes from	
		rabbits	mice
Peritoneal leukocytes	0	4	4
	2	128	128
	5	4096	1024
	8	4096	1024
	12	4096	1024
	24	8192	512
Blood leukocytes	0	4	4
	2	4	4
	5	16	32
	8	1024	512
	12	512	512
	24	1024	64

duced more interferon, but synthesized it much more rapidly than
blood leukocytes. It can accordingly be considered that mobilized
monocytes are more active producers of interferon than circulating
blood leukocytes.

During the study of exudates obtained after 24 h differences
were noticed between the dynamics of production of interferon by
the leukocytes used immediately after removal from the peritoneal
cavity and by leukocytes kept in a refrigerator at 4°C for 18-20 h.

As Table 48 shows, keeping leukocytes at 4°C in medium 199
with 10% blood serum (peritoneal leukocytes) or keeping whole
blood with heparin or 5% versene solution (10% of the total volume)
altered both the quantity of interferon produced by them and the
dynamics of its formation. Peritoneal leukocytes and circulating
blood leukocytes, infected with virus immediately after explanta-
tion, produced 4-8 times more interferon than the corresponding
leukocytes kept for 18-20 h before infection. In addition, interferon production by the leukocytes infected immediately reached
virtually its maximum 3 h before the corresponding interferon
production by stored leukocytes. Consequently, the changes were
similar in character to those in the two types of leukocytes kept
in different media, which suggests that they are independent of the

TABLE 48. Dynamics of Interferon Formation by Rabbit and Mouse
Leukocytes Kept for Different Periods

Material	Time of keeping before infection with virus, h	Time of taking blood, h	Interferon titer with leukocytes from	
			rabbit	mice
Peritoneal leukocytes 24 h after irritation of peritoneium	0	0	8	n.i.
		2	128	
		5	2048	
		8	1024	
		11	1024	
		24	2048	
		48	2048	
	24	0	4	n.i.
		2	32	
		5	32	
		8	32	
		11	128	
		24	256	
		48	n.i.	
Blood leukocytes	0	0	<4	4
		2	<4	16
		5	16	32
		8	1024	512
		12	512	512
		24	512	128
		48	1024	128
	24	0	<4	16
		2	<4	16
		5	15	8
		8	128	32
		12	256	256
		24	256	256
		48	n.i.	128

Note: n.i., not investigated.

composition of the medium. The changes were evidently due to other causes.

Because of these results, it was decided to compare the dynamics of interferon formation in primary cultures of myodermal tissue from a rabbit embryo, cultivated *in vitro* for 1 month, with the dynamics of interferon formation by leukocytes obtained freshly and stored at 4°C for 18 h. With the same multiplicity of infection the interferon titers in the culture fluid of the rabbit fibroblasts did not reach their maximum until 24-48 h after infection, i.e., interferon production was retarded even more. Similar results were obtained with suspensions of leukocytes and with mouse tissue cultures (Table 48).

4.2. Interferon Production by Monkey Blood Leukocytes

At the beginning of our investigations it had been reported in the literature that interferon prepared in a culture of monkey kidney cells inhibits multiplication of vaccinia virus in human skin. These findings indicated that monkey interferon possesses definite antiviral activity in man. It had also been reported that the species specificity of interferon is not absolute and that it is also active in cells of closely related species. The study of interferon production by monkey leukocytes was therefore of special interest.

As stated above, leukocytes were obtained from the blood of rhesus monkeys. Ability to produce interferon was determined after their whole blood had been kept with heparin at 4°C for 18-20 h.

These experiments showed that the quantity of interferon produced is directly dependent on the concentration of leukocytes in the suspension and on the dose of virus added. Optimal ratios between the dose of added virus and the concentration of leukocytes were obtained in experiments in which for each leukocyte there was about 1 TCD_{50} of Chikungunya and vesicular stomatitis viruses or 10-100 TCD_{50} of Newcastle disease virus (Tables 50 and 51).

TABLE 49. Dynamics of Interferon Production in Cultures of Rabbit and Mouse Cells

Species	Type of cells	Duration of keeping or cultivation before infection with virus	Time of maximum of interferon content after infection with virus, h	Interferon titer
Rabbit	Peritoneal leukocytes	0 h	5	1024
	Peritoneal leukocytes	24 h	24	128
	Embryonic fibroblasts	about 30 days	24	256
Mouse	Peritoneal leukocytes	0 h	5	1024
	Peritoneal leukocytes	24 h	12	256
	Transplanted line	not known	24	256

TABLE 50. Effect of Concentration
of Monkey Leukocytes on
Interferon Production

Number of leukocytes 1 ml of suspension	Interferon titer
2,000,000	32
450,000	16
146,000	8
80,000	4

TABLE 51. Effect of Dose of Virus on
Interferon Formation in Suspensions of
Monkey Leukocytes

Inducing virus	Multiplicity of infection, TCD_{50}	Interferon titer
Chikungunya	1	16-32
	0.1-0.3	4-8
Vesicular	1	32
stomatitis	0.1	4
NDV	10-100	32-64
	1	16

The interferon-inducing activity of the three viruses used
was about equal (Table 51). If anything, slightly higher titers
were obtained with NDV. Certain properties of the preparations
of monkey leukocytic interferon were studied. They were stable
for not less than 48 h at pH 2.0, resistant to heating at 56-60°C
for 1 h, and they were completely inactivated at 80°C after 60 min.

Experiments on homologous and heterologous cells demonstrated their marked species specificity. Activity of the interferon
preparations was most evident in cells of the homologous series.
In heterologous cells, notably cultures of mouse and chick fibroblasts, they had no inhibitory action on the viruses. It is important to emphasize that interferon induced by monkey leukocytes
was active in cultures of strains of human diploid cells and in
monolayer cultures of human fibroblasts and kidney cells. In
heterologous human cells, however, the activity of monkey interferon was much lower, only 10-15% of that found in monkey cells.

Consequently, monkey leukocytes proved to be active producers of interferon, and in this respect they were more active than somatic kidney cells.

To sum up the results of the experiments with animal leukocytes, it was found that the principles governing the formation of leukocytic interferon are similar for animals of different species. Animal leukocytes possess high interferon-producing ability. On the basis of a more detailed study of interferon production by human leukocytes a technique for the large-scale preparation of human leukocytic interferon has been developed.

4.3. Interferon Production by Suspension of Human Leukocytes

The packed leukocytes obtained as described above consisted of a suspension of leukocytes in plasma with 10% preserving solution. It also contained a certain number of erythrocytes. Determination of the number of leukocytes in the suspension during keeping in fact began 24 h after the blood had been taken from the donor. This suspension was described as the original suspension. The possibility of keeping a suspension of leukocytes in medium 199 with 10% bovine serum and the effect of keeping at different temperatures (37, 22, and 4°C) also were studied. During keeping changes were found in the number of leukocytes and in their ability to produce interferon. This latter effect was established under adequate conditions. In all experiments the leukocyte concentration was adjusted to 1 million/ml and NDV was added with a multiplicity of 10. The inhibitory activity of the culture fluid was determined after incubation for 24 h at 37°C. The results are given in Tables 52 and 53.

The optimal conditions for keeping leukocytes were found to be in plasma with preserving solution 7b. The storage temperature had no significant effect. Comparatively rapid destruction of the leukocytes took place in medium 199 with serum. Less than 30% of the original number of leukocytes still remained in the suspension after 48 h.

In view of these results, in the subsequent work the leukocytes were kept in plasma or whole blood and used in the experiments not later than 48 h after the blood had been taken from the donor. Under these conditions the "yield" of leukocytes and interferon was relatively standard in character.

TABLE 52. Effect of Duration of Keeping on Concentration of
Human Leukocytes

Keeping medium	Keeping temperature	0 h	24 h	48 h	72 h	96 h	120 h
Plasma	37°	21×10^6	15×10^6	11×10^6	9×10^6	3.5×10^6	3.5×10^6
+7b	22°	21×10^6	14×10^6	11×10^6	9×10^6	2.5×10^6	2.5×10^6
	4°	21×10^6	15×10^6	12×10^6	9×10^6	3.5×10^6	2.5×10^6
199 + 10% serum	37°	21×10^6	10×10^6	6×10^6	2×10^6	1.5×10^6	1.5×10^6
	22°	21×10^6	11×10^6	6×10^6	3×10^6	1.5×10^6	1.0×10^6
	4°	21×10^6	11×10^6	6×10^6	3×10^6	1.5×10^6	1.0×10^6

TABLE 53. Effect of Duration of Keeping on Intensity of Interferon Production by Leukocytes

Keeping medium	Keeping temperature	0 h	24 h	48 h	72 h	96 h
Plasma + 7b	37°	512	128	32	32	4
	4°	512	256	256	256	64
199 + 10%	37°	512	256	32	4	<4
serum	4°	512	256	64	4	<4

4.3.1. Importance of the Blood Group

Blood from donors of groups O(I), A(II), and B(III) was tested.
If the original concentrations of leukocytes (10^6/ml) and the multiplicity of infection with NDV (1 TCD_{50}) were the same, identical
results were obtained (Table 54).

Consequently, the blood group had no significant effect on
the yield of interferon.

4.3.2. Effect of Incubation Medium for Leukocytes with Virus on Quantity of Interferon Formed

In the first experiments medium 199 was tested with different
concentrations of human blood plasma. To prevent the plasma from

TABLE 54. Ability of Leukocytes of Different Blood Groups to Produce Interferon

Blood group	Interferon titer
O(I)	128-512
A(II)	128-512
B(III)	128-512

TABLE 55. Effect of Plasma Concentration in Medium 199 on Interferon Production by Human Leukocytes

Plasma concentration, %	Interferon titer
0.1	<4-4
1	8-32
5	128-512
10	128-512
20	128-512

clotting after addition of the virus-containing allantoic fluid, heparin was first added to the incubation medium (10 units/ml). The results showed that the presence of plasma is of decisive importance in interferon production by leukocytes. The absence of plasma led either to complete inability of the cells to produce interferon, or the titers obtained were extremely low. Optimal conditions were created by the addition of 5-10% plasma to medium 199 (Table 55). The possibility of replacing plasma by homologous and heterologous serum was next studied. It was found that replacement of the plasma by serum and the origin of the serum had no significant effect on the interferon yield (Table 56).

The effect of the composition of the incubation medium on interferon production also was studied.

The following media were tested: Tyrode-cystine-peptone fluid, Eagle's medium, medium 199, and 0.5% solution of lactalbumin hydrolysate. 5% Bovine serum was added to all the media. The yield of interferon was the same in all media. In the subsequent experiments medium 199 with 5-10% serum accordingly was used.

4.3.3. Effect of Leukocyte Concentration in Suspension on Interferon Production

Experiments to determine the role of leukocyte concentration were carried out as follows. The number of leukocytes was counted in the original material and suspensions with an equal leukocyte concentration were obtained from it by successive double

TABLE 56. Effect of Species
of Serum on Interferon
Production by Human
Leukocytes

Species of blood serum or plasma	Interferon titer
Human plasma	256
Human serum	256
Bovine serum	256
Monkey serum	256

Note: In these experiments 5% serum
or plasma was added to the medium 199.

dilution. The number of leukocytes was again counted in each
suspension, which was then poured in volumes of 5 ml into tubes.
The NDV was then added with a multiplicity of 1 and the tubes were
incubated at 37°C for 24 h. The inhibitory activity of the culture
fluids was determined.

The results in Table 51 show that within certain limits the
amount of interferon produced by leukocytes is directly proportional to the concentration of leukocytes in the suspension.

An increase in the concentration of leukocytes above the optimal level does not increase, but decreases the yield of interferon.

4.3.4. Effect of Reaction of the Medium

In these experiments the pH was measured after infection
of the leukocytes with virus.

Optimal conditions for interferon production by the leukocytes
were obtained at pH 7.3-7.5 (Table 58). An acid or strongly alkaline
medium depressed the ability of the leukocytes to produce interferon.

4.3.5. Effect of Incubation Temperature

The optimal temperature of interferon production by human
leukocytes was 36.5-37°C. A decrease to 35 or below or an increase to 38°C led to a marked decrease in interferon production
(Table 59).

TABLE 57. Effect of Concentration of Human Leukocytes on Interferon Production

Number of leukocytes in 1 ml of suspension	Interferon titer
5,000,000	16
2,600,000	32
1,200,000	256
653,000	64
152,000	8
16,000	<2

TABLE 58. Effect of pH of Medium on Interferon Production by Human Leukocytes

Initial pH of medium	Interferon titer
5.0	<2
6.0	8
6.5	32
7.0	128
7.3-7.5	256
7.8	128
8.0	32
9.0	<2

4.3.6. Importance of the Species of Inducing Virus and the Multiplicity of Infection

The interferon-inducing activity of vesicular stomatitis, influenza A and A2, parainfluenza type 1, Sendai, NDV, Sindbis, and vaccinia (dermovaccine strain MNIIVP and ovovaccine strain Mastykova) was tested. Comparative tests showed that Newcastle disease, vesicular stomatitis, and Sendai viruses possessed the greatest, and approximately equal, ability to induce interferon formation; in the other viruses tested this ability was weak (Table 60). In these experiments the multiplicity of infection was 1 for all viruses.

The results given in Table 60 for NDV were obtained with strain N. Tests of ability to induce interferon carried out on other strains (V1 and K) gave similar results.

The role of multiplicity of infection was studied by the use of Newcastle disease virus. Just as with monkey leukocytes, an increase in the multiplicity of infection led to a marked increase in interferon production (Table 61). The largest amount of interferon was produced by a multiplicity of 10-100.

As was pointed out above, no differences in the ability of strains of NDV of different virulence to induce interferon could be detected. However, in subsequent experiments strain N was mainly used. This strain accumulates in high titer (10^8-10^9) in the al-

TABLE 59. Effect of In-
cubation Temperature on
Interferon Production by
Human Leukocytes

Incubation temperature	Interferon titer
22°	<4
33°	32
35°	64
37°	256
39°	64

TABLE 60. Interferon-
Inducing Activity of Dif-
ferent Viruses in Sus-
pensions of Human
Leukocytes

Inducing virus	Interferon titer
NDV	256
Vesicular stomatitis	256
Sendai	128
Influenza A	32
Influenza A2	32
Ovovaccine	8
Dermovaccine	8
Sindbis	<4

TABLE 61. Effect of Multiplicity
of Infection on Interferon
Production by Human Leukocytes

Dose of virus (in TCD_{50}) calculated per leukocyte	Interferon titer
10-100	256
1	128
0.1	32
0.01	4
0.001	2

lantoic fluid of infected chick embryos, it possess a well-marked
cytopathic action (making it convenient for titration), and it is a
safe virus with which to work.

4.3.7. Dynamics of Interferon Production by Human Leukocytes

The first point to make is that the dynamics of interferon
production was determined with suspensions of leukocytes kept at
room temperature for 18-20 h. The suspension was prepared in
a volume of 100 ml and in a concentration of 10^6 cells/ml, NDV
was added with a multiplicity of 10, a sample was taken, and the
suspension was incubated at 37°C. Later, 5-ml samples of culture

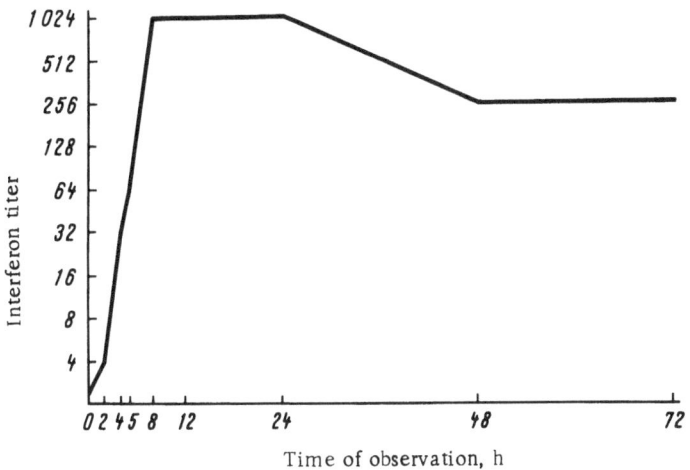

Fig. 4. Dynamics of interferon production by human leukocytes.

fluid were taken from the flask after 1, 2, 4, 6, 8, 12, 24, and 48 h
and replaced by an equal volume of nutrient medium. The dynamics
of interferon production by the leukocytes is illustrated in Fig. 4.
The first interferon was found in the medium after incubation of
the leukocytes with virus for 2 h and a maximum was reached after
8 h. Further incubation of the suspension led only to a very
slight increase in the interferon titer. For practical purposes,
collection of the culture fluid 18-20 h after infection of the leukocytes
gave the optimal yield of interferon and was most suitable for its
subsequent treatment. The possibility of obtaining further interferon from leukocytes which had already produced it previously
also was studied. After collection of the first culture fluid the
leukocytes were washed and resuspended in a fresh batch of medium
199 with 10% serum, the concentration was adjusted to 10^6 cells/ml,
and the suspension was divided into three parts. One part was
incubated without further treatment with virus, the second part
was reinfected with NDV, and the third part was infected with
vesicular stomatitis virus with a multiplicity of 1. In some experiments the second interferon inducer was added in a dose 10
times greater than that used the first time, i.e., the multiplicities
of infection were 1 and 10, respectively.

As Table 62 shows, a second yield of interferon was not obtained from leukocytes when reinfected with homologous or
heterologous viruses.

TABLE 62. Interferon Production by Leukocytes in
Response to Repeated Action of Inducers

First inducer of interferon	Interferon titer	Second inducer	Interferon titer
NDV	128	Not added	4
NDV	128	NDV	<4
NDV	128	Vesicular stomatitis virus	<4
Vesicular stomatitis virus	128	NDV	<4
Vesicular stomatitis virus	128	Not added	<4
Not added	<4	NDV	256
Not added	4	Vesicular stomatitis virus	128

TABLE 63. Interferon Production by Human Leukocytes in Response to Consecutive Addition of Virus and Nonvirus Inducers

Nature and dose of first inducer	Interferon titer	Nature and dose of second inducer	Interferon titer
NDV, 1 TCD_{50} per cell	128	Pyrogenal, 25 $\mu g/10^6$ cells	<4
Not added	—	Pyrogenal, 25 $\mu g/10^6$ cells	16
Pyrogenal, 25 $\mu g/10^6$ cells	16	NDV, 1 TCD_{50} per cell	32
NDV, 0.01 TCD_{50} per cell	4	NDV, 10 TCD_{50} per cell	32
Not added	—	NDV, 10 TCD_{50} per cell	256
NDV, 1 TCD_{50} per cell per cell	128 128	NDV, 10 TCD_{50} per cell	<4

It will also be noted that an increase in the dose of inducer
did not lead to further substantial production of interferon. Consequently, the refractory state of the leukocytes could not be overcome even by a tenfold increase in the dose of the inducing virus.

Different results were obtained by the consecutive use of
viral and nonviral (pyrogenal) inducers. In these experiments

the virus was added with a multiplicity of 10 and pyrogenal in a dose of 25 μg per 10^6 leukocytes and the mixtures were incubated for 18-20 h.

The yield of interferon was reduced if the virus inducer was added after pyrogenal. Presumably the pyrogenal, being a weaker inducer of interferon, exhausted only some of the interferon-producing capacity of the leukocytes and for this reason the refractory state after the addition of pyrogenal was only partial. This hypothesis is supported by results obtained with homologous inducing virus (NDV) when small (0.01 TCD_{50} per cell) and large (10 TCD_{50} per cell) doses were added consecutively (Table 63).

It is concluded from the results of these experiments with repeated exposure to interferon inducers that the highest yield of interferon was obtained in response to a single exposure to the optimal dose of interferon inducer virus.

4.3.8. The Properties of Leukocytic Interferon

The properties of native preparation of leukocytic interferon were studied. Cells and other large particles were removed from the incubation medium 18-20 h after addition of the inducer by centrifugation at 2500 rpm for 15 min. To inactivate the virus the supernatant was treated with 40% hydrochloric acid solution to pH 2.0. After the fluid had been kept for 4 days at 4°C the pH was adjusted with 50% NaOH to 7.4 and the properties of the resulting inhibitor were studied. It was not precipitated by centrifugation at 100,000 g for 2 h, it was stable at pH 2.0 for not less than 7 days, and it lost about 70% of its activity by heating for 1 h at 60°C and by treatment with 0.1% trypsin solution at 37°C for 30 min.

Experiments on homologous and heterologous cells revealed the well-marked species specificity of interferon. The activity of interferon in homologous cells was exhibited against vesicular stomatitis virus down to dilutions of 1:256 to 1:512 in assay by cytopathic effect and to dilutions of 4096-8192 in assay by Dulbecco's plaque method in strains of diploid cells of human myodermal tissue. In heterologous cells and, in particular, in cultures of mouse and chick fibroblasts, leukocytic interferon had no inhibitory action on viruses. Meanwhile, it was active in monkey kidney cells. However, the titers of its inhibitory activity were from 8 to 16 times lower than in homologous cells.

TABLE 64. Characteristic Properties
of Leukocytic Interferon

Method of treatment	Interferon titer after treatment
Untreated	64
pH 2.4 for 7 days	64
Heating to 60°C for 60 min	16
Heating to 80°C for 30 min	4
Trypsin, 0.1%, 30 min	8
Centrifugation at 100,000 g for 2 h	64
Treatment with anti-NDV serum	64
Keeping at 4°C for 8 months	64
Lyophilic drying and keeping for 18 months	64
Keeping at 20°C for 12 months	32

Antiserum against Newcastle disease virus did not reduce the antiviral activity of leukocytic interferon. It inhibited multiplication of vesicular stomatitis, smallpox, and vaccinia viruses, i.e., it did not exhibit virus specificity. The results of a study of the properties of leukocytic interferon are shown in Tables 64 and 65.

4.4. Interferon Production in Growing Cultures of Human Leukocytes

Results for interferon production in leukocyte suspensions were described in the previous sections. Interferon production in

TABLE 65. Determination of Species
Specificity of Human Leukocytic Interferon

Species and type of cell culture	Titer of inhibitory activity
Human fibroblasts	32
Monkey kidney cells	4
Chick fibroblasts	<2
Mouse fibroblasts	<2

the experiments described above was due to the action of a "shock" dose of virus. It was therefore interesting to study interferon formation during reproduction of virus in leukocytes growing *in vitro*.

It has been shown that NDV reproduces in suspensions of human leukocytes [274, 551]. However, since reproduction of the virus was only slight in degree and interferon was produced early and in large quantities, the authors cited above linked these two phenomena and so explained the resistance of the leukocytes to NDV. A similar hypothesis was put forward to explain the inability of Sendai virus to reproduce in human leukocytes.

In experiments conducted jointly with Barinskii and Dement'ev, we tested St. Louis encephalitis, herpes simplex, and Coxsackie A11 viruses.

Phytohemagglutinin (obtained from Bulgaria) was added to the medium to stimulate growth and reproduction of the leukocytes. Knowing the ability of phytohemagglutinin to induce interferon formation, as a first step tests were made to see if it stimulated the inhibitor in the growing leukocytes. In none of the experiments was the culture fluid found to have inhibitory properties. It must also be stated that, although the general term "leukocytes" is used, in the experiments now described the cells were evidently monocytes or lymphocytes. However, since the composition of the cells in the cultures was not identified, they can best be described as leukocytes.

To prepare the culture of lymphocytes, 15 ml of venous blood from adult donors was transferred immediately after taking into test tubes with 0.1 ml liquid heparin in a dilution of 1 : 10 and incubated for 1-2 h at 37°C to sediment the cells. Each tenfold dilution of the test material collected at various times after infection of the leukocyte cultures was used to infect four cultures in a dose of 0.1 ml each. Titration was carried out by Kerber's method. Coxsackie A11 virus was titrated by the plaque method and assayed in plaque-forming units (p.f.u.). In each dish 0.3 ml of virus in known dilution was applied to the cell monolayer.

In the control experiments samples of the original virus-containing suspensions were tested at the corresponding times; they were diluted 1 : 2 with nutrient medium and incubated along with the experimental cultures. All tests were repeated twice. To assay the interferon the test material was treated with hydrochloric acid and alkali. Interferon was titrated in a monolayer culture of

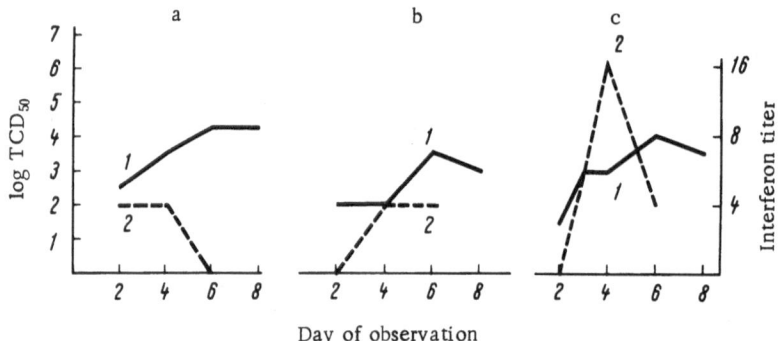

Fig. 5. Reproduction of viruses and interferon formation in a culture of human blood leukocytes: a) herpes virus; b) St. Louis encephalitis virus; c) Coxsackie A11 virus; 1) dynamics of reproduction of virus; 2) dynamics of interferon formation. Abscissa, days after infection; ordinate on left, titer of virus (log $TCD_{50}/0.1$ ml or log p.f.u./ml); ordinate on right, interferon titer in reciprocals of dilution.

human embryonic myodermal tissue (a strain of diploid cells after 8–9 subcultures).

The results of the study of reproduction of the viruses and interferon formation are given in Fig. 5. This shows that the titers of herpes virus rose slowly in the culture of lymphocytes to reach a maximum (4.0 log TCD_{50}) by the 6th–8th day after infection (the period of observation in these experiments). The heat-inactivation curve of·strain L_2 at 37°C shows that by the 4th day the titer of the virus had fallen sharply (from 5.0 to 2.0 log TCD_{50}), and by the 6th day no biologically active virus could be found on the basis of its cytopathic effect in the test experiments. No visible cytopathic changes in the cells of the leukocyte culture could be found in un-stained preparations under a magnification of 80 times.

During reproduction of herpes virus in the lymphocyte cul-tures, the interferon content in the culture medium reached a maximum 48 h after infection, i.e., considerably before the maximum of virus accumulation.

In the experiments to study reproduction of St. Louis en-cephalitis virus the titers of this virus in a culture of human blood leukocytes rose slowly to reach a maximum on the 6th day after infection (3.5 log TCD_{50}), and remained at approximately the same level for some days longer. The interferon content in the culture medium, as in the preceding experiment, reached its maximum before accumulation of the virus.

The heat-inactivation curve of the virus at 37°C shows absence of biologically active virus after 48 h.

St. Louis encephalitis virus reproduced more rapidly in the culture of chick fibroblasts to reach its maximal titers on the 3rd day (4.5 log TCD_{50}), and it produced almost total destruction of the cells of the monolayer.

Reproduction of Coxsackie A11 virus and interferon formation in the culture of lymphocytes showed a slow increase in the titer of the virus beginning on the 3rd day after infection and reaching its maximum on the 6th day (2.64×10^4 p.f.u./ml). By the 8th day the titer of the virus had begun to fall (2.61×10^3 p.f.u./ml). The dynamics of interferon formation in this case was approximately the same as in the preceding experiments, but a maximum was reached later than during reproduction of herpes simplex virus and St. Louis encephalitis virus (after 96, 48, and 72 h, respectively, with accumulation of the test viruses reaching its maximum at approximately the same times).

In a culture of human kidney tissue Coxsackie A11 virus reproduced up to high titers (2.06×10^5 p.f.u./ml) as early as 24 h after infection and the titer reached a maximum after 48 h (3.96×10^6 p.f.u./ml). A marked cytopathic effect developed 24 h after infection, and the cells of the culture were completely destroyed 48 h after infection.

A study of heat inactivation of Coxsackie A11 virus showed that the titers fell sharply at 37°C within 3 days. However, small quantities of biologically active virus still remained on the 6th day, as shown by the formation of single plaques beneath the agar. On the 8th day of keeping the virus no longer formed plaques, indicating its complete inactivation by heat.

To sum up these results it must be emphasized that all the tested viruses accumulated slowly in cultures of leukocytes, and the secretion of interferon into the medium reached its maximum considerably sooner than the maximum of virus reproduction.

4.5   Conclusion

Our experiments showed that the leukocytes of human and animal blood and the peritoneal leukocytes are active producers of interferon. These results are in agreement with those obtained by other workers.

New and very interesting results were obtained to show the effect of the origin of the leukocytes on their ability to produce interferon. It was first shown that mononuclear and polynuclear cells of the peritoneal exudate are more active producers of interferon than leukocytes obtained from the circulating blood.

Blood leukocytes also produced interferon more slowly than peritoneal leukocytes. It can accordingly be concluded that mobilized leukocytes are more interferon-competent than intact circulating blood leukocytes. This conclusion is supported by the results of several investigations. It has been shown [576] that peritoneal macrophages differ in several of their properties from circulating monocytes and that mobilization of leukocytes leads to differentiation of the monocytes, with the appearance of changes in morphology, cytochemistry, and biochemistry by comparison with the remaining monocytes [252].

Another change which must be added to this list is evidently an increase in the ability of the cells to produce interferon. Leukocytes from an inflammatory focus presumably not only produce more interferon, but they also produce it more quickly than leukocytes of the circulating blood.

Interesting results have also been obtained by the study of the effect of the time of testing the ability of leukocytes to produce interferon after their removal from the body. In the first place, a marked quantitative difference was found. Freshly obtained leukocytes produced 8-16 times more interferon than leukocytes kept for 18-20 h at 4°C. A marked difference also was observed in the dynamics of interferon production by freshly obtained and stored leukocytes. The former produced interferon much more rapidly and its titer reached a maximum 4-5 h after addition of the virus, whereas if the leukocytes were stored, their interferon production only reached its maximum 24 h after infection.

It will thus be noted that the formation of serum interferon after intravenous infection of viruses reached its maximum at the same time as in the case of induction of interferon production by freshly obtained leukocytes.

Analysis of these results suggests that the development of an inflammatory focus, especially if the virus enters the organism by peripheral pathways, thereby stimulating the ability of the leukocytes to produce interferon, is a phenomenon which benefits the organism. Phagocytosis, by mobilizing the leukocytes, evidently also increases their interferon-producing ability. This, in turn, inhibits reproduction of the virus. Other evidence in support of this hypothesis is given by the results of a study of interferon production in growing leukocytes.

A number of general principles observed in our experiments must be mentioned. The slow accumulation of all the tested viruses in cultures of leukocytes, and also the fact that their titers were lower than during reproduction on other sensitive tissues, will be noted. The infectivity of viruses in cultures of human blood leukocytes remained at a moderate level until the 8th day after infection (the period of observation), indicating the development of a state of dynamic equilibrium between heat inactivation and reproduction of the viruses at 37°C. Finally, a study of heat inactivation at 37°C showed that all strains of viruses used in the investigation, in the concentrations used to infect the cultures of leukocytes, completely lost their biological activity in the course of 8 days.

Cultures of human blood leukocytes infected with virus remained outwardly unchanged in these experiments throughout the period of observation when native preparations were examined (with the MBR microscope, magnification 80 times). However, to investigate this problem more thoroughly, cytological and cytochemical observations are essential.

The study of the dynamics of interferon formation showed that this process is not so much the result of the action of a "shock" dose of the inducer as the result of reproduction of the virus. In the case of a shock dose the accumulation of interferon reached a maximum 7-8 h after infection. In growing leukocytes the liberation of interferon into the medium reached a maximum long before the maximum of virus reproduction. This earlier formation of interferon by the blood leukocytes, as was pointed out above, may be of great importance in the pathogenesis of infection. Consequently, irrespective of the ability of a virus to reproduce in leukocytes, its penetration into the blood stream and its phagocytosis stimulate the early formation of interferon which, on reaching sensitive cells, may increase their resistance to the virus. The possibility cannot be ruled out that the reduced ability of viruses to reproduce in culture of leukocytes by comparison with cultures of chick fibroblasts and human kidney cells is connected with the early formation of interferon, before reproduction of the virus.

An important part of our investigations was the study of the optimal conditions for interferon production by human leukocytes. The necessity for the study of this problem is dictated by the species specificity of interferon. To test its action in man, an accessible tissue which actively produces interferon must be available. Attempts to utilize diploid cells for this purpose led to the production of interferon preparations with comparatively low activity. Leukocytes were found to be the most suitable cells in these experiments. Since leukocytes are essentially waste products during the preparation of plasma and packed red cells, the production of interferon on a large scale is a problem of real significance. In turn, the wider availability of interferon would enable its potential value in the prevention and treatment of virus infections to be properly assessed. Without large-scale observations it is impossible to reach reliable conclusions regarding the prophylactic and therapeutic value of interferon.

The rules for interferon production which we developed and applied in practice are considered to provide a solid basis for the large-scale production of leukocytic interferon.

PART II

Effect of Exogenous Interferon and Stimulators of Endogenous Interferon on Virus Infections

Effect of Exogenous Interferon
on Virus Infections

5.1. Action of Exogenous Interferon on Exper-
imental Virus Infections

The effect of exogenous interferon on the origin and course
of virus infection has been studied by numerous investigators. Originally experiments were carried out on rabbits infected with vaccinia and herpes viruses. The first experiments were carried
out by Isaacs and co-workers, who injected chick interferon intradermally into rabbits 24 h before infection with vaccinia virus
with the result that the development of the cutaneous lesions was
restricted [429]. Much better results were obtained by using rabbit
interferon in experiments of various types [377]. The interferon
was injected: a) on the day before infection; b) at the same time
as the virus; c) on the day after infection. The intensity of the
protective action of the interferon depended on the dose of vaccinia
virus used. If 10^4-10^5 infective doses of vaccinia virus were used
for infection complete protection was observed if the interferon was
injected the day before the virus, but not if it was injected with or
after the virus. Interferon gave complete protection when injected
simultaneously with the virus provided that the infective dose of
the virus was reduced by half. No protection was found if the interferon was injected after infection with the virus regardless of its
dose. Rabbit interferon has been used for the treatment of vac-
cinial and herpetic keratitis [242]. After infection via the scarified
cornea interferon was injected subconjunctivally six times a day.
In the case of infection by herpes virus, interferon had no therapeutic

action despite its use for 4 days, but it was effective against vac-
cinial keratitis. Repetition of these experiments by Hirst and Finter
(cited in [289]) revealed a well-marked therapeutic effect in herpetic keratitis, but only if partially purified preparations of homologous interferon were used.

The effect of exogenous interferon on reproduction of vaccinia virus also was studied in experiments on monkeys [196]. A
preparation obtained from monkey kidney cells prevented the
development of necrosis after intradermal infection with vaccinia
virus. The effect of exogenous interferon on virus lesions of the
eyes also was studied by Ermol'eva and co-workers [67] and by
others [1, 3, 4, 104].

The protective action of exogenous interferon is also manifested in infections by arboviruses and other agents. Hitchcock
and Isaacs [342] observed the protective action of intraperitoneally
injected exogenous homologous interferon in mice infected extra-
neurally with Bunyamwera virus. These workers found that interferon acts for a short time and that endogenous interferon has no
effect on antibody formation. The prophylactic effect of concentrated
homologous interferon, injected into animals before infection
with Sindbis, Semliki forest, and encephalomyocarditis viruses,
has been described [236, 284, 288].

The protective action was more marked if the number of
injections was increased, evidence of the brevity of action of the
interferon. For example, to protect mice against intraperitoneal
infection with encephalomyocarditis or Semliki forest viruses
it was necessary to give interferon in doses of between 3000 and
5000 units repeatedly by intramuscular or subcutaneous injection.

Baron and co-workers [212] studied the prophylactic action
of intravenously injected mouse interferon after intracerebral
infection with encephalomyocarditis and vesicular stomatitis viruses
and intraperitoneal infection with Germiston virus. The most
definite protection was found in the case of infection with the last
virus. Even a single injection of 133 units of interferon prolonged
the life of the animals and led to survival of more than 10% of them.
In the experiments with the other two viruses, an increase in the
protective action was found with an increase in the number of injections of interferon. Eight injections, each of 200 units of interferon, gave the best results. A marked protective action also was

obtained against infection by encephalomyocarditis and vesicular stomatitis viruses in doses of 30 and 80 LD_{50}, respectively.

The effectiveness of interferon in experimental infection of mice with tick-borne encephalitis virus was studied by Chumakov and co-workers [186-188]. Concentrated preparations of homologous interferon were used and were injected intramuscularly. The animals were infected intraperitoneally. Interferon had mainly a prophylactic action and led to survival of 38-62% of the animals if injected daily during the first 4 days of the incubation period. Interferon had a weaker action during the second half of the incubation period.

Andzhaparidze and co-workers [5] studied the effect of homologous interferon on reproduction of tick-borne encephalitis virus in mice (intraperitoneal infection). Intravenous or intracerebral injection of interferon into the mice 24 h before their infection with tick-borne encephalitis virus in a dose of 100 LD_{50} prevented death of 50% of the animals. The protective effect was observed for 2-3 days after the injection of interferon and repeated injections potentiated its action.

The action of exogenous interferon in experimental influenza was studied in experiments on animals [61, 494, 556]. Intranasal injection of interferon into mice before infection with the virus prevented death of about 30% of the animals and significantly inhibited reproduction of the virus in the lung. Link and co-workers [432] showed that homologous interferon, if injected three times, inhibits reproduction of virus in the lung. A single intranasal injection had no effect on the course of influenza infection. Exogenous interferon was also effective against herpetic infection of mice and in fowl plague [31, 108, 229, 378, 410]; the prophylactic action of the interferon was found to depend on its concentration and dose and on the frequency and site of its injection. The action of interferon on virus RNA was observed after its intraperitoneal injection into chickens, and in the case of RNA of poliovirus, in the case of intracerebral injection. No poliovirus could be found in the brain of the birds [601].

Ovsyannikova and Zeitlenok [117] studied the effect of exogenous interferon on the development of an infection in cotton-tail rats due to peroral infection with Coxsackie ABIV-Coxsackie A7 virus. A single prophylactic injection of interferon (before infection of

the animals with the virus) and repeated injections of homologous
interferon after infection led to a significant decrease in mortality.
With an increase in the duration of the incubation period and in
the number of repeated injections of interferon, the decrease in
mortality among the experimental animals became more marked:
heterologous chick interferon, under identical experimental conditions, had no protective action. Incidentally, in experiments on
mice infected with tick-borne encephalitis virus, Chumakov and
co-workers [188] had previously shown that chick interferon has
no protective action.

There are reports in the literature of a prophylactic action
of interferon preparations against tumors.

For instance, an increase of between 2 and 5 times in the
survival period of hamsters infected with polyoma virus, if
treated previously with homologous interferon, has been described
[198]. The prophylactic action of interferon has also been demonstra
ted against infection with other oncogenic viruses: Rous sarcoma
[62, 175, 410, 525], Shope fibroma [396, 397], and Ehrlich's ascites
carcinoma [172] viruses. Gresser and co-workers [323] used interferon for the prevention of splenomegaly in mice infected with
Friend's virus. A positive effect was observed if frequently daily
intraperitoneal injections of the interferon were given. Similar
results have been obtained by other workers [135]. When these
results are evaluated, attention must be paid to certain special
features and general rules established by the study of the action of
exogenous interferon *in vivo*.

The first matter to which consideration must be paid is that not
only homologous, but also heterologous preparations of interferon
have antiviral activity; heterologous activity is most frequently
shown by native allantoic interferon. Its purification abolished its
activity in animals of heterologous species. Considering the marked
species specificity of interferon, it can be presumed that the effectiveness of heterologous interferon, when native preparations are
used, is due to their content of interferon-like or interferon-inducing
substances.

The next matter to be emphasized is the predominantly
prophylactic action of interferon. Injection of interferon beforehand, 3-24 h before infection, proved to be more effective than
administration together with or after the virus. Injection of interferon into tissue infected with virus is also more effective and

smaller quantities of interferon are required under these circumstances than for its administration by other routes. The effectiveness
of exogenous interferon is directly dependent on the antiviral activity of the preparation. The use of a highly active preparation
for prophylactic purposes was found to be effective not only against
localized, but also against systemic virus infections. Increasing
the dose or the number of injections of interferon potentiated its
protective action. This confirms the view that its action is of
short duration because of its elimination or destruction in the body.
This was confirmed experimentally by the work of Subrahmanyan
and Mims [553], who studied the rate and path of spread of intravenously injected interferon in mice. They found that most of the
interferon disappears from the bloodstream in 5 minutes, but at
the end of this time much of it can be found in the liver, lungs, and
kidneys. No interferon was ever found in the brain and spleen.
The rapid disappearance of intravenously injected interferon from
the bloodstream has also been described by other workers [54,
211]. Gresser and co-workers [326] compared the rate of elimination of interferon from the bloodstream when injected intravenously and intraperitoneally. They found that by the second method of administration interferon appeared quickly in the bloodstream
and remained at a high level for 5 h. Rapid disappearance of interferon when injected intravenously is explained by its excretion with
the urine. Intraperitoneal injection leads to slower elimination of
interferon from the body. At the same time, the fact that interferon
can no longer be detected in the bloodstream soon after its administration evidently does not mean that its antiviral action is
at an end. In view of the mechanism of action of interferon (induction of the synthesis of antiviral protein) it can be assumed
that the tissues of the body still retain their resistance to viruses
for some length of time after its disappearance from the bloodstream. This is shown, in particular, by the fact that the resistance of an animal to viruses is in some cases even more marked
24 h after injection than 1 h after injection of interferon.

The prophylactic action of exogenous interferon was
studied by us in experiments carried out jointly with Gumennik. Albino mice, some newborn and others weighing 7–8 g, were
used for the experiments and were infected with influenza or ectromelia virus. The choice of these viruses was determined by the
fact that influenza in mice is an infection which attacks predomi-

nantly the respiratory organs, while ectromelia is a typical systemic infection.

Influenza A virus, strain PR-8 was injected intranasally and
ectromelia virus intraperitoneally. In most experiments the viruses
were infected in a dose of 10-100 LD_{50}.

Preparations of exogenous homologous interferon were obtained by intravenous infection of mice weighing 25-30 g with Newcastle disease virus. The animals were exsanguinated 4 h later,
the serum was separated, and the residual virus in it was inactivated by treatment with acid to pH 2.0. Activity of the serum
interferon was assayed in a system of transplanted mouse L cells
with vesicular stomatitis virus. During titration in this system
the activity of the interferon was 1024-2048 units/ml. The unit
of activity was taken to be the smallest quantity of interferon with
an inhibitory action on 100 TCD_{50} of vesicular stomatitis virus in
transplanted mouse L cells. The interferon was injected in the
same way as the virus or intramuscularly. By the intranasal route
each mouse received 50-100 units of interferon, and by the intramuscular route about 400 units. In some experiments a single
injection of interferon was given, while in others it was injected
repeatedly, before and after infection.

Observations on the animals were continued for 2 weeks after
infection.

In the first series of experiments the effect of exogenous
interferon was studied on experimental influenza. The mice of
one group received homologous interferon intranasally and those
of another group received a placebo (normal serum). Batches
of 10 mice from each group were then infected either at once or
after intervals of 24 and 48 h.

The results of these experiments are given in Table 66.

A single injection of interferon had a protective effect which
was more marked against infection with a dose of 10 LD_{50}. After
infection with 100 LD_{50} the action of interferon was used. The
greatest protection was obtained in experiments in which interferon was injected 24 h before infection. Simultaneous injection
of interferon and virus gave a less marked effect.

The effect of the number of injections of interferon in the
course of 3 days, followed by infection of the mice with 10 LD_{50}

TABLE 66. Effect of Exogenous Interferon on Experimental Influenza in Mice

Group	Infecting dose	Interval between injection of interferon and infection, h	Number of mice which died
Receiving interferon	100	0	8/10[*]
		24	7/10
		48	10/10
	10	0	6/10
		24	4/10
		48	9/10
	100	0	10/10
		24	10/10
		48	10/10
	10	0	10/10
		24	9/10
		48	9/10

[*]The numerator shows number of mice which died; the denominator, the total number of mice infected.

of virus, also was investigated. These experiments were carried out on 100 animals divided into two groups: 50 mice received interferon and 50 the placebo. Among the group of animals receiving interferon 23 mice (46%) survived, while all 50 infected mice in the control group died (100%).

Consequently, prophylactic injection of interferon daily for 3 days gave the same protection as a single injection 24 h before infection.

The action of interferon when injected subcutaneously also was studied. In these experiments a less active preparation of interferon with a titer of 1:64 was used, but it was injected in a dose of 0.25 ml daily for 7 days. The first injection of interferon coincided with the time of infection with 10 LD_{50} of influenza virus. Daily subcutaneous injection of interferon for 7 days into 25 mice prevented death of 28% of the animals, compared with a 4% survival rate in the control group, which also consisted of 25 animals.

In the next series of experiments the action of exogenous interferon was studied on the course of ectromelia in mice. Interferon with an initial titer of 1:1024 was injected intraperitoneally

TABLE 67. Effect of Four Injections of
Interferon on Mortality among Mice from
Ectromelia

Group	Number of mice which died	Survival rate, %
Receiving interferon	7/16	56.3
Control	15/16	6.3

TABLE 68. Action of Interferon on Infection with Coxsackie A6 Virus in Mice of Different Ages

Age of mice	Dose of virus, LD_{50}	Number of animals remaining healthy in experiment	Number of animals remaining healthy in control
48 h	10	0/18	0/15
48 h	1	12/34	9/51
12 days	10	54/77	17/69
12 days	100	2/30	0/30

Note. Here and in the subsequent tables the numerator shows the numbers
of animals which survived and the denominator, the total number of animals
in the experiment.

in a dose of 0.5 ml. Consequently, at each injection each mouse
received about 500 units of interferon.

If a single injection of interferon was given, this was done
on the day before infection with virus. The only result was that
the incubation period of the disease was doubled. For instance,
whereas all the animals in the control group died between the 4th
and 7th day, in the group receiving interferon the animals developed
the disease and died between the 9th and 14th day.

In the next experiments interferon was injected 4 times: on
the day before infection, on the day of infection, and the next 2
successive days. Consequently, each mouse received over 2000
units of interferon intramuscularly. The virus was injected intraperitoneally. The animals of the control group received normal
serum at the same times and observations continued for 2 weeks.
The results are given in Table 67.

These results show that an increase in the dose of interferon given by daily injections considerably increased its protective effect. In the group of animals receiving interferon 43.7% of the mice died, compared with over 93% in the control group; the mortality in the latter group was therefore approximately twice that in the former group.

In a joint investigation with Gutman, we also studied the effect of interferon on the development of the disease in mice infected with Coxsackie A6 virus. Experiments were carried out on mice aged 2 and 12 days which were infected intramuscularly with 1 or 10 LD_{50} of virus.

In the 12-day mice, interferon, when injected intramuscularly, gave a well-marked positive effect: from 55 to 87% of the animals showed no signs of infection; in those animals which did become ill the incubation period was doubled. The best results from interferon were obtained by its injection 3 h before infection, followed by daily administration during the incubation period, 4 or 5 times in all.

However, in the mice aged 2 days, interferon had no protective action when given in the same way (Table 68).

The dynamics of reproduction of the virus and of the formation of endogenous interferon and antibodies in the infected mice also was studied (Fig. 6). A corresponding experiment was car-

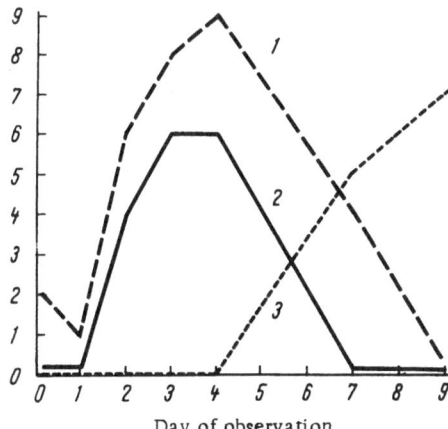

Day of observation

Fig. 6. Dynamics of reproduction of virus and formation of endogenous interferon and antibodies in mice infected with Coxsackie A6 virus: 1) virus; 2) interferon; 3) antibodies.

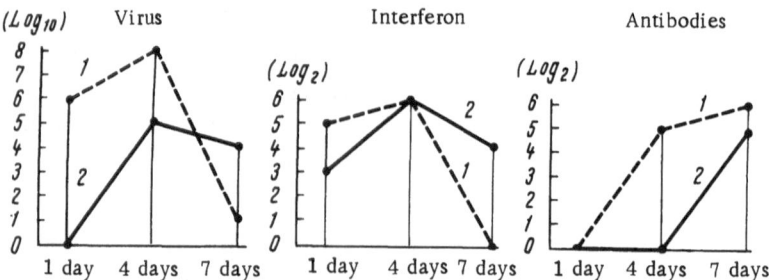

Fig. 7. Dynamics of reproduction of virus and formation of endogenous interferon and antibodies in mice infected with Coxsackie A6 virus and receiving exogenous interferon: 1) mice infected with Coxsackie A6 virus; 2) mice infected with Coxsackie A6 virus and receiving exogenous interferon.

ried out on mice receiving repeated injections of interferon by the above scheme (Fig. 7).

The following conclusions can be drawn from these experiments:

1. To demonstrate the effectiveness of interferon in enterovirus infections not only must the preparation used have a high interferon content, but it must also be administered repeatedly. The age of the animals is significant: in newborn mice the action of interferon is much weaker than in animals 12 days old.

2. The dynamics of reproduction of Coxsackie A6 virus in the blood reaches a maximum on the 5th day after infection, which coincides with the development of symptoms of the disease. The formation of endogenous interferon corresponds to the dynamics of virus reproduction and is complete on the 7th day. Meanwhile the content of virus falls sharply: on the 9th day neither virus nor interferon can be found in the blood of the surviving mice. Antibodies appear in the blood on the 7th day and reach their maximum titer on the 9th day, when both virus and interferon are completely absent.

3. In infected mice treated with exogenous interferon, the content of virus in the bloodstream is lower. Interferon is found from the 1st to the 7th day, which coincides with the time of appearance of antibodies in the bloodstream.

The intensity of the antiviral action can thus be explained by the combined effect of exogenous interferon and of endogenous interferon which is produced in the course of the infection.

In our experiments with ectromelia virus the effectiveness of interferon also was compared in two groups of mice of different ages. Newborn mice aged 24-48 h and mice over 1 year old, weighing 25-30 g, were used. Four injections of interferon were given, by the scheme described above. The newborn mice received 0.2 ml interferon per injection, the adult mice 0.5 ml.

The results in Table 69 show that the effectiveness of interferon in ectromelia is independent of the animals' age.

5.2. Clinical Trials of Exogenous Interferon

The first clinical trials for prophylactic and therapeutic purposes were conducted mainly with preparations of heterologous interferon.

The first trials of exogenous interferon in man were carried out in England [528]. Interferon prepared in monkey kidney tissue was injected intradermally in a dose of 0.1 ml into 38 volunteers. Next day vaccinia virus was introduced into the same areas of the skin. The opposite arm of the same volunteers, into which a placebo was similarly injected, served as the control. A typical vaccination reaction developed in the areas first treated with interferon in 6 volunteers, a weakly positive reaction was observed in 8, and a negative reaction in 24 volunteers. Meanwhile, the typical vaccination reaction developed in the control areas in 37 volunteers.

TABLE 69. Effectiveness of Interferon Against
Ectromelia in Mice of Different Ages

Group	Age or weight	Number of mice which died	Survival rate (in %)
Receiving interferon	25-30 g	8/16	50
	Newborn	7/14	50
Receiving normal serum	25-30 g	15/16	6.3
	Newborn	14/14	0

Exogenous interferon was found to be effective in the treatment of keratitis complicating vaccination [385].

Interferon obtained in chick embryos and cultures of chick fibroblasts has been used with some success in the treatment of virus diseases of the human eyes and skin. In particular, Ermol'eva and co-workers [67] used chick allantoic interferon for the treatment of patients with adenovirus keratoconjunctivitis. Altogether 53 patients were treated by instillation of interferon into the eyes every 2 h throughout the day until recovery was complete. In patients treated with interferon the duration of the disease was reduced by one half to two thirds by comparison with the control group. Similar results were obtained in the treatment of keratitis caused by herpes simplex virus.

Allantoic interferon has been tested in dermatological practice for the treatment of diseases caused by the viruses of herpes simplex, herpes zoster, and vesicular stomatitis [67]. Administration of interferon in liquid form or as an ointment 2-3 times a day led to a more rapid recovery. Ermol'eva and Furer [275] described successful local application of interferon obtained in human diploid cells and leukocytes for the treatment of virus diseases of the eyes and skin. Leukocytic interferon was particularly effective in skin diseases caused by herpes simplex virus. In some cases recovery was observed on the second day after the beginning of treatment.

In a review of experience gained over 5 years in the treatment of herpes of the eyes with human leukocytic interferon, Kasparov [615a] describes its high efficacy when injected subconjunctivally. Clinical recovery in patients treated with interferon was accompanied by a five- to sixfold decrease in the frequency of detection of herpetic antigen on immunofluorescence testing of conjunctival scrapings.

Other workers [8, 123, 172] also obtained good results by the treatment of patients with skin lesions of herpes simplex and herpes zoster with interferon. In other dermatoses of virus etiology interferon ointment gave little or no therapeutic effect. For instance, not a single cure was obtained in 20 patients with molluscum contagiosum.

Considering the short duration of action of interferon, Fadeeva and co-workers [176] prepared a long-acting preparation by mixing interferon with polyvinylpyrrolidone. After initial reports of successful trials with this preparation it was later found to be toxic [177].

Preparations of homologous and heterologous interferon have been used for the prevention and treatment of virus diseases.

Ermol'eva and co-workers [63] described the successful use of chick interferon in the treatment of influenza. However, these results were not confirmed by subsequent clinical observations.

Zalmanzon and co-workers [82] reported that intranasal administration of exogenous chick interferon reduces the incidence of influenza in man by half. More reliable data concerning the use of human leukocytic interferon for the prevention of influenza in children's institutions are given by Zlatkovskaya and co-workers [89]. The preparation was given in a dose of 0.2 ml intranasally 3 times a day for 4 days. The use of interferon was found to be of prophylactic value and it limited the spread of influenza. The results of the use of interferon in diseases regarded as incurable are of great interest [276, 277].

In an influenza epidemic in 1970, Kursinova et al. [615b] made observations on the treatment of Hong Kong influenza by aerosol inhalation of an improved interferon preparation. Patients with the typical symptoms of influenza were chosen in the first 24 h after the onset of the illness. The group of patients treated with interferon consisted of 112 persons, and the control group consisted fo 48 persons receiving ordinary medicinal treatment.

Interferon treatment abolished the toxic manifestations and fever in most patients during the first day and had a favorable effect on local inflammatory changes in the upper respiratory tract. In 13 patients a subfebrile temperature persisted for more than 3 days after treatment. In these patients there was evidence of concomitant disease (pneumosclerosis, chronic laryngotracheitis, tonsillitis).

These workers consider that aerosol inhalation is the most suitable method of interferon administration in influenza. The reason is because the massive introduction of the aerosol into the respiratory organs gives the most rapid effect.

Similar results for the early treatment of influenza patients with leukocytic interferon were obtained by Sapozhnikov et al. [619a].

However, in their observations they used native interferon and not
the partially purified and concentrated preparation.

Human leukocytic interferon was used in the treatment of 11
patients with acute myeloblastic leukemia, 7 patients with acute
lymphatic leukemia, 2 leukemic patients with herpes zoster, 7
newborn infants with cytomegaly, and 1 newborn infant with generalized herpetic infection. Several patients with leukemia were treated in the course of a year by intraveous injection of up to 3 liters
of interferon, with a visible improvement in their condition. All
patients with cytomegaly were cured. Usually this disease is lethal
in the newborn. The infants received up to 40 ml of interferon
daily by intravenous injection. Although no definite conclusions
were drawn regarding the effectiveness of interferon in the treatment of virus infections the results nevertheless provide sufficient
grounds for clinical trials of more active and more highly purified
preparations of interferon.

Unsuccessful attempts to use monkey interferon for the prevei
tion of diseases in man caused by rhinovirus and also by Coxsackie
A21 and type 1 parainfluenza viruses have also been reported [531].
In these observations interferon was first injected intranasally into
volunteers who were then infected with one of the viruses mentioned
The absence of a prophylactic effect was presumably due to the low
activity of the heterologous interferon preparation. However, these
workers attribute their results to the rapid removal of the preparation from the surface of the mucous membrane of the respiratory
tract by the ciliated epithelium covering it.

Most of the clinical trials of exogenous interferon have accordingly shown that it is most useful for the prevention and treatment of virus infections giving rise to predominantly local lesions.
At the same time, because of the species specificity of interferon the
question arises of the nature of the active principle of the antiviral
activity of heterologous interferon preparations. Further research
is essential to provide the correct answer. However, as was mentioned above, the prophylactic and therapeutic effect of preparations obtained in heterologous systems may be due to other interferon-like inhibitors or inducers which they contain.

A method of obtaining human leukocytic interferon has been
described earlier in this book. The effectiveness of preparations

of human leukocytic interferon obtained by the present writer was tested in experiments conducted jointly with Porubel' on 357 volunteers. Interferon with a titer of not less than 1 : 64 was used in order to determine its activity on strains ot human diploid cells of myodermal tissue.

The effect of preparations of exogenous human interferon on immunological reactions of persons vaccinated with living influenza vaccine from strain A2/M21/65 and on the survival of the virus in the upper respiratory tract was determined in these experiments.

Observations were made on volunteers between 18 and 45 years of age. After preliminary testing for antibodies against influenza A2 virus, persons in whom the antibody titer in the hemagglutination inhibition test was 1 : 20 were selected. Leukocytic interferon was injected in a dose of 0.25 ml into each nasal passage by means of an atomizer. The control group received medium 199 as a placebo. The preparations for testing were marked only with identification numbers.

After administration of the interferon the volunteers were vaccinated with influenza virus A2/M21/65 in a dose of 10^6 $ID_{50}/0.25$ ml. Daily for 4 days the content of the virus in nasopharyngeal washings was determined by the method of reisolation in chick embryos.

Immunological changes in the vaccinated volunteers were analyzed on the basis of a fourfold or greater increase in the titer of antibodies in two specimens of serum taken just before the experiment and 14 days after injection of the living virus.

For the comparative study a preparation of interferon obtained by infection of a monolayer culture of chick fibroblasts also was used. Activity of the human and chick interferons was identical and they contained 64-128 units when assayed by inhibition of the cytopathic effect on homologous cells. Observations were made initially on 157 volunteers, divided in 3 groups. A group of 47 subjects received human interferon by intranasal injection. The second group of volunteers (51) received interferon obtained from chick cells. The third group, consisting of 59 persons, acted as the control and received medium 199 instead of interferon intranasally. All the volunteers were vaccinated 1-2 h after receiving

TABLE 70. Effect of Leukocytic Interferon on Immunological Responses of Volunteers When Given 2 h
before the Virus

Preparation given before vaccination	Number of persons vaccinated	Survival of virus shown by			
		isolation in chick embryos		increase in antibody titer	
		abs.	%	abs.	%
Human interferon	47	11	23.4	18	38.3
Chick interferon	51	25	49.0	31	60.7
Medium 199	59	37	62.8	30	50.8

the interferon or placebo, and the content of virus was then determined in nasopharyngeal washings (Table 70).

This interval between administration of the interferon and
virus was chosen on account of experimental results obtained with
tissue cultures showing that this period is sufficient for interferon
to exhibit a reliable prophylactic action. The prophylactic action
is seen particularly clearly if the excretion of the virus is compared in chick embryos. Persons receiving preliminary treatment with human interferon excreted the virus 2.5 times less
frequently than the controls.

However, according to the serological tests, the prophylactic
action of interferon was weak and was manifested in only 30% of
the vaccinated subjects.

It should be mentioned that in this group of volunteers there
were no reactions to vaccination although there were in the control
group. These experiments confirmed our findings with regard to
the species specificity of interferon obtained in tissue culture experiments. Intranasal injection of the preparation of chick interferon had only a very slight effect on the survival of the virus.
When survival of the virus was assessed by the increase in titer
of antibodies the chick interferon had no protective action what-
soever.

In later experiments other schemes of administration of
preparations of the leukocytic interferon and virus to the volunteers were used in order to determine the duration of the prophylactic action of the interferon when given once or repeatedly.

Different groups of volunteers received interferon 2, 24, 48, and 72 h before infection.

The results of these observations are shown in Table 71. The best protective action of interferon was found when two injections were given, the first 24 h and the second 2 h before infection. Of 25 volunteers, none showed survival of the virus and an increase in the antibody titer was observed in 5 persons, or 20%.

Similar results were obtained in the case of infection with virus 24 h after injection of interferon and a further injection of interferon 24 h after the virus. Survival of the virus, as shown by isolation in chick embryos, was observed in 8.9-18.1% of volunteers, and as shown by an increase in antibody titer, in 22.7-29% of volunteers. No prophylactic action of interferon was observed if it was given 72 h before the virus.

It can be concluded from these observations that the prophylactic action of the interferon tested does not exceed 48 h in duration and that repeated administration gives a higher protective effect. It is relevant to mention here that in trials of the prophylactic value of leukocytic interferon prepared by us, conducted jointly with the Central Institute of Epidemiology, Ministry of Health

TABLE 71. Effect of Exogenous Interferon on Survival of Influenza Vaccine Virus When Administered under Various Conditions

| Scheme of administration of interferon and virus | Number of volunteers | Survival of virus shown by | | | |
| | | isolation in chick embryos | | increase in antibody titer | |
		abs.	%	abs.	%
Medium 199 (control)	51	24/50	48.0	21/47	44.7
Interferon, virus after 24 h	56	5/56	8.9	16/55	29.0
Interferon, virus after 24 h, interferon again after a further 24 h	22	4/22	18.1	5/22	22.7
Interferon twice in 1 day, virus 24 h later, preceded by interferon again (2 h beforehand)	25	0	0	5/25	20.0
Interferon, virus 48 h later	22	12/22	54.5	6/22	27.2
Interferon, virus 72 h later	24	12/24	54.1	11/24	45.7

of the USSR, during an influenza A2 epidemic at the beginning of 1967, results confirming these observations on volunteers were obtained.

According to Bolotovskii and Nefedova leukocytic inteferon was given to groups of adults and to groups of children between the ages of 7 and 9. Each group consisted of about 100 persons, and the same number of subjects received a placebo in an experiment in which the substances given were identified by codes. Interferon was injected three times at three-day intervals.

By the frequency of catarrhal symptoms and fever the number of persons falling ill was smaller in the experimental group than in the control, but because of the difficulty in making a precise clinical diagnosis of influenza, the results of interferon treatment were based on laboratory serological tests. Persons who had received interferon developed influenza between 3 and 4 times less frequently than those of the control group.

The most marked effect of interferon was found in children: 7.7% developed influenza compared with 42.5% in the control group.

During an epidemic of Hong Kong influenza human leukocytic interferon was tested for prophylactic purposes in several institutions. Results obtained by the Central Institute of Epidemiology are given in Table 72. They show that intranasal administration of the preparation reduced the incidence of influenza by 2.4–3.5 times.

The interferon content in nasal washings from the volunteers after intranasal injection of leukocytic interferon also was studied. These investigations were carried out on 37 volunteers. Nasal washings were obtained before administration of the interferon and 24 and 48 h later. The material obtained was treated with HCl to pH 2.4 for 48 h and then with NaOH to pH 7.4. The inhibitory activity of the nasal washings in a dilution of 1 : 2 to 1 : 16 was determined in a strain of diploid cells of myodermal tissue of a human embryo with vesicular stomatitis virus. No inhibitor could be detected in any of the washings obtained from the volunteers.

The possibility of using exogenous interferon raised the question of possible side effects of interferon on the cells and tissues of the body.

TABLE 72. Prophylactic Value of Human Leukocytic Interferon against Hong Kong Influenza (from data of the Central Institute of Epidemiology, Ministry of Health of the USSR)

Preparation	Number of cases	Incidence abs.	%	Effectiveness K	E%
Adults (Moscow)					
Interferon	2994	231	7.7	2.4	56.3
Placebo (control)	3129	551	17.6		
Children aged 7-16 years (Moscow)					
Interferon	1917	119	6.2	3.5	69.2
Placebo (control)	2055	413	20.1		
Children aged 2-6 years (Donetsk)					
Interferon	463	22	4.7	2.4	59.3
Placebo (control)	454	53	11.6		

$$K = \frac{\text{Incidence of influenza in group receiving placebo (B)}}{\text{Incidence in group receiving interferon (A)}}$$

$E = 100 (B-A)/B.$

According to some investigators interferon has no toxic action on the body as a whole or on cells cultivated *in vitro*. Wagner and Levy [586], for instance, found no changes in the mitotic activity of chick fibroblasts treated with interferon.

Ermol'eva and co-workers [65, 71] did not observe a toxic action of chick interferon on primary trypsinized and transplanted tissue culture cells. No degenerative or other changes likewise were found after three injections, each of 0.5 ml, of the same preparation into albino mice. After subcutaneous or intramuscular injection moderately severe signs of irritation appeared, in the form of slight hyperemia and migration of polymorphs and some increase in the number of histiocytes.

As a result of their investigations, Zhdanov and co-workers [77, 78] even state that interferon stimulates growth of the cell culture. Interferon not only accelerated the formation of the cell monolayer but prolonged the life of the culture.

Meanwhile there are reports of the opposite character. Cocito and co-workers [253, 254], for instance, stated that unpurified preparations of interferon inhibit the synthesis of protein and nucleic acids in rat cells. An adverse action of interferon on cell metabolism has also been observed by other workers [121, 334, 424, 425, 484, 541].

Critical analysis of these investigations into the action of interferon on the metabolism of uninfected cells does not provide evidence of their complete reliability. The possibility cannot be ruled out that purified preparations of interferon would be completely harmless. Ho [345] considers that the inhibitory action of interferon on cell reproduction is nonspecific and is due to interferon-like substances.

Confirmation of this is given by recent work carried out with highly purified preparations of interferon [220, 423]. It was found that they had no effect on the rate of synthesis of RNA, DNA, and protein in the cells of the chick embryo. The rate of synthesis of these cell components was measured by the incorporation of valine into protein or of uridine into fast- or slow-labeled RNA.

Finally, according to results obtained by Fadeeva and co-workers [179], interferon does not possess sensitizing properties when injected intravenously into albino mice, guinea pigs, or rabbits.

In conclusion, it can be said that the prophylactic value of interferon is no longer in doubt but the effectiveness of this compound in the treatment of virus infections, especially of the generalized type, is not yet clear.

5.3. Conclusion

The results of experiments on mice have shown that exogenous interferon of homologous origin has a well-marked prophylactic effect in experimental influenza, enterovirus infection, and ectromelia. This action is well defined in the case of infection with a dose of 10 LD_{50} and less marked against infection in a dose of 100 LD_{50} or more. An increase in the infecting dose greatly reduces the effectiveness of interferon. The protective action of a single injection of interferon lasts not much more than 24 h and it is more clearly defined in those experiments in which it is given before infection with the virus. The intensity of the protective action is directly dependent on the dose of interferon given. This was demonstrated particularly clearly in experiments with ectromelia virus, when four injections of interferon gave a much stronger protective action than a single dose. It thus follows that one of the chief ways in which the effectiveness of interferon can be increased is by injecting it more frequently, and another way is by the production of more active and more concentrated preparations. The results obtained by us are in agreement with those described by other workers [212, 284, 288].

It is important to emphasize that interferon has been found to be effective against infections involving principally the respiratory organs, against systemic infections, and against infection caused by myotropic enterovirus.

A study of the effectiveness of action of interferon in mice of different ages infected with ectromelia revealed no difference. However, age differences were significant in mice infected with Coxsackie A6 virus.

Before we began our investigations no reports of the effect of human interferon on human virus infections had been published. One reason preventing extensive trials of interferon as a prophylactic and therapeutic agent is its marked species specificity. Only by the use of human leukocytes for interferon production has it become possible to obtain sufficiently active preparations for use in experiments on volunteers. Observations have shown that leukocytic interferon has a marked protective action, especially if administered repeatedly.

Several factors must of course be taken into account when the action of leukocytic interferon is assessed: the optimal dose of the preparation, the frequency and method of its administration, the character and nature of the infectious process, the sensitivity of the virus against which the interferon is being used. Further improvement of the method of production of leukocytic interferon with the object of obtaining sufficient material for its large-scale use with the least expenditure of effort is a particularly important aspect of the problem.

It will probably soon be possible to obtain the active principle in an optimal concentration, which will mean that minimal volumes of the preparation can then be injected. It is also necessary to standardize human interferon, so that the results obtained in different laboratories can be compared.

Despite these difficulties and the existence of many unsolved problems we are confident that human leukocytic interferon or interferon obtained in some other human tissue will find its due place in the armamentarium for the control of virus infections.

Chapter 6

Effect of Stimulators of Endogenous Interferon on Experimental Virus Infections

6.1. Stimulation of Endogenous Interferon by Intravenous and Other Methods of Injection of Inducers of Virus Origin

In 1963, Baron and Buckler [209] found that the intravenous injection of various viruses into mice leads to the formation of interferon which can be found in the animals' serum. The interferon appeared in the serum within 1 h and reached its highest concentration 4 h after infection. In order of diminishing interferon-inducing activity the viruses tested were arranged as follows: Newcastle disease, Sindbis, Sendai, and vaccinia viruses. These workers showed that interferon formation is induced by the virus in the material injected and is not due to its reproduction. The concentration of the inducing virus was of essential importance to the detection of the serum interferon. Interferon could be induced by a single intravenous dose containing not less than 10^6 p.f.u. of infective virus.

Later the method of intravenous injection of virus into mice to induce interferon was used by many workers [35, 45, 225, 548], and intravenous injection of NDV into animals became the standard procedure for the induction of serum interferon.

Sindbis virus has been widely used for the induction of serum interferon in rabbits [347, 354, 356, 405].

Interferon formation in the serum of chickens, hamsters, and monkeys has been induced by intravenous injection of NDV [170,

211, 603], Powassan [413], influenza, Sindbis [603], and herpes simplex [557] viruses, and also inactivated Semliki forest virus [39].

Some workers regard rats and chickens as poor producers of interferon [548]. However, by intravenous injection of large doses of NDV [513] and Sindbis virus [268] considerable quantities of interferon were induced in the serum and spleen of rats.

The possibility of inducing interferon formation in cockerels, mice, and man by administration of heated Semliki forest virus (HSV) was studied by Vil'ner, Zeitlenok, and co-workers [39].

Intravenous injection of this inducer into cockerels and mice was followed by the formation of serum interferon, the maximum titer being reached after 3-4 h. Similar results were obtained by intramuscular injection of HSV inducer into human volunteers.

Comparative studies of interferon formation in the serum and organs of mice after intraperitoneal injection of living and inactivated influenza virus showed that interferon appears in the serum after 2 h and reaches its maximum after 5 h, falling there-after until 24 h. The interferon titer in the organs rose until 24 h and interferon could be detected until the 4th day. The dynamics of interferon formation was similar after injection of the living and inactivated viruses [15]. Most of the authors cited above state that interferon induced by intravenous injection of viruses disap-pears from the blood stream comparatively quickly. Interferon circulating in the blood could usually be detected for no more than 24-36 h.

There is no reliable information regarding the site of for-mation of the serum interferon in the body. The claim has how-ever been made that the chief producers are the cells of the reticulo-endothelial system (RES): leukocytes and phagocytes of the pe-ripheral blood, the spleen, and other organs of the RES.

The role of leukocytes in interferon production can be deduced from the results of investigations which have demonstrated their ability to synthesize this inhibitor *in vitro* [277, 280, 313, 319, 549].

Kono and Ho [405] reported that rabbit spleen cells, when infected *in vitro* with Sindbis virus, produce interferon more quickly than the cells of other organs. They also found that after intravenous

injection of large doses of this virus into rabbits the highest concentrations of interferon are found in the spleen. Similar results
were obtained in rats in which the interferon concentration in the
spleen was 40 times higher than in the serum [513]. De Somer and
Billiau [268] consider that cells of the RES and, in particular, of
the spleen are the most active producers of interferon. According
to their findings the interferon concentration in the spleen 6 h after
injection of Sindbis virus into rats reached almost 20,000 units per
gram tissue. If the virus was injected into these animals and
splenectomy was then performed, the spleen produced almost as
much interferon as *in vivo*. These results were confirmed
by those of other workers [301, 470, 553] who found that splenectomy
leads to a marked decrease in the production of virus-induced interferon. Admittedly in the experiments of Borecky and co-workers
[228] and of De Somer and Billiau [268] splenectomy was not followed
by a decrease in the production of serum interferon. Other evidence
of the important role of the RES in interferon production is given by
experiments in which it was blocked by thorotrast [556] and a more
recent investigation which showed that leukocytes of the peritoneal
exudate of rabbits produce interferon much more quickly than other
types of cells [539]. This may evidently explain why interferon is
produced most quickly of all by intravenous injection of viruses.

So far as the rapid decrease in the interferon concentration
in the spleen is concerned, it is not yet completely clear whether
this is due to its elimination or to its deposition in the organs.

Experiments have shown that after intravenous injection of
exogenous interferon it can still be detected in the organs even
after it has disappeared from the bloodstream [358, 553]. Nevertheless it is evident that most interferon, whether exogenous or
endogenous, is eliminated with the urine [223, 269, 326, 357].

In some experiments the interferon concentration in the urine
was 5 times higher than in the spleen.

In the investigations cited above insufficient attention was
paid to the dynamics of interferon formation in the organs of the
animals in relation to the virulence and tropism of the viruses.

With these considerations in mind, we made a comparative
study of the ability of certain viruses to induce interferon formation
when injected intravenously.

Viruses pathogenic to mice (influenza A and ectromelia) and nonpathogenic viruses (Newcastle disease), differing in their tropism, were used. It was especially sought to determine the correlation between the concentration of serum and "organ" interferon and its dependence on the tropism of the viruses. Another factor of great interest was the study of the dynamics of serum interferon formation in the blood of different species of animals in response to injection of the same inducer. The interferon-inducing activity of strains of NDV with different virulence to birds also was studied.

Noninbred mice weighing 15-18 g and chinchilla rabbits weighing 2.5-3 kg were used.* An epizootic strain K and vaccine strains V1 and N of Newcastle disease virus, strain PR-8 of influenza A virus, and Western equine encephalomyelitis (WEE) viruses were used as inducers.

Newcastle disease and influenza viruses were administered in the allantoic fluid of infected chick embryos, and WEE virus in the culture fluid of a monolayer of chick fibroblasts after degeneration under the influence of this virus. The virus was injected intravenously into mice in a dose of 10^7-10^8 TCD_{50} in a volume of 1 ml, and into rabbits in a volume of 5 ml. Blood was taken from the animals at different times and the concentration of virus and interferon determined over a period of time. At each time of investigation 10 mice were used and their sera were pooled before titration. The interferon concentration in the mouse sera was determined by testing serial twofold dilutions of serum on a primary trypsinized culture of mouse embryonic tissue or on L cells of clone 929. The rabbit interferon was titrated in rabbit embryonic fibroblasts which had been subcultured 5-10 times *in vitro* in medium 199 with 10% bovine serum.

Before titration of the interferon the virus in the serum and organs was inactivated by addition of 6N HCl to pH 2.0 followed by induction at 4°C for 96 h. Preliminary tests showed that at this hydrogen ion concentration in the medium the strains of NDV used are inactivated in organ suspensions within 48 h. After inactivation of the virus the pH of the serum was adjusted to 7.2-7.4 with 5N NaOH. The test virus was added in the titration in a dose of

---

*Some of the investigations described in this section were carried out jointly with Yu. B. Fedorova.

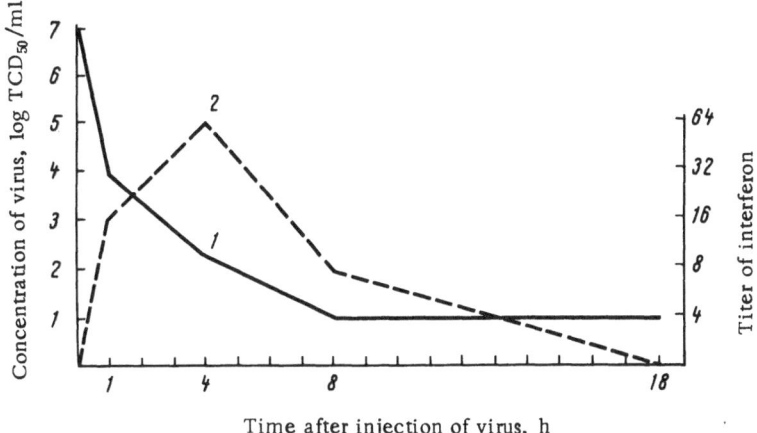

Fig. 8. Relationship between concentrations of interferon and virus
in the blood of mice after intravenous injection of NDV: 1) virus;
2) interferon.

100 TCD_{50} in a volume of 0.1 ml. Inhibition of the cytopathic effect
of the virus was used as the indicator for titration.

In the initial experiments the correlation between the concentrations of NDV virus and interferon was studied in the blood
of mice. One hour after intravenous injection of NDV in a dose of
10^7-10^8 TCD_{50} its concentration in the serum was 10^3-10^4 TCD_{50},
and after 18 h the virus could no longer be found. Interferon,
however, in most cases was detected in small quantities after 1 h
and its maximal titer (1:16 to 1:64) was reached after 4 h. Its
concentration then fell rapidly, and after 8 h it was found in the
blood in a dilution of 1:8.

In individual cases a decrease in the interferon titer was
observed after 8 h. No interferon could be detected in the serum
24 h after injection of the viruses (Fig. 8).

In experiments on mice the interferon-inducing activity of
epizootic strain K and vaccine strains N and V1 was studied after
intravenous injection.

The interferon-inducing activity of epizootic strain K and
vaccine strains N and V1 when given by intravenous injection was
studied in experiments on mice. Equal doses (10^7) of these viruses,

TABLE 73. Titers of Interferon
in Serum of Mice 4 h after Intravenous Injection of NVD

Strain	Virulence for birds	Interferon titer
K	Virulent	16,384
N	Vaccine	8,192
VI	Vaccine	16,384

in the form of allantoic fluid of chick embryos, were injected into
the mice in a volume of 1 ml. All the mice were exsanguinated
4 h later and the interferon titer was determined in cells with
vesicular virus.

The results (Table 73) show that, irrespective of their
virulence for birds, the interferon-inducing activity of the strain
of NDV in mice is similar.

In the next experiments the dynamics of interferon formation
were studied after intravenous injection of viruses differing in
their tropism but pathogenic for mice. In this way correlation
between the serum and organ interferon could be established. It
was important to discover whether a pneumotropic virus, when
injected intravenously, induces interferon in the lungs more intensively than in other organs, and whether WEE virus behaves
similarly in the brain. NDV, which is nonpathogenic for mice,
was used for comparison. All three viruses were injected intravenously in a dose of 10^7 TCD_{50} in a volume of 1 ml. The blood,
kidneys, lungs, and brain were taken 2, 4, 6, 8, 12, and 24 h later
and, after inactivation of the viruses by treatment with acid, their
interferon content was determined. It will be remembered that
the organs were taken after exsanguination of the animals. Interferon was detected in L cells which, under these experimental
conditions, were more sensitive to interferon than primary mouse
fibroblasts. The dynamics of the interferon content in the serum
and organs of the mice is shown in Table 74.

The results given in Table 74 show that the dynamics of
interferon formation after intravenous injection of the viruses is
independent of the properties of the virus. The only differences
between the viruses were quantitative, in the intensity of their

TABLE 74. Dynamics of Interferon Content in Serum
and Organs of Mice after Intravenous Injection
of Viruses

Virus	Time of taking material, h	Interferon titer in			
		serum	lung	kidney	brain
N	2	2,048	320	40	40
	4	16,192	640	640	320
	6	4,096	n.i.	n.i.	n.i.
	8	64	320	320	160
	18	<8	40	20	40
PR-8	2	54	<20	<20	<20
	4	512	80	40	<20
	6	32	80	80	<20
	8	16	20	160	<20
	18	<8	<20	20	<20
WEE	2	32	<20	<20	<20
	4	256	80	40	<20
	6	32	80	80	<20
	8	8	20	160	<20
	18	<8	<20	20	<20

Note: n.i., not investigated.

inducing activity. NDV possessed the highest and WEE virus the
lowest activity; influenza virus occupied an intermediate position.
Regardless of which of the three viruses was injected, interferon
was found in detectable quantities in the serum after 2 h and its
content reached a maximum after 4 h, when it began to decrease
rapidly. Approximately the same dynamics was observed in the
organs tested. Consequently, the tropism of the virus was unim-
portant as regards the distribution of the interferon. Nevertheless,
it must be noted that interferon appeared and disappeared in the
organs later than in the spleen. Interferon disappeared latest of
all from the kidneys. The reason for this is evidently that serum
interferon is formed outside the organs studied and is partially
absorbed in them. Presumably the interferon detected in the
organs is this absorbed interferon. The interferon found in the
kidneys, on the other hand, is that destined for excretion in the
urine. To verify this hypothesis 1 ml NDV with a titer of 10^7 TCD_{50}
was injected intravenously into each of a group of mice weighing

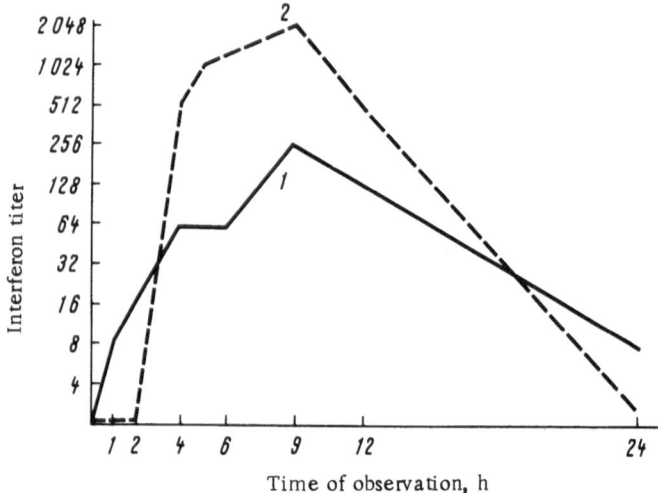

Fig. 9. Correlation between interferon concentrations in the serum and urine of mice after injection of NDV: 1) blood serum; 2) urine.

18-20 g. The mice were placed on Petri dishes after 1, 2, 4, 8, and 18 h and micturition was induced by mechanical stimulation. The same procedure was carried out with a control group of mice, which did not receive the virus. The samples of urine thus obtained were treated in the usual way with acid and alkali and titrated in L cells. The results given in Fig. 9 show that the interferon concentration in the urine was considerably higher than its concentration in the serum, as a result of both the filtration and the concentration functions of the kidneys. At the same time these results show that interferon is excreted with the urine almost simultaneously with its formation.

It should also be noted that NDV proved to be a highly active inducer of interferon when injected intravenously not only in mice, but also in rabbits.

As already stated above, NDV with a titer of 10^8 TCD_{50} was injected intravenously into rabbits in a volume of 5 ml and blood was taken from the auricular vein 1, 2, 4, 6, 8, and 24 h later. The serum was treated in the usual way and titrated in rabbit fibroblasts with vesicular stomatitis virus. The results (Table 75) show that the dynamics of interferon formation in rabbits is similar to that

TABLE 75. Dynamics of Accumulation of Serum Interferon in Rabbits

Rabbit No.	Time of taking blood, h	Interferon titer
1	1	512
	2	2,048
	4	>16,384
	6	16,384
	8	8,192
	24	32
2	1	<4
	2	4,096
	4	8,192
	6	>16,384
	8	n.i.
	24	128

Note: n.i., not investigated.

in mice. The only difference was that interferon was found for a longer time in the serum; its titer even after 24 h was still 1 : 32 to 1 : 128.

To determine the effect of splenectomy on serum interferon production, N. R. Gutman, working in our laboratory, carried out a series of experiments on splenectomized mice. Two conditions were found to be of decisive importance: the time of injection of the inducing virus and its properties. For instance, a sharp decrease in interferon production took place regularly if Newcastle disease virus was injected intravenously 24 and 48 h after the operation. Three days after splenectomy the experimental and control mice behaved identically. If influenza A2 virus was injected as the inducer, 7 days after the operation interferon production in the experimental mice was 4-6 times lower than in the control. An important factor in this result was evidently that mice are susceptible to influenza virus but not to NDV. Another noteworthy feature of these experiments was the rate of development of compensatory processes in the animals. Only a comparatively short time was needed for the normal functions of the lymphoid tissue, responsible for interferon formation, to be restored.

Splenectomy had an even more marked action if accompanied by injection of the serum of rabbits immunized with the lymph glands taken from mice.

TABLE 76. Effect of Splenectomy and Antilymph-Gland
Serum on Production of Serum Interferon

Inducing virus	Titer of serum interferon in mice after			
	splenectomy	injection of serum	splenectomy and injection of serum	control
NDV	256	64	0	4,000
Influenza A2	64	16	0	256

As an example the results of one experiment will be described
in which NDV was injected one day after splenectomy and influenza
virus 7 days after the operation (Table 76).

Clearly the antilymph-gland serum had a marked depressant
effect, further evidence of the important role of lymphoid tissue
in interferon production.

6.2. Effect of Virus Inducers of Interferon Formation on Experimental Virus Infections

The ability of biologically active and inactivated viruses to
induce interferon formation when administered by different routes
provided the basis for the study of the possible use of stimulators
of endogenous interferon for the prevention and treatment of virus
infections.

This problem was originally studied in experiments on
animals, in most cases with the aim of investigating the effect of
stimulators of endogenous interferon on experimental influenza
and arbovirus infections. These experiments showed that intranasal administration of influenza A virus had a well-marked prophylactic action against subsequent infection with Bunyamwera virus
[342]. In the control group 86% of the infected animals died, whereas in the experimental group a lethal infection was observed in
only 33% of the animals.

Denys and co-workers [267] and other investigators [60, 530]
have described the prophylactic action of influenza virus inactivated by ultraviolet radiation (UV-vaccine) in mice infected experimentally with influenza virus. Intranasal injection of the UV
vaccine gave protection against influenza virus for 48-72 h.

Prophylactic (24 h beforehand) intraperitoneal injection of vaccinia virus, inactivated by ultraviolet radiation, prevented death of animals after intracerebral infection with vesicular stomatitis virus [313].

After the intensive and rapid production of interferon after intravenous injection of NDV into mice had been discovered, this method of stimulation of endogenous interferon was used by many investigators [212]. This method was shown to ensure the survival of 65% of mice after intracerebral infection with encephalomyocarditis virus. A similar effect was observed with Germiston virus (an arbovirus of the Bunyamwera group), in which case marked protection was observed not only when the interferon inducer was injected before the arbovirus or simultaneously with it, but also when injected 2 h after infection [212]. Similar results were obtained by intravenous and intraperitoneal injection of NDV into mice 24, 18, and 4-6 h before infection with encephalomyocarditis virus in a dose of 1000 LD_{50}. Survival of 70-80% of the animals was observed. Influenza viruses A2/M21/65 and B (Lich) inactivated by ultraviolet radiation [181, 182] had a similar action.

In the study of the prophylactic effect of virus inducers of interferon against arbovirus infection in mice [136], NDV and heat-inactivated Semliki forest virus were used as inducers. Preliminary intravenous injection of NDV gave a marked protective effect against tick-borne encephalitis virus. Injection of the inducing virus as late as 2 days after infection of the mice with 50-100 LD_{50} of the encephalitis virus led to the survival of 23.8% of the animals compared with only 4.4% in the control group [136]. Swine influenza virus, inactivated by ultraviolet radiation, has also been used to induce interferon. The UV vaccine, injected intranasally or intraperitoneally 3 or 24 h before infection of mice with 10-100 LD_{50} Eastern equine encephalomyelitis (EEE) virus, protected them against the disease. Injection of UV vaccine 48 h before infection was less effective [16, 101, 133].

The protective action of endogenous interferon against experimental influenza has been studied in experiments of various types [33]. Preliminary injection of interferon inducer (NDV), 18-20 h beforehand, completely protected mice from death after injection with 100 LD_{50} influenza A virus (strain PR-8), gave partial protection against infection in a dose of 1000 LD_{50}, but was ineffective against infection with 10,000 LD_{50} [145, 147, 148, 177].

Intranasal infection of albino mice with influenza A1 virus led to the development of an asymptomatic infection in the animals, accompanied by marked accumulation of interferon in the lungs. Superinfection of these animals with a highly pathogenic strain of influenza A virus (PR-8) reduced the mortality. On histological investigation the almost complete absence of edema of the lungs characteristic of the toxic action of influenza A virus was found. The same paper also describes experiments to study the effect of NDV, injected intravenously into rabbits, on smallpox infection. Complete inhibition of reproduction of vaccinia virus was found for 3 days after injection of the interferon inducer. Vaccinia virus, when injected later, reproduced less intensively than in control animals [148].

The results of these experiments thus provide a basis for the use of nonpathogenic viruses, effective in inducing interferon, for prophylactic and therapeutic purposes. Calculations have shown that injection of interferon inducers, especially intravenously, is accompanied by the formation of large quantities of interferon in the body. In particular, Baron and co-workers [211] calculated that after intravenous injection of the highly active interferon inducer NDV into a mouse more than 100,000 units of interferon are formed. According to Ho and Postič, the formation of between 5 and 150 million units of interferon is induced after intravenous injection of the same virus into a rabbit weighing 1 kg [357, 358].

It must also be remembered, however, that the antiviral effect obtained by injection of an interferon inducer is of short duration. Repeated injection of the inducers is therefore necessary in order to obtain a long effect. However, if this is done the antigenicity of virus suspensions (viruses themselves and tissue substrates) on the one hand, and tolerance to repeated injection of interferon inducers of similar type, on the other hand, must be borne in mind.

6.3. Stimulation of Endogenous Interferon by Double-Stranded RNAs and Their Effect on Virus Infection

The search for active interferon inducers led to the conclusion that homologous single-helical RNAs are weak inducers

of interferon. In the case of infection of cells by RNA-viruses
the true active principle is considered to be the replicative form
of RNA, formed at a certain stage of virus reproduction [645, 646].

It has now been established that besides replicative forms
of viral RNAs, double-stranded viral RNAs and double-stranded
RNAs of synthetic origin can also induce interferon formation. In
particular, interferon-inducing activity has been found in the viral
RNA of rheoviruses and in replicative forms of RNA-viruses of
animals and of mutant coliphages MS 2 and MU 9 [644-646, 668,
669, 690]. The ability to induce interferon formation has recently
been demonstrated in replicative forms of chickenpox [619], Mengo
[642], and vaccinia [636] viruses.

The analogous ability of statolon and helenine, containing
replicative forms of viruses infecting molds, has been mentioned
earlier.

The dynamics of interferon formation after intravenous injection of the substances into animals was similar to that found
with viruses. It was shown experimentally that statolon protects
animals infected with MM, encephalomyocarditis, and vesicular
stomatitis viruses [100]. Helenine also has a protective action in
mice infected with different viruses [522]. Aksenov et al. [607]
described the interferon-inducing activity of double-stranded RNA
found in ribosomal RNA, and also of an RNA obtained by incomplete
alkaline hydrolysis of total yeast RNA.

The synthetic coiled double-stranded complexes of self-
polymers have recently attracted particular interest for their
interferon-inducing activity [655-657]. These compounds are
looked upon as the most promising stimulators of endogenous interferon. Artificial synthesis of these polymers yields a chemical-
ly pure product and excludes the presence of impurities. One of the
most important advantages of the artificial copolymers is the absence of antigenic properties, so that repeated and prolonged
stimulation of interferon formation *in vivo* is possible.

Of the synthetic double-stranded self-polymers, a synthetic
complex of polyriboinosinic and polycytidylic (poly I:C) acids has
been found to be the most powerful inducer [645, 646]. This complex in small doses, measured in micrograms, stimulates interferon formation in animals when injected intravenously and makes
them resistant to virus infections [644-647]. Complexes of poly-

adenylic and polyuridylic acids (poly A : U) and also of polyinosinic acid with cytidylic acid dinucleotide (poly I : di C) proved to be less active. A complex of synthetic self-polymers has been tested successfully on rabbits and monkeys [615].

The highest blood level of interferon after intravenous injection of double-stranded RNAs is found 2 h after the injection. Injection of preparations of poly I : C, previously treated with DEAE-dextran, into albino mice enhances interferon production by 4-8 times [623].

In response to treatment with double-stranded RNAs, interferon synthesis in the cells takes place *de novo*. Preliminary treatment of the cells with actinomycin D completely inhibits interferon formation, even in the presence of DEAE-dextran [692]. However, there is also evidence that the poly I : C complex stimulates the liberation of preformed interferon in cell cultures.

Vilcek et al. [693] have recently shown that the antiviral action of the poly I : C complex occurs in two stages. In the first stage interferon is synthesized, while in the second stage the newly formed interferon induces the formation of specific antiviral protein. Addition of actinomycin D after completion of transcription of interferon mRNA by poly I : C completely abolished the protective action of the copolymer, despite the formation of adequate quantities of interferon.

The interferon-inducing activity of the poly I : C copolymer has also been studied clinically in the treatment of 20 patients with cancer [647], who received the preparation by intravenous injection in doses of between 2 and 4000 μg/kg body weight. In 14 of 20 patients interferon was found in the blood after not less than 2 h, and it reached its maximal concentrations between 12 and 48 h after injection of the copolymer. In some patients the inhibitor could be detected in the blood serum for up to 72 h.

Double-stranded RNAs and, in particular, poly I : C copolymer possess a broad spectrum of antiviral activity. In cell cultures they inhibit replication of rhinoviruses, the viruses of vesicular stomatitis, vaccinia, and herpes [655, 656], as well as Sindbis virus, fowl plague virus, and Venezuelan encephalomyelitis virus [618]. Contact between cells and polynucleotide complex for 1 h leads to adsorption of the preparation in sufficient amount to produce a near-maximal antiviral effect. The greatest inhibition of viral reproduction by the polymer is found in the presence of DEAE-dextran. According to Novokhatskii [618], this dose for vesicular stomatitis virus is 4-5.5, for Sindbis virus 5-5.5, for Venezuelan equine encephalomyelitis virus 5.5-6, and for fowl plague virus 3-3.5, log p.f.u./ml. The doses of poly I:C and of DEAE-dextran inducing the most active inhibition of virus replication were 10-40 μg/ml and 60-100 μg/ml, respectively. The dynamics of development of the antiviral effect differed for different viruses. It must be emphasized that interferon production by cell cultures treated with poly I:C as a rule was weaker than the antiviral effect. The presence of DEAE-dextran has a stimulating action on interferon formation.

In mice [657] the preparation was most effective against mouse pneumonia, Columbia SK, and vaccinia viruses, moderately effective against type 1 parainfluenza, and weakly effective against infection with rabies and influenza B viruses. No protective action was found against infection of mice with influenza A and A2 viruses or with yellow fever and Marek viruses.

In observations on volunteers, poly I:C has a marked protective effect against rhinovirus infection and a somewhat less marked effect against infection with influenza A2 (Hong Kong) 68 virus [653]. It must be borne in mind that interferon can be found in human blood serum after deep inhalation of poly I:C [681].

Doses of the copolymer giving marked protection of mice differ for different infections. Complete, 100% resistance to pneumonia virus was produced by administration of 8 μg per mouse, and to Columbia SK virus by injection of 30 μg of the poly I:C complex. Its action was not merely prophylactic, but also therapeutic. A single injection of 100 μg of the polymer intraperitoneally lowered the titer of Venezuelan equine encephalomyelitis virus in the mouse brain by 3.5-4.5 log LD_{50}. Repeated injection of poly I:C led to the almost complete protection of the animals; the titer of the virus in the brain could not be determined for 4-5 days after infection [623].

A protective effect of the poly I:C copolymer was discovered in rabbits with a severe form of herpes of the eyes [685] and in rabbits infected with street rabies virus [643]. Injection of the interferon inducer in a dose of 1 mg/kg, even 3 h after infection

of the rabbits with 25-30 LD_{50} of the virus, gave 100% protection
of the animals. Injection of poly I:C 24 h after infection protected
66% of the rabbits against the disease. It is important to emphasize
that, despite the absence of signs of the disease, the animals nevertheless produced antibodies, as a result of which the rabbits became
resistant to subsequent infection by the same virus.

The poly I:C complex also had some degree of protective
action against infection of chickens and hamsters with oncogenic
viruses (type 12 adenovirus, Rous sarcoma, Moloney, and Friend
viruses [670, 672, 687]). Injection of poly I:C complexes, nontoxic to animals, into mice before or after infection with mouse
sarcoma virus completely or partly protected the mice [673]
against the development of tumors, while in tissue culture the number of foci of transformation was reduced.

The mechanism of the antitumor action of the double-stranded
RNAs is unknown. The view is held that the antitumor effect of interferon is not connected with its antiviral activity, for it is also exhibited against nonviral tumors. Interferon possibly potentiates the
immunological responses of the body to the tumor cells. The possibility cannot be ruled out that activity of synthetic double-stranded
RNAs is connected with their direct cytotoxic action on the tumor
cells. This hypothesis is supported by the embryotoxicity of the
poly I:C complex, which may even cause complete adsorption of
rabbit embryos, in the final stages of pregnancy. In their degree
of differentiation and rate of growth, tumor cells correspond to
embryonic cells.

Turning to the possible clinical use of artificial stimulators
of interferon, an extremely important aspect is the study of its
safety, i.e., the absence of side effects. The safety of the poly
I:C complex has been tested in cell cultures and *in vivo* in animals
and man. In particular, Baugh et al. [631] showed that poly I:C,
when tested in diploid cultures of human fibroblasts, did not change
the rate of growth of the cells nor did it prevent their aging. Moreover, cells subcultured in the presence of this copolymer did not
induce tumor formation when introduced into the retrobuccal pouch
of hamsters treated with cortisone.

The toxicity of the copolymer has been tested in mice, rats,
dogs, and monkeys when injected by different routes [655, 656].
The complex was most toxic for dogs, and when injected intra-

venously into these animals changes were found in the small blood vessels, the liver, and the hematopoietic organs. These changes were minimal or absent on subcutaneous and, in particular, on intranasal injection. The toxic effect was less marked in mice, rats, and monkeys. The authors cited also emphasized that in experiments on mice injections of poly I:C accelerate the appearance of autoimmune diseases of the systemic lupus erythematosus type in man. Because of the severe changes detected in dogs, intravenous injection of poly I:C in man was permitted until recently by American investigators only in patients with inoperable forms of cancer [655]. For the prevention of respiratory virus infections in man, it is considered that only intranasal administration is acceptable. It has already been mentioned that in a recent study Field et al. [647] tested the poly I:C complex on 20 patients with cancer, in whom the only clinical response to the preparation was a rise of temperature. Laboratory tests revealed no appreciable changes in liver, kidney, and bone marrow functions. The coagulability of the blood likewise was unchanged.

The presence of toxic properties of the poly I:C copolymer stimulated the search for methods of overcoming them. In particular, it was recently suggested that one way of achieving this result was to reduce its molecular weight by sonication [657]. However, Morahan et al. [678a] found that, irrespective of their molecular weight, poly I:C complexes inhibit metabolism of the drugs hexobarbital and amidopyrine in mice. These workers conclude that the inhibition of the ability of the body cells to detoxicate foreign chemical substances by poly I:C is a serious side effect of this substance which is independent of the molecular weight of the complex.

It has also been shown recently that poly I:C aggravates the course of experimental infection in mice caused by the fungi Candida albicans, C. immitis, and C. neoformans when injected intravenously [694a]. The number of colonies in the kidney tissue of mice treated with poly I:C on the 3rd-5th day after infection with C. albicans was 40-300 times greater than in the controls.

6.4. Stimulation of Endogenous Interferon by Other Nonviral Inducers and Its Effect on Experimental Virus Infection

The ability to induce the formation of endogenous interferon is a property possessed by bacteria, bacterial endotoxins [347,

548], rickettsias [391, 590], chlamydozoans [458], mycoplasmas [548], and the protozoan Toxoplasma gondii [293, 520]. Toxoplasmas stimulated interferon formation when injected intraperitoneally into mice. The inhibitor was found in the blood serum and peritoneal fluid of these animals. The interferon-inducing activity of the chlamydozoans was detected as a result of intravenous injection into mice.

Interferon formation in mice has also been induced by means of the antibiotic cycloheximide [606]. However, the dose of antibiotic required to induce interferon led to irreversible suppression of protein synthesis and to death of the animals.

Interferon-inducing activity has thus now been discovered in a number of different nonviral agents. Borecky and Lackovic [226] mention 22 nonviral agents capable of inducing the formation of interferon-like substances. Of all these agents, the interferon-inducing properties of bacteria and products of microbial origin have received the most study. The evidence to be presented later in this book will therefore have been obtained mainly by the study of these agents. They exhibit maximal activity in experiments on animals.

The ability of bacteria and their products to induce interferon formation when injected intravenously was demonstrated by Youngner and Stinebring [548] and by Ho [347] in experiments on chickens and mice as the result of intravenous injection of Brucella abortus, Serratia marcescens, and Salmonella typhimurium [347, 548, 603], and also after injection of Bordetella pertussis into mice [225]. Interferon formation takes place in rabbits _in vivo_ under the influence of Escherichia coli and its endotoxins, while intravenous injection of the endotoxins of S. marcescens and S. typhimurium is accompanied by the early appearance of an inhibitor, whose titer reaches a maximum after 2 h.

Interferon induction in rabbits takes place under the influence of the endotoxin of typhoid bacteria [474, 475]. Interferon-inducing activity of the polysaccharides prodigiosan and acetoxan, which were isolated in 1960 by Ermol'eva and Vaisberg [181], has also been demonstrated. It was shown, in particular, that prodigiosan inhibits interferon formation in mice, chick embryos, and cultures of chick fibroblasts.

It has been shown that mannan, a polysaccharide isolated from Candida albicans, can induce interferon formation when injected intravenously into mice [228].

The interferon-inducing activity of synthetic polyanions which have the property of stimulating activity of cells of the RES in the liver, spleen, and lymph glands and which exhibit antiviral properties has recently received intensive study [84, 454, 455, 504]. It has been shown that polyanions with a molecular weight of not less than 17,000 can induce interferon formation. The ability of these polyanions to induce interferon has been demonstrated not only in animals (mice and rabbits), but also in man.

These results indicate that many substances possess the property of inducing interferon. Bacteria and products of microbial origin constitute the largest group of these substances. The most important component responsible for the interferon-inducing activity of these agents is evidently polysaccharide in nature. Interferons induced by viruses have been shown to be not completely identical with those induced by products of microbial origin and by bacteria. These differences are found by the study of the dynamics of interferon formation induced by them and they are also reflected in the properties of the interferons themselves. As was shown above, virus inducers stimulate maximal quantities of interferon between 4 and 12 h after intravenous injection. Bacterial endotoxins and certain bacteria, on the other hand, induce rapid formation of interferon, which reaches a maximum 2 h after injection. The rate of formation of interferon induced by viruses and by endotoxins is independent of the species of the animal and is determined principally by the properties of the inducing agent.

Differences are also found between interferons induced by viruses and bacterial endotoxins. Interferon induced by bacterial endotoxins possesses a higher molecular weight (89,000-90,000) [329], it is sensitive to pH 2.0, and is thermolabile – it is completely inactivated by heating to 65°C for 30 min [227, 346-348]. Interferon synthesized *in vivo* after injection of synthetic polyanions intraperitonially into mice possesses similar properties. Its titer in the serum reaches a maximum 18 h after injection of the inducer [454].

Statolon possesses most of the properties characteristic of virus interferon inducers: it can induce interferon both in tissue

culture and *in vivo* ; the dynamics of formation of the interferon
induced by it is similar to that of formation of virus interferon
[398-402]. It is interesting to note that the molecular weight of
interferon from tissue cultures inoculated with statolon (about
30,000) is identical with the molecular weight of virus interferon
[452, 453].

The molecular weight of interferon formed by human leukocytes under the influence of phytohemagglutinin is 18,000.

Interferon induced by B. abortus [329] and by trachoma-
inclusion conjunctivitis (TRIC) virus has a molecular weight of
about 50,000 [458].

Interferon induced by nonviral agents has so far received
little study. There is no clear idea regarding the mechanism or
site of its formation. On the basis of the ability of bacterial endotoxins to stimulate interferon formation *in vitro* only in leukocytes
and of the sharp decrease in interferon production after splenectomy, it has been postulated that the cells of the RES are the main
and, perhaps, the only producers of this interferon [225, 227, 358].
This hypothesis is confirmed by the discovery of an inhibitor after
intravenous injection of bacteria and their endotoxins not only
into the blood, but also in large numbers into the spleen [268, 358].

In view of the different times of appearance of virus and
nonvirus (endotoxin) interferons, Stinebring and Youngner [548]
postulated that the former, which reaches a maximum level in the
blood after 6-12 h, is synthesized *de novo*, while the latter, which
reaches its maximum 2 h after injection, is already present in the
organism and is liberated from the cells by the endotoxin. This
hypothesis was tested by administering puromycin and cycloheximide
substances which inhibit protein synthesis *in vivo*. As a result,
interferon formation induced by the viruses was inhibited, but there
was no appreciable effect on the rate of formation or the quantity
of interferon produced in response to injection of bacterial endotoxins [393, 606]. Actinomycin D likewise had no effect on interferon formation induced by endotoxins [350].

The facts described above can be summed up in the statement that inducers of different nature cause the formation of interferons which differ from each other in certain essential features
but which share the most important biological property, namely,
antiviral activity.

The antiviral activity of bacterial lipopolysaccharides was discovered before they were known to possess interferon-inducing properties. However, the mechanism of their action remained unknown. It was only after the work of Ho, Youngner, and Stinebring that the protective action of bacterial endotoxins and lipopolysaccharides could be explained by stimulation of endogenous interferon. It must be mentioned here that some of the investigations cited above were carried out before 1964, at a time when the antiviral activity of endotoxins had been demonstrated but their interferon-inducing properties were not mentioned.

In the experiments of Hook and Wagner [360], for instance, an endotoxin isolated from Salmonella abortus equi and injected in a dose of 1 μg intravenously or intracerebrally into mice protected some of the animals against lethal infection by the virus of equine encephalomyelitis or of encephalomyocarditis. Gledhill observed that a filtrate from S. typhimurium, when injected intraperitoneally, greatly increased the period of survival of mice infected with ectromelia virus [316]. Repeated intranasal administration of yeast or plant nucleic acids to mice considerably reduced the mortality among animals infected 24 h previously with influenza or encephalomyocarditis virus [555].

Results providing evidence of the protective action of microbial polysaccharides and lipopolysaccharides are of special interest. Some of these compounds have a protective action when administered in concentrations which have no toxic action on the body.

The preventive effect of the polysaccharide prodigiosan was described by Furer and co-workers [181]. In the course of 4-7 days, about 20% of mice in the group treated with prodigiosan died compared with 100% mortality in the control series.

Oh and Gill [475] observed that the rabbit's cornea is resistant to the toxic action of NDV (when injected into the anterior chamber of the eye) if the rabbit received a preliminary intravenous injection of 10 or 100 μg typhoid endotoxin. Pollikoff [492] studied the effect of intraocular injection of an endotoxin isolated from S. marcescens on herpetic keratitis in rabbits. It was found that a prophylactic injection of 20 μg of the endotoxin 18 or 72 h before infection, or a similar injection 72 h after infection significantly inhibited reproduction of the virus and reduced the severity of the disease.

Reports of the antiviral activity of copolymers of vinyl-pyrrolidone [84, 454, 455, 504] are of great interest. Zeitlenok and co-workers [84] studied the activity of 12 copolymers with crotonic acid, crotonic aldehyde, and maleic acid anhydride. Most of the tested copolymers had a protective effect and reduced the concentration of virus in the blood and brain of animals infected with tick-borne encephalitis virus. Regelson [504] showed that a pyran copolymer induces adequate quantities of interferon and has a preventive and therapeutic action against infection with leukemia virus.

It must, however, be pointed out that pyran is evidently of theoretical interest only, because of the large doses required to induce interferon and because of the thrombocytopenia which it produces as a side effect [678].

Several papers have thus now been published in which the antiviral activity of stimulators of endogenous interferon has been demonstrated. When only one injection was given, bacterial endo-toxins and the other substances had mainly a prophylactic effect. Repeated injections of endotoxin in some cases proved harmful because of their toxic action. Only polyanions (statolon, etc.) had an interferon-inducing action when given in nontoxic doses.

The pyrogen of Soviet manufacture most widely used in clinical practice is pyrogenal, which has proved effective in several diseases [36]. However, the action of pyrogenal in virus infections has not been studied. Since it is a bacterial lipopolysaccharide, we investigated the effect of pyrogenal on virus infections and on interferon induction.

Pyrogenal was obtained from the N. F. Gamaleya Institute of Epidemiology and Microbiology, Academy of Medical Sciences of the USSR, as a sterile solution in ampules. The concentration of pyrogenal was 10-100 μg/ml. Noninbred mice weighing 25-40 g were used in the tests. Pyrogenal was injected into the caudal vein of the animals or intramuscularly into the thigh in a volume of 0.1-0.2 ml. Groups of at least four mice were exsanguinated after various time intervals and their serum was obtained and tested for the presence of inhibitor

To begin with the interferon-inducing action of pyrogenal was tested on mice, chick embryos, and tissue cultures.

In these experiments pyrogenal was injected intravenously
or intramuscularly into the mice in a dose of 1 μg per animal
and the animals were exsanguinated after 1, 2, 4, 6, 12, 18, and
24 h. The dynamics of the serum inhibitor concentration depended
on the method of injection of the pyrogenal (Fig. 10). A characteristic feature of intravenous injection was the rapid formation
of large quantities of interferon, reaching a maximum after 2 h.
When the intramuscular route was used the titer of inhibitor did
not reach its maximum until 12 h. In both cases the interferon
concentration in the serum 18 h after injection was minimal (Fig.
10).

In additional tests the minimal dose of pyrogenal stimulating
interferon formation in mice was determined. This was found to
be 0.001 μg by intravenous injection.

The ability of pyrogenal to induce interferon formation was
also studied in chick embryos, tissue cultures, and suspensions
of human leukocytes. For this purpose pyrogenal was injected
into the allantoic cavity of 12-day chick embryos in doses of 0.01,
0.1, 1, and 10 μg per embryo. Each dose was tested on five embryos.
The allantoic fluid was collected after 48 h, pooled, and titrated

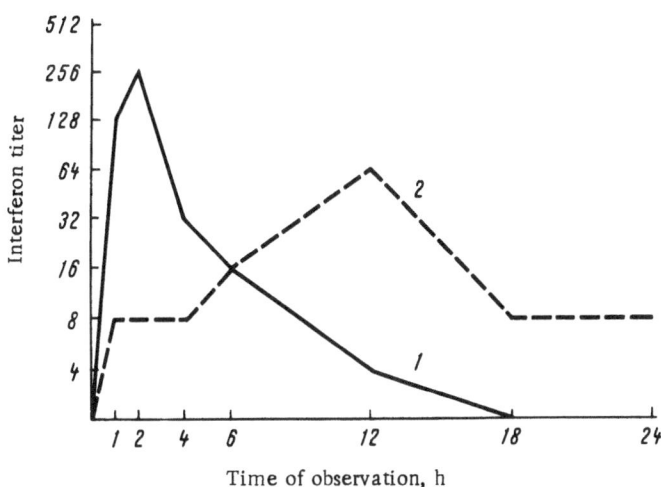

Fig. 10. Dynamics of interferon formation after injection
of 1 μg pyrogenal: 1) intravenously; 2) intramuscularly.

on chick fibroblasts with Chikungunya virus. No interferon could be detected in any of the experiments.

Attempts to induce interferon formation by pyrogenal in monolayer cultures of chick fibroblasts and transplanted mouse L-929 cells also proved unsuccessful. Doses from 0.01 to 50 μg were tested in 100-ml Pavitskaya flasks with monolayer cultures. No inhibitor was found in any of the test samples over a period of 5 days. Combined administration to monolayer cultures likewise did not stimulate the interferon-inducing action of NDV.

Pyrogenal thus did not induce interferon formation in primary cultures of chick embryonic cells and transplanted line L-929 growing *in vitro*. Nevertheless, it did exhibit this property in human leukocytes. A suspension of human leukocytes containing 1 million cells/ml was used. Pyrogenal was added at the rate of 1 μg to 1 ml of suspension. The culture fluid collected after 24 h showed inhibitory activity against VSV in a titer of 1 : 16. In these experiments a strain of diploid cells of myodermal tissue after 25 subcultures was used for titration.

The properties of the inhibitor found in the serum of mice after intravenous injection of pyrogenal were studied next. Species-specificity was determined in experiments on mouse and chick cells and virus specificity in experiments with VSV and smallpox virus. The results of the study of these and other properties are shown

TABLE 77. Properties of Interferon Induced
by Pyrogenal

Method of testing	Characteristic properties
Titration in homologous and heterologous cells	Active only in homologous cells
Inhibitory activity against VSV and smallpox virus	Inhibits both viruses
Sedimentation at 100,000 g for 2 h	Not sedimented
Resistance to 0.1% trypsin at 37°C for 1 h	Reduces antiviral activity
Resistance to heating at 56°C for 1 h	Antiviral activity lost completely
Resistance to acid at pH 2.0 for 18-20 h	Activity reduced

in Table 77. The inhibitor induced by pyrogenal is indistinguishable
from interferons induced by bacterial endotoxins from E. coli.
Meanwhile the inhibitor formed under the influence of pyrogenal
differed in some of its properties from the interferon induced by
viruses. The former is more thermolabile and its activity is reduced if kept at pH 2.0 for 18-20 h. The molecular weights of interferons induced by viruses and by lipopolysaccharide agents [329]
and the dynamics of their formation also are different.

Having regard to these differences in properties and also,
evidently, in the mechanism of formation, we suggest that interferons
induced by viral agents and formed *in vivo* may be suitably named
α-interferons, while those induced by bacteria and bacterial polysaccharides, possibly preexisting in the body, may be called β-inter-
ferons. This may facilitate the classification of the interferons and
also be of practical value.

In the next experiments a more detailed investigation was
made of the interferon-inducing action of pyrogenal.

Pyrogenal, of course, has a pyrogenic action and raises the
body temperature of animals. In mice, however, it is less active
in this respect. According to Martynov [112], 0.1 μg pyrogenal
raises the body temperature of mice by only 1.1°C 1 h after intravenous injection, and the normal body temperature is restored
after 3-4 h. An increase in the dose of pyrogenal does not potentiate
its pyrogenic action. Consequently, the time of elevation of the
temperature and of the maximum of interferon production after
intravenous injection of pyrogenal coincides. This coincidence
is of definite interest in connection with the observed increase
in interferon production under the influence of a raised temperature.

A study of the correlation between the dynamics of the serum
interferon titer and the circulating leukocyte count proved negative.
The maximal leukocytosis was not accompanied by any increase
in interferon production (Table 78). Differences in the interferon-
inducing activity of different batches of pyrogenal were observed
in experiments on mice. To rule out the possibility of accidental
factors possibly influencing the manifestation of the interferon-
inducing activity of pyrogenal, 12 batches of pyrogenal were tested
simultaneously on the same group of mice.

TABLE 78. Correlation between Interferon Concentration
and Leukocyte Count in the Blood of Mice after Injection
of 1 μg Pyrogenal

Time of testing blood after injection of pyrogenal, h	Method of injection of pyrogenal			
	intravenously		intramuscularly	
	leukocyte count	interferon titer	leukocyte count	interferon titer
Control	9,500	<4	9,500	<4
1	8,300	64	9,000	4
3	3,000	256	6,900	8
12	24,000	4	14,600	64
18	27,500	44	20,900	8
24	20,800	4	11,800	8

Each batch of pyrogenal was tested on a group of six mice
which received 1 μg of the pyrogenal intravenously. The animals
were exsanguinated after 2 h. The sera of the animals receiving
the same batch of pyrogenal were pooled and titrated on L cells
with VSV.

Equal doses of different batches of pyrogenal were found
to differ in their interferon-inducing activity. The titer of interferon induced by different batches of pyrogenal varied from 1:16
to 1:128. In other words, eightfold differences in the interferon-
inducing activity of the pyrogenal batches were obtained.

No data which could possibly explain these differences are
yet available. The possibility cannot be ruled out that substances
determining the interferon-inducing activity, but not the pyrogenic
activity, of the pyrogenal preparations occur in the Salmonella
typhosa cell.

To continue the study of correlation between the pyrogenic
and interferon-inducing action of bacterial polysaccharides, pyrogen:
was compared with prodigiosan. The reason for this comparison
was that the substances are obtained from different bacteria and
are isolated by different methods. As was mentioned earlier,
prodigiosan was obtained by Ermol'eva and Vaisberg from cells
of Bacterium prodigiosum. Furer and co-workers [118] found
that this polysaccharide has interferon-inducing activity in experiments on animals, chick embryos, and tissue cultures. The
writer studied its ability to induce interferon formation by intravenous injection into mice weighing 15-18 g. The dynamics of

interferon formation induced by prodigiosan was found to be the same as that in response to injection of pyrogenal. However, the interferon-inducing activity of prodigiosan was less than that of pyrogenal for an equal pyrogenic effect. Whereas the serum interferon concentration in mice after injection of 1 μg pyrogenal was 256 units, after injection of between 1 and 100 μg prodigiosan not more than 16 units of activity could be found.

The interferon-inducing doses of pyrogenal and prodigiosan were thus different. The reasons are evidently differences in the methods of obtaining these substances and differences in their chemical composition.

Subsequent experiments were carried out to determine the interferon-inducing action of pyrogenal in rabbits weighing 3 kg. Pyrogenal was injected intravenously in doses of 1, 10, 25, and 100 μg. Each dose was tested on two rabbits. Blood was taken for interferon titration after 1, 2, 6, 12, and 24 h. The serum was titrated in cultures of rabbit fibroblasts after the 7th subculture *in vitro*. The test virus was VSV.

The interferon concentration reached its maximum 2 h after injection of the pyrogenal. The optimal interferon-inducing dose for rabbits was 10 μg. A similar result was obtained after injection of 25 μg. A decrease in the dose to 1 μg or its increase to 100 μg did not increase the interferon production.

In no case was the serum interferon titer higher than 1:32. These differences found during the study of the intensity of interferon-inducing action could be explained by differences in the sensitivity to interferon of the mouse and rabbit cells used to titrate the interferons. However, this explanation must evidently be ruled out because similar results were obtained during titration of serum interferons induced by viruses on the same cells.

The interferon-inducing action of the endotoxin (lysate) of Shigella flexneri type I also was studied experimentally by us. The purpose of this investigation was to examine the possible effect of bacterial agents and their disintegration products on the activity of viruses in the intestine. The endotoxin was prepared by I. M. Ambarnikov,* who studied the effect of bacterial endotoxins on viruses *in vitro*.

---

*A graduate student working in our laboratory.

The method of preparing the lysate of S. flexneri was as follows. The bacteria were grown on plain agar. A 48-h culture of bacteria was washed off the agar with sterile physiological saline and rinsed three times with the same solution to remove traces of agar. The bacteria were sedimented by centrifugation at 1500 rpm for 1 h. The total number of bacterial cells in the residue was counted and twice distilled water added to give a suspension containing 7 billion bacterial cells in 1 ml. The bacterial suspension was frozen to -20°C and thawed to 37°C in a water bath 10 times. The disintegrated bacteria and debris were sedimented by centrifugation at 5000 rpm for 1 h. The supernatant, containing products of thermolysis of the bacteria, was used in the experiments as the endotoxin of the dysentery bacteria. The ability of the resulting preparation to induce interferon formation was tested *in vivo* and *in vitro*.

The interferon-inducing ability *in vitro* was determined in experiments on cultures of chick fibroblasts. The lysate was added to 100-ml Pavitskaya flasks in a volume of 1 ml and samples were taken daily for 3 days for determination of their interferon content. None of the samples of the bacterial lysate tested revealed any inhibitory properties.

To study interferon-inducing activity *in vivo*, 1 ml of the bacterial lysate was injected into a series of mice and the animals were exsanguinated five at a time after 1, 2, 4, 6, 8, and 18 h. The results of titration of samples of serum obtained from these mice are given in Table 79, which shows that the dynamics of interferon formation induced by lysate of S. flexneri cells is indistinguishable from that following injection of pyrogenal.

A comparative study of inhibitors induced by pyrogenal and by the bacterial lysate also was undertaken. Their properties proved to be identical. They possessed species specificity, they were virus-nonspecific, they were destroyed by heating to 56°C for 1 h, and their activity was reduced slightly if kept at pH 2.4 for 24 h.

In addition to preparations obtained from bacteria by a special method (pyrogenal), products of bacterial breakdown obtained by thermolysis thus also possess an interferon-inducing action. Presumably the presence of these substances in the intestine has some effect on the viability of viruses in the human intestinal tract.

TABLE 79. Dynamics of Interferon Formation after
Intravenous Injection of Lysate of S. flexneri Cells
into Mice

Time of taking samples, h	Interferon titer	Time of taking samples, h	Interferon titer
1	64	6	<4
2	128	8	<4
4	16	18	<4

The object of the next experiments was to determine the effect of certain factors on interferon production induced by pyrogenal.
There is comparatively little information in the literature on this
question.

In experiments on rabbits, Postic and co-workers [500] were
unable to detect any increase or decrease in interferon production
at 37°C or at 4°C. They concluded that in rabbits the optimum
temperature for interferon formation induced by E. coli endotoxin
is lower than that for the formation of virus-induced interferon.
The same authors studied the effect of cortisole and adrenalectomy on interferon production induced by endotoxin. Cortisole
had an inhibitory action. Conversely, adrenalectomy increased
interferon production induced by endotoxin.

We studied the effect of the external environmental temperature of animals and of internal irradiation on interferon formation in experiments on mice.

No previous attempts had been made to study the effect of
these factors on interferon formation induced by bacterial lipopolysaccharides in mice. No reports of any investigations into
the induction of interferon by lipopolysaccharides in animals
receiving external or internal irradiation could be found. To
determine the effect of the environmental temperature, mice
weighing 25-30 g were divided into 3 groups with 10 in each group
and kept at 4, 22, and 37°C. After the mice had been kept for
18-20 h at this temperature 1 μg pyrogenal was injected intravenously and the mice were kept for a further 2 h at the same temperature. Blood taken from each group of animals was then pooled
and the serum obtained from it was titrated on L cells with

TABLE 80. Effect of External Environmental Temperature of Animals on Interferon Formation Induced by Pyrogenal

Environmental temperature	Interferon titer
4°	64
22°	256
37°	128

Table 81. Effect of Internal Irradiation on Interferon Formation Induced by Pyrogenal

Group of animals	Interferon titer
Unirradiated	256
Irradiated	16-32

vesicular stomatitis virus. The results of these experiments are given in Table 80.

These results show that room temperature is optimal for interferon production induced by pyrogenal. Elevation of the temperature to 37°C led to a small decrease in interferon production. However, lowering the environmental temperature of the animals to 4°C led to a fourfold decrease in interferon production.

Cooling the body thus adversely affects interferon production induced by pyrogenal.

Since the experiments with internal irradiation were carried out on mice weighing 16-18 g, each animal received P^{32} in a dose of 34 μCi. The irradiated and control mice each received an intravenous injection of 3 μg pyrogenal 2 weeks after the injection of P^{32}. The animals were exsanguinated after 2 h and the serum interferon titer determined (Table 81).

These results show that irradiation with P^{32} sharply inhibited interferon production by the mice. The interferon concentration in the serum of the irradiated animals was 8-16 times lower than in the serum of the unirradiated controls.

Factors reducing the resistance of the organism, notably cooling and internal irradiation, thus reduced the ability of mice to produce interferon in response to induction by the bacterial lipopolysaccharide pyrogenal.

6.5. Tolerance or Hyporeactivity in Interferon Production

Workers studying the formation of interferon have encountered a phenomenon which has been called tolerance or hyporeactivity

[354]. These terms have been used to describe a temporary absence of response of tissues to repeated injection of an interferon-inducing agent.

The phenomena of hyporeactivity were first discovered in experiments on tissue cultures [241, 428, 551], and later in experiments on animals. Tolerance has been found to develop, in particular, in rabbits during the period of 12 h after injection of E. coli endotoxin or of Sindbis virus. The state of tolerance lasted 6 days. The cells of the animal then reacquired the ability to respond as before by producing interferon [354]. Tolerance to the repeated injection of endotoxin has been described in mice [604] and to repeated infection with Sindbis virus in rats [513]. Besides tolerance to a homologous interferon inducer, tolerance to a heterologous inducer of interferon formation has also been described.

Treatment of animals with endotoxin, followed by infection with virus 48 h later (or in the reverse order: virus first and endotoxin later) led to a marked decrease in interferon production [604, 605].

Partial heterologous tolerance has been observed in mice by the action of Newcastle disease virus after preliminary injection of B. pertussis [225]. Similar relationships have been observed after the consecutive administration of statolon and NDV, and vice versa [481].

However, no heterologous tolerance has been discovered between statolon and endotoxin in whatever order they were administered [605].

Tolerance in animals can be explained on the basis of the appearance of a factor in the serum which inactivated the interferon-inducing activity of the endotoxin. A study of the properties of this factor has shown that it is inactivated by heating to 56°C for 1 h and that it is not an antibody [356].

Repeated injection of homologous or heterologous interferon inducers thus revealed the complete or partial tolerance of the cells to the second injection. It should be noted, however, that the results so far obtained are contradictory.

Nevertheless, a clear understanding of the phenomenon of tolerance would not only be of theoretical importance but would also facilitate the choice of preparations for possible use as inter-

TABLE 82. Tolerance to Repeated Injection of Pyrogenal

Method of first injection	Interferon titer	Method of subsequent injections	Interferon titers from repeated injections after						
			1 day	2 days	4 days	5 days	6 days	7 days	8 days
Intravenously	256	Intravenously	<4	<4	<4	<4	32	256	256
Intramuscularly	64	Intravenously	<4	<4	<4	<4	16	256	256
Intravenously	256	Intramuscularly	<4	<4	<4	<4	16	64	64

TABLE 83. Tolerance to Repeated Injection of Interferon-Inducing Virus

Interval between injections, days	Interferon titer after repeated injection of NDV
control	4096
1	<4
2	<4
3	<4
4	16
5	128
6	1024
7	4036

TABLE 84. Serum Interferon Concentration after Repeated Injection of Interferon Inducers

Method of injection	Dose of first injection of pyrogenal, g	Interval between injections, h	Method of injection and dose of second interferon inducer	Interferon titer
Intravenously	1.0	Control	Not injected	512
Intravenously	1.0	24, 48, 72 96, 120 144, 168	NDV, 10^8	8,192 16,384
Intramuscularly	-	Control	NDV, 10^8	16,384

feron inducers in practice. It was therefore decided to study the effect of tolerance to pyrogenal (Table 82), to Newcastle disease virus (Table 83), and to prodigiosan. Experiments were carried out on mice weighing 35-40 g into which the interferon inducers were injected intravenously and intramuscularly. The animals were exsanguinated 4 h after injection of pyrogenal.

In the next experiments the appearance of tolerance was studied during consecutive injection of virus and nonvirus inducers of interferon. As the results in Table 84 show, injection of the virus inducer, even if given 24 h after the pyrogenal, led to the formation of interferon in high titers in the blood of the mice.

These results indicate that tolerance to pyrogenal does not extend to the subsequent injection of a virus inducer (NDV).

However, if the virus and pyrogenal were given in the opposite order complete tolerance was observed when the pyrogenal was given 24 h after the virus. The state of tolerance disappeared by the 7th day after primary induction (Table 85).

An attempt also was made to discover the mechanism of tolerance by investigating the serum of tolerant animals. For this purpose mice were injected with pyrogenal and blood taken from them 2 h later. The serum was mixed with an equal volume of interferon inducer and injected in a volume of 1 ml intravenously into animals in which the interferon was titrated after 2 h.

TABLE 85. Serum Interferon Concentration after Consecutive Intravenous Injection of Virus and Pyrogenal

Interferon inducer injected	Interval between injections, h	Method of injection and dose of pyrogenal, μg	Interferon titer
NDV	Control	–	8192
Pyrogenal	Control	–	256
NDV	24-120	Intravenously, 1.0	<4

TABLE 86. Effect of Serum of
Tolerant Animals on Interferon-Inducing Activity
of Pyrogenal

Material injected	Interferon titer
Pyrogenal + serum of tolerant mice	4
Pyrogenal + serum of normal mice	64

Animals injected with a mixture of normal serum and the interferon inducer were used as the control. The results are given in Table 86.

They show that in the period of tolerance the serum contains a factor which inhibits the interferon-inducing activity of pyrogenal. This is in agreement with the findings of Ho and co-workers [356], who obtained similar results with endotoxin.

The effect of internal irradiation on the state of tolerance during successive administration of different inducers of interferon also was studied. In these experiments the interferon inducer was first injected into the mice, and this was followed by internal irradiation by injection of P^{32} in a dose of 2 μCi/g body weight.

Animals receiving the interferon inducer or P^{32} alone were used as the controls. The interferon inducer was injected into all the animals 2 weeks after receiving the radioisotope, and 2 h later serum was obtained from the animals and its interferon concentration estimated (Table 87).

It will be clear from Table 87 that internal irradiation inhibits interferon production induced by pyrogenal. The irradiated animals produced from 8 to 32 times less interferon than the controls. Irradiation of the animals had no significant effect on the duration of tolerance. It will be noted that preliminary administration of pyrogenal before irradiation reduced the inhibitory effect of irradiation on interferon production induced by the subsequent injection of the polysaccharide. The preliminary injection

TABLE 87. Intensity of Tolerance in
Mice Subjected to Internal Irradiation

Group of mice	Interferon titer
Pyrogenal repeated after 14 days	256
Pyrogenal + irradiation + pyrogenal	32
Irradiation + pyrogenal	8
+ pyrogenal	256

of the bacterial lipopolysaccharide evidently had a protective effect on the cells producing interferon which are vulnerable to irradiation.

It is interesting to compare these results with those obtained by Klemparskaya [100], who demonstrated the protective action of bacterial lipopolysaccharides on the course of radiation sickness.

The results of the present investigation are at the same time further evidence in support of the humoral nature of tolerance. If tolerance had been due to a temporary loss of the ability of the cells to synthesize particular proteins, interferon production in animals which had received a preliminary injection of the inducer would have been suppressed to a greater degree than in the mice receiving irradiation only. Presumably the humoral factor of tolerance disappears gradually from the body with the corresponding restoration of its ability to produce interferon.

6.6. Conclusion

Our experiments to study the ability of viruses to induce interferon formation when injected intravenously confirmed results of other workers relating to the efficacy of this method of induction. They also showed that interferon formation is not connected with reproduction of the virus. A gradual decrease in the concentration of virus was observed in the serum of the animals. The decrease in concentration of virus during the first hour after infection is probably due to its adsorption by the animal's cells [224]. Interferon production after maximal adsorption of virus by the cells took place most intensively over a period of 4-8 h. Its concentration in the blood then fell in conjunction with a general decrease

in the concentration of virus in the body. Consequently, interferon
production reaches a maximum at a time corresponding to the
highest concentration of virus in the resistant animal also. No
differences were found in the dynamics of interferon formation
after intravenous injection of viruses differing in their pathogenicity
for mice. The distribution of interferon among the organs depended
on the tropism of the viruses. These results indicate that the same
cells participate in interferon production after intravenous injection of viruses of whatever tropism. In the viremic phase of the
infection cells of the organs to which the inducing virus exhibits
tropism probably do not play the decisive role in the production
of serum interferon. Presumably interferon produced by the RES
and adsorbed by the tissues is found in the organs. Evidence that
interferon eliminated quickly and intensively with the urine is not
produced by the kidney cells is given by its lower concentration
in the kidney tissues than in the urine itself.

When injected intravenously into rabbits NDV proved to be
a highly active inducer of interferon. The fact that interferon was
found in the serum for a longer time may perhaps be explained
by differences in the sensitivity of the cells on which the interferon in the sera was titrated.

As was mentioned above, conflicting results were obtained
regarding the effect of splenectomy on virus-induced interferon
production. Our findings can evidently explain some of these contradictions. In particular, the intensity of interferon production
in splenectomized mice was found to depend both on the time
elapsing after the operation and on the properties of the inducing
virus. At the same time, the decrease in interferon production
after splenectomy is evidence of the important role of the lymphoid
tissue in interferon formation. This is confirmed by the results
of the present experiments: injection of cytotoxic antilymph-gland
serum sharply reduced interferon production.

Interesting results were obtained in the study of pyrogenal.
According to Veselkin [37] pyrogenal induces a febrile reaction,
stimulates energy metabolism, and increases protein synthesis
and phagocytic activity. To these and, possibly, other changes
taking place in the body under the influence of pyrogenal must be
added yet another property of the substance which we have described,
that is, its action in inducing interferon production. The fact that

bacterial endotoxins and polysaccharides such as pyrogenal are inducers of interferon explains the hitherto unknown mechanism whereby these substances stimulate nonspecific resistance to virus infections as demonstrated in a number of investigations [59, 316, 331, 360]. It is interesting to note that in a series of investigations into this problem bacterial endotoxins and polysaccharides gave only a prophylactic and comparatively brief effect in experiments with ectromelia, influenza, and mouse pneumonia viruses. However, it may be that the treatment by means of irritants, which many physicians used with benefit before the antibiotic era, of pneumonia and certain other diseases is also based on a similar mechanism of action.

Our experiments showed for the first time that bacterial lipopolysaccharides exhibit interferon-inducing activity when administered not only intravenously but also intramuscularly. The only differences between the two methods are in the dynamics and intensity of interferon formation. Probably the later occurrence of the maximum of the interferon concentration in the blood is due to its gradual liberation into the blood stream.

No correlation could be found between the dynamics of the serum interferon concentration and the leukocyte count in the circulating blood. This finding is of particular importance, first, because leukocytes are active producers of interferon *in vitro*, as shown by experiments with interferon-inducing viruses, and second, because, as Budnitskaya [36] found, 90-95% of the pyrogenal administered is fixed to the surface of the blood leukocytes. The intensity of interferon production is evidently independent of the leukocyte count and is determined by other factors.

Experiments to compare pyrogenal and prodigiosan showed that there is no parallel between their pyrogenic and interferon-inducing activity. Of course bacterial lipopolysaccharides of different origin and obtained by different methods differ in their ability to induce interferon synthesis.

Before our investigations, interferon-inducing activity had been found in lipopolysaccharides obtained from E. coli, B. prodigiosum, S. typhosa, and other microorganisms. We demonstrated for the first time that S. flexneri also possesses this property and that the dynamics of interferon formation induced by pyrogenal and by a lysate of S. flexneri cells is similar. The possibility cannot be ruled out that the breakdown products of bacteria in the intestinal tract influence the vital activity of viruses. In particular, the low sensitivity of the enteroviruses to interferon enables them to overcome this protective barrier and to reproduce in the intestinal wall.

The results of a study of the effect of the external environmenta temperature of mice on interferon formation induced by pyrogenal confirm the results obtained on rabbits by Postic and co-workers [500] to the effect that a temperature of 37°C does not lead to an increase in interferon production. At the same time we showed that, by contrast with rabbits, keeping mice at 4°C leads to a marked decrease in interferon production. It was shown for the first time that internal irradiation of animals leads to marked inhibition of interferon synthesis induced by lipopolysaccharide, probably because of a decrease in the general ability of the organism to synthesize proteins.

The phenomenon of tolerance, described by us and by other investigators, is unquestionably an important factor which will provide fresh information about inducers of endogenous interferon.

Tolerance arising in animals to the repeated injection of pyrogenal plays a significant role in determining the number of injections of interferon inducers which must be given for prophylactic and therapeutic purposes. It is important to note, from this standpoint, that tolerance to pyrogenal does not extend to virus inducers of interferon (in our experiments to fowl plague virus). This phenomenon can evidently be accepted as firmly established since other investigations, yielding identical results, have also been published [604].

The practical importance of tolerance is particularly great because a single injection of inducers can rarely be sufficient on account of their very short action. If there are to be any prospects for therapeutic application, interferon inducers must be injected repeatedly. The rational combination of inducers which will potentiate, rather than block, interferon production must therefore receive careful attention of research workers.

Our results show that interferon formation induced by a virus and by pyrogenal differs in its mechanisms. The rate of formation of interferons suggests that after injection of a virus

interferon is synthesized *de novo* . The possibility cannot be ruled
out that the interferon induced by pyrogenal already exists in the
body and is rapidly liberated into the bloodstream after intravenous
injection of the lipopolysaccharide. This hypothesis is also supported by the ability of pyrogenal to induce interferon formation
by leukocytes *in vitro* while not inducing its formation in growing
chick fibroblasts and chick embryos. Since the organism is constantly
exposed to the action of interferon inducers, and especially of bacteria and their breakdown products and also of viruses, presumably
the interferon which they induce accumulates in cells of the RES,
including leukocytes. It is therefore possible that at the moment
of their removal from the body leukocytes contain interferon which
they liberate into the medium under the influence of pyrogenal.
In tissue cultures and in chick embryos, on the other hand, this
exposure to interferon-inducing agents is absent and, consequently,
no interferon accumulates in them and none is liberated.

Other evidence of differences between the mechanisms of
interferon formation induced by viruses and by lipopolysaccharides
is the absence of tolerance during consecutive injection of pyrogenal
and virus. The reason why tolerance is present if the injections
are given in the opposite order is evidently that interferon already
existing in the body and liberated through the action of the interferon-
inducing virus is also utilized for the synthesis of virus-induced
interferon. This hypothesis is supported by results showing the
appearance of an early "heavy" interferon with a molecular weight
close to that of the interferon induced by bacterial lipopolysaccharides. Perhaps the virus initially liberates the preexisting
interferon and then induces synthesis of new interferon.

In the light of results obtained by us and other workers it
can be safely concluded that there are at least two inhibitors possessing antiviral action and until now grouped together under a
common name. We suggest that one of them be called α-interferon
and the other β-interferon, on the basis of the properties of interferons induced *in vivo*. The α-interferon appears in the tissues
through the action of virus inducers proper, the second through
the action of bacteria, bacterial substrates, and other inducing agents
of a nonviral nature. α-Interferon has a molecular weight of
20,000-30,000 and is thermostable. β-Interferon has a higher
molecular weight (70,000-90,000), it is thermostable, and it does
not give rise to complete tolerance to virus inducers.

Chapter 7

Clinical Trials of Stimulators
of Endogenous Interferon

7.1. Stimulation of Endogenous Interferon in Man and Its Effect on Virus Infections

Interferon formation in man is known to take place both in natural virus infections and after artificial introduction of viral and nonviral agents into the body [455, 594, 597]. It was evidently Isaacs [366] who first pointed out the desirability of using stimulators of endogenous interferon for the prevention and treatment of virus infections. Many other workers have subsequently shown that the course of virus infections can be influenced by administration of interferon inducers of viral and nonviral origin [11, 39, 82, 83, 84, 86, 126, 128, 136, 189, 288-290]. However, most investigations have been carried out in the form of animal experiments. Comparatively few clinical studies of interferon induction in man have been undertaken. The first report of interferon production in man in response to injection of inactivated viruses was made by Wheelock and Dingle [596]. To treat a patient with acute myeloid leukemia they injected large doses of various inactivated viruses intravenously and repeatedly at intervals of 4-14 days, and in some cases they found interferon in the blood. The patient received consecutive injections of NDV, influenza virus, and Semliki forest virus and a marked but transient improvement in his condition was observed.

Interferon production was also studied in volunteers inoculated with vaccine strain 17-D of yellow fever virus [598]. Interferon was found in the serum of 10 of the 15 inoculated volunteers from

178

the 4th to the 7th day after inoculation, the titer reaching a maximum on the 6th day. Since the interferon was observed 24 h after
the development of viremia, termination of the viremia can be
regarded as the result of interferon formation.

A study of the effect of living measles vaccine showed that
interferon is found in the blood of vaccinated persons from the
6th until the 10th day after vaccination [488]. The effect of this
vaccine on reproduction of vaccinia virus, which differs considerably
from measles virus, was investigated *in vivo*. Children aged
from 11 to 36 months were vaccinated with smallpox vaccine at
different times after measles immunization. Interferon was found
in the serum of 87% of the 131 children on the 9th-10th day after
measles vaccination. Maximal protection against vaccinia virus
was observed in the period when the serum interferon level was
maximal. Protection after measles vaccination was shorter in
duration and lower in intensity if highly virulent smallpox vaccine
was used. The protective action of interferon could be overcome
by a large dose of virus. It is interesting to note that six children
whose blood contained no detectable amount of interferon were
also protected against vaccinia virus. In these authors' opinion
this shows that amounts of interferon adequate to secure protection
against a virus infection may be present in the body even though
it cannot be found in the serum. During the first days and beyond
the 20th day after immunization with measles vaccine, a typical
reaction to smallpox vaccine developed in persons vaccinated
against smallpox in this period [489].

In experiments of 30 volunteers Jao and co-workers [379]
studied interferon production after intranasal infection with influenza A2 virus. Twelve subjects developed influenza. Interferon was found in the nasopharyngeal washings and blood of
6 of them, in the serum only in 5, and in the nasal washings only in
1 volunteer. Excretion of the virus always preceded the detection
of interferon. Interferon was found in one volunteer without excretion of the virus.

Priimyagi and co-workers tested poliomyelitis and measles
vaccine viruses as stimulators of interferon formation in man.
The maximal interferon titer was determined on the 7th-8th day [126].
The presence of interferon in washings from the nasal mucous

membrane after intranasal administration of influenza vaccine has
also been confirmed by other workers [3].

Some particularly interesting results have been obtained
concerning the stimulation of endogenous interferon whose formation was not connected with reproduction of the injected agents in
the body. Extensive studies of the effectiveness of the interferon
inducer IVS as a stimulator of the endogenous interferon of arbovirus vaccine [9, 39, 84, 97, 98, 134]. This preparation has been
shown to induce interferon production in cell cultures and also
in man and animals [9, 39, 97, 98].

Reports [455, 460] of the induction of interferon in man by
means of a synthetic polyanion of known composition are also
very interesting. It is claimed that polyanions with a molecular
weight of over 17,000 and, in particular, synthetic double-stranded
polyribonucleotides can be used in clinical practice.

Although the facts described above indicate that interferon
can be induced *in vivo* with the aid of various agents, preliminary
calculations show that large doses of the inducer must be injected
in order to stimulate a sufficiently high interferon concentration
in the body. In particular, according to Chumakov and co-workers
[189], to obtain a well-marked effect in a generalized virus infection about 10^{10} p.f.u. of Newcastle disease virus must be injected (intravenously) into a human patient. The injection of such
large doses of the virus must entail a risk to the patient. At the
present stage of knowledge the local administration of interferon
inducers thus appears to be the most rational course. It is in
this direction that the most encouraging results have been obtained.
Zalmanzon and co-workers [80-82] used swine influenza virus,
inactivated by ultraviolet radiation, for the prevention of
influenza at the height of an epidemic and observed a three to
fourfold decrease in the morbidity during the epidemic in 1965.
Admittedly Zalmanzon and co-workers [83], using the same virus,
were later unable to obtain statistically significant proof of its
efficacy. However, the use of living influenza and measles vaccines under the same conditions reduced the incidence of the
disease by 2-3.7 times. According to other reports intranasal
administration of UV-inactivated virus has a marked protective
effect against influenza.

Other workers have used stimulators of endogenous interferon for the prophylaxis of influenza and have obtained positive results [89, 127, 128, 275].

The interferon inducer IVS has also been tested therapeutically [39] for the treatment of patients with diseases of the skin and eyes of virus etiology. It has been given as lotions, repeated instillations, and by subconjunctival and intramuscular injections. Rakhmanov and co-workers [134], for instance, found that IVS has a marked therapeutic effect against herpes simplex and herpes zoster accompanied by lesions of the skin, including in recurrent cases. Other workers obtained good results in the treatment of herpes simplex and herpes zoster [9] and of herpetic keratitis [97]. Similar results have been obtained in the treatment and prevention of adenovirus infections of the eyes [98, 111] and of trachoma [10].

Interferon formation in man in response to injection of virus and nonvirus agents was studied by us in experiments conducted jointly with L. A. Porubel'. In most cases interferon formation by cells of the upper respiratory tract was found after intranasal injection of the inducers. Living and killed vaccine strains of influenza virus as well as some other inactivated viruses were used for this purpose. Newcastle disease virus, inactivated by ultraviolet radiation, and pyrogenal also were tested as inducers of interferon.

In experiments on 479 volunteers the effect of some of these interferon inducers on survival of vaccine strain A2/M21/65 of influenza virus also was investigated.

To determine the dynamics of interferon formation after injection of living influenza virus, volunteers were infected intranasally with vaccine virus A2/M21/65 in a dose of 10^6 $ID_{50}/0.25$ ml. The inactivated viruses were prepared in different ways. As virus-containing material the allantoic fluid (influenza viruses and NDV) or chorioallantoic membrane (vaccinia virus) of infected chick embryos in a titer of 10^7-10^8 ID_{50}/ml for chick embryos was used. Heated interferon inducers of influenza viruses A2/M21/65 and B (Lich) and vaccinia virus were obtained by heating virus suspensions at 56°C for 30-60 min. Besides the heated influenza and vaccinia viruses, influenza virus A2/M21/65 inactivated by for-

malin in a concentration of 1 : 4000 or by ultraviolet radiation
(BUV-15 lamp, distance from source of light 15 cm, thickness of
layer of liquid 3 mm, exposure 10 min) also were used. However,
in some experiments inactivation under these conditions was not
sufficiently effective. In some cases some of the virus remained
infectious. For this reason, results on interferon formation in
volunteers receiving completely and partially inactivated influenza
virus will be described below.

Influenza virus B (Lich) inactivated by ultraviolet radiation
as described above, and the same virus inactivated by γ-rays in
a dose of 10^6 R also were tested on two groups of volunteers.

The method of irradiation was as follows. The allantoic
fluid was centrifuged for 10-15 min and poured into ampules each
containing 4 ml. These were irradiated on a γ-ray apparatus
with Co^{60} with a total activity of 20 kCi. The dose rate of irradiation was 2000 R/min. Under these conditions the virus lost its
infective properties but retained its hemagglutinating and antigenic
properties [17].

Completeness of inactivation of the viruses was judged on
the basis of two consecutive subcultures in chick embryos.

For 3-4 or more days after injection of the interferon inducer the survival of the virus (in the case of injection of the infectious virus) in the nasal cavity and pharynx was determined
by the method of reisolation of the vaccine strain in chick embryos.
To determine the dynamics of interferon formation nasal washings
were obtained at the same times.

Immunological changes in the infected volunteers were
estimated on the basis of a fourfold or greater increase in the
antibody titer in pairs of sera.

7.2. Interferon-Inducing Properties of Living Influenza Vaccine Virus

The dynamics of interferon formation by cells of the upper
respiratory tract after vaccination with living influenza vaccine
was studied in experiments on 30 volunteers. Daily for 4 days
after vaccination and again on the 7th day after administration
of the virus the interferon and virus content was determined in
the nasal washings.

TABLE 88. Correlation between Survival of Virus and Detection of Interferon

Number of volunteers	Number in which virus survived	Number in which interferon was found	Agreement between survival of virus and detection of interferon	Virus isolated but interferon not found	Virus not isolated but interferon found
30	14	13	12	2	1

TABLE 89. Interferon Titers in Nasal Washings of Volunteers Observed on Particular Days

Day of observation	Interferon titers							Mean interferon titers
	1:2	1:2	1:4	1:8	1:16	1:32	1:64	
1	1	2	3	2	2	3	0	12.3
2	1	1	2	3	3	3	0	13.7
3	1	1	2	3	2	4	0	14.3
4	6	5	1	1	0	0	0	1.7
7	12	0	0	0	0	0	0	6.1

Results showing correlation between survival of the virus and detection of interferon are shown in Table 88.

It is clear from Table 88 that survival of the virus coincided with detection of interferon in 12 of the 14 volunteers. In two volunteers although the virus survived no interferon was found, and in one survival of the virus could not be demonstrated either by reisolation of the virus or by a rise in the antibody titer, but the inhibitor was found in the nasal secretion. Consequently, a direct correlation between survival of the virus and detection of interferon was not present in every case.

Interferon could be found in the nasal washings after 24 h and its concentration reached a maximum after 48–72 h, when it began to fall rapidly, disappearing after 96 h. Before vaccination the inhibitor was found in four volunteers in whom survival of the virus was not observed.

The quantity of interferon in the nasal washings of the volunteers varied. Its titer varied from 1:2 to 1:32 at different times of investigation (Table 89).

TABLE 90. Correlation between Survival of Influenza Virus and Detection of Interferon in Nasal Washings of Vaccinated Volunteers

Total number of volunteers with interferon	Time of investigation (in hours)	Number of volunteers with		
		virus	increase in titer of antibodies	interferon
13	24	5	0	11
	48	7	0	12
	72	7	0	12
	96	4	0	1
	2 weeks	-	6	-
Total:		8	6	13

The results in Table 89 show that the mean interferon titers were almost identical during the first 3 days, with a slight tendency to rise at the end of this period. On the 4th day after vaccination interferon was found in fairly low titers and in only a limited number of volunteers. It will be noted that reisolation of the virus was possible at these same times (Table 90).

It will be clear from Table 90 that interferon could be found in the nasal washings of some volunteers despite negative results of the virus reisolation test. Subsequently survival of the virus in this group of vaccinated volunteers was confirmed when paired samples of serum were tested. Consequently, interferon formation after vaccination with influenza virus proved to be a unique indicator of survival of the virus. However, it must be remembered that not all cases of survival of the virus were accompanied by interferon formation. In these observations coincidence was not observed in 2 of the 14 volunteers.

In 12 of the 14 volunteers survival of the virus coincided with the detection of interferon. Interferon could be found in the nasal washings after 24 h and its concentration reached a maximum after 48-72 h. Before vaccination the inhibitor was found in low titer in four volunteers in whom survival of the virus was not observed.

The level of interferon in the nasal washings of the volunteers varied. Its titer varied from 1 : 2 to 1 : 32 at different times of investigation (Table 88).

TABLE 91. Interferon in Nasal Washings after Administration of
Partially Inactivated A2 Influenza Virus

Preparation given to volunteers	Number of volunteers	Number of persons with interferon on successive days of observation			
		before vaccination	1	2	3
Partially inactivated		3	47	24	7
influenza virus	71	(4.2%)	(66%)	(33.8%)	(9.8%)
Normal allantoic		2	3	3	2
fluid	· 40	(5%)	(7.5%)	(7.5%)	(5%)

7.3. Interferon-Inducing Properties of Partially UV-Inactivated A2 Influenza Virus

The inducing action of influenza A2 virus, partially inactivated by ultraviolet radiation, was investigated in experiments on 111 volunteers. This investigation was carried out in two stages: the first in March and the second in July, 1966. In March, the interferon inducer was given to 41 volunteers and a placebo (normal allantoic fluid) to 20 volunteers; in July the inducer was given to 30 volunteers and the placebo to 20. Nasal washings were tested before administration of the inducer or the normal allantoic fluid and daily after their administration for 3 days. The results of the tests for interferon in the nasal washings are summarized in Table 91. Survival of the virus was not determined in these experiments.

Interferon was found in more than half of the volunteers 24 h after vaccination, but the percentage of those with interferon in their nasal washings after 72 h had fallen to 10. Evidently survival of the virus was of short duration and the interferon therefore disappeared rapidly from the nasal washings. The interferon titers in the nasal washings were four times lower than after administration of the living virus. In addition, three noteworthy features were observed during the tests. First, the rate of survival of the virus (on the basis of detection of interferon) was 82.9% in March but only 43% in July; second, all cases (10 of the 111 volunteers) in which the inhibitor was present before vaccination concerned volunteers whose nasal washings were tested in July; third, the titers of interferon in July were on the average

TABLE 92. Interferon in Nasal Washings of Volunteers Receiving Partially Inactivated Influenza Virus

Time of investigation	Group of volunteers	Total number of volunteers	Number of volunteers with interferon					Mean interferon titer
			below 1:2	1:2	1:4	1:8	1:16	
March	Experimental	41	7	25	6	3	–	2.7
	Control	20	20	–	–	–	–	<2.0
July	Experimental	30	17	2	5	6	–	5.5
	Control	20	18	–	–	–	–	<2.0

TABLE 93. Interferon-Inducing Properties of Viruses Inactivated by Various Methods

Virus and method of inactivation	Number of volunteers	Detection of inhibitor on successive days of observation				Titer of inhibitor
		1	2	3	total	
Influenza A2 virus, ultraviolet radiation	22	12	2	0	12	2–4
Vaccinia virus, heating to 56°C	10	2	0	0	2	2
Influenza B virus, ultraviolet radiation	10	3	1	0	3	2
Influenza B virus, γ-radiation	10	3	0	0	3	2
Normal allantoic fluid	10	0	0	0	0	<2

twice as high as in March. The results for the two groups of volunteers are compared in Table 92.

Analysis of the results in Table 90 shows that the mean titers of the inhibitor found in March were approximately 1 : 2.7, whereas in July they were 1 : 5.5. In addition, the inhibitor was found in July in 10 volunteers even before vaccination. It is difficult to decide what is the nature of this inhibitor because its low titers and the small number of washings tested prevented any study of its properties.

7.4. Interferon-Inducing Properties of Inactivated Viruses

The interferon-inducing properties of influenza A2 and B viruses and of vaccinia virus when inactivated by various methods were next investigated (Table 93).

Intranasal injection of inactivated viruses was followed by interferon formation and in most volunteers interferon could be detected during the first 24 h after administration of the inducer. Later the interferon disappeared quickly. After 48 h it could be found only in individual subjects, and after 72 h it was no longer found in any of the washings.

The results of determination of the interferon-inducing activity of viruses in volunteers can be summarized in the statement that it was highest in the case of the living vaccine strain of influenza virus, followed by the same virus when partially inactivated by ultraviolet radiation; the interferon-inducing activity of viruses completely inactivated by various methods was weaker still. Among this last group, the ability to stimulate interferon formation was most marked in the case of influenza A2/M21/65 virus. However, since the tests with inactivated viruses were carried out on a limited number of volunteers and at different seasons of the year, it is impossible to draw any hard and fast conclusions. Further investigations are necessary. It can, however, be said that the use of pyrogenal on 15 volunteers by intranasal administration failed to demonstrate any interferon-inducing activity.

7.5. Effect of Stimulators of Endogenous Interferon on Survival of Influenza Vaccine Virus

On the basis of results showing the dynamics of interferon formation by cells of the upper respiratory tract the effect of

TABLE 94. Effect of Stimulators of Endogenous Interferon on Survival
of Influenza Vaccine Virus Injected 24 h after the Interferon Inducer

Group	Virus stimulating endogenous interferon	Number of volunteers in group	Survival of influenza virus as shown by			
			isolation in chick embryos		increase in antibodies	
			abs.	%	abs.	%
1	Influenza A2 virus inactivated by formalin	22	n.i.	n.i.	8	36.3
2	Influenza A2 virus inactivated by heat	15	4	26.6	5	33.0
3	Influenza A2 virus inactivated by UV radiation	19	3	15.7	3	16.6
4	Influenza B virus inactivated by UV radiation	10	5	50.0	7	70.0
5	Influenza B virus inactivated by γ-radiation	10	6	60	6	60.0
6	Vaccinia virus inactivated by heat	16	6	37.5	8	50.0
7	Normal allantoic fluid	90	48	53.3	57	63.3

Note: n.i., not investigated.

various stimulators of endogenous interferon on the survival of
influenza A2/M21/65 vaccine virus was studied. Considering that
interferon is found 24 h after administration of the stimulator,
the volunteers were infected 18–20 h after intranasal administration
of the inducer.

Before administration of the vaccine virus nasal washings
were taken and their interferon content determined.

The effect of the various stimulators of endogenous interferon on survival of influenza A2 virus was studied in tests on 182
volunteers. Besides UV-inactivated viruses, other interferon inducers were used.

As Table 94 shows, the interferon inducers tested differed
in their prophylactic action. The almost complete absence of
prophylactic action of influenza B virus when activated by various
methods will be noted.

The survival of influenza A2 vaccine virus in these groups of
volunteers was virtually on the same level as in the control group.

Only a very slight prophylactic effect was observed in the group of volunteers receiving inactivated vaccinia virus. Influenza A2 viruses inactivated by formalin and by heat possessed an appreciably prophylactic effect. The most marked prophylactic action on the survival of the influenza vaccine virus was shown by influenza A2 virus inactivated by ultraviolet radiation. In this group of volunteers the rate of survival of the influenza virus was 3.5 times less than in the control, as shown both by isolation in chick embryos and by the increase in antibody titer.

These differences in the effectiveness of the interferon inducers used depended, it was concluded, on the quantity of interferon induced by them. The interferon concentration in the nasal washings was found to be inversely proportional to the rate of survival of the virus. The rate of survival of the virus was also found to depend on the presence of inhibitor in the washings before administration of the interferon inducer (Table 95).

As Table 95 shows, when the inhibitor was present in the nasal washings in a titer of 1 : 2 or higher, the survival rate of the virus fell considerably. The prophylactic action was particularly marked if the interferon titer was 1 : 4 to 1 : 8. Nevertheless, the presence of interferon in the nasal washings does not completely prevent survival of the influenza vaccine strain although it reduces it considerably.

The prophylactic effect of the viruses used thus depends on their interferon-inducing activity. However, the effect of the homologous or heterologous antigenic structure of the interferon

TABLE 95. Relationship between Survival
Rate of Influenza Virus and Interferon Titers
in Nasal Washings

Number of volunteers and interferon titer	Survival rate of virus as shown by			
	isolation in chick embryos		increase in antibody titer	
	abs.	%	abs.	%
Total number 56, with titers as follows				
< 1 : 2-32 persons	15	46.8	20	62.5
1 : 2-12 persons	4	33.3	3	25
1 : 4-1 : 8-12 persons	1	8.3	1	8.3

inducer and the virus tested for survival cannot be completely ruled out.

Be that as it may, administration of inactivated homologous virus produced immunity to influenza in a large proportion of persons within 24 h.

In the next experiments, which were conducted jointly with L. A. Porubel' and G. S. Churkin, the interferon inducers and prophylactic action of UV-inactivated influenza virus was studied during an outbreak of adenovirus infection.

The method of conducting the observations on the volunteers has been described by the writer previously [163]. On this occasion the only difference was that the tests were carried out on two separate groups of people with identical working and living conditions.

The control group initially received normal allantoic fluid by the intranasal route, while the experimental group received the inducer. Living influenza virus was administered to the subjects of both groups 24 h later. Only those subjects who were free from clinically manifest forms of acute respiratory diseases during the month before the experiment began were included in the tests.

Pairs of sera were tested in the hemagglutination inhibition test (HIT) with influenza A2/M21/65 antigen and in the complement fixation test (CFT) with adenovirus antigen prepared from the strain isolated in the group of subjects studied from a patient during an outbreak of acute respiratory infection before the investigation.

The first sera of the pairs were obtained in the group 11 days before the beginning of the experiment, during an outbreak of acute respiratory infection. The second sera were obtained from the same persons 40 days after the first (3.5 weeks after the beginning of the experiment).

The HIT was performed by the usual method with chick erythrocytes. Two doses of antigen and two doses of complement were used in the CFT. Contact between the dilutions of serum and the antigen and complement took place at 4°C for 16-18 h. Before the reaction the serum was treated with carbon dioxide. It must first be pointed out that 20 days before the beginning of the experiment an outbreak of acute respiratory infection had occurred in the experimental group 20 days before the experiment began and it lasted for 10 days. By the beginning of the experiments the number of cases had decreased but the outbreak was not completely at an end.

Eight cytopathogenic agents identified in the CFT as adenoviruses were isolated from the nasopharyngeal washing of 13 patients in transplanted HEp-2 cells. In the first sera of all 23 subjects who had had the infection a fourfold or greater increase in titer of antibodies against adenoviruses was found. In the same sera tested in the HIT a diagnostic increase in antibody titer against influenza viruses was detected in only three cases (one each against types A2, B, and C).

Consequently, the adenovirus etiology of the outbreak was proved conclusively. It is important, however, to emphasize the differences between the incidence of the disease in the two groups studied. In one of them the incidence of acute respiratory infection was twice as high as in the other. The possibility could not therefore be ruled out that the adenovirus infection may have affected the rules of the experiment. Accordingly the observations in each group were conducted separately, with segregation of experimental and control groups in each of them.

For convenience of description the group with the lower incidence of acute respiratory infection will subsequently be described as group A and that with the higher incidence as group B.

TABLE 96. Presence of Interferon and Survival Rate of Influenza Virus in Group A

Preparation administered	Number of subjects with interferon in nasal washings		Survival rate of influenza virus as shown by			
			isolation in chick embryos		increase in antibody titer	
	abs.	%	abs.	%	abs.	%
Interferon inducer	11/23	47	6/21	28.6	7/21	34
Normal allantoic fluid	2/22	9	12/19	63.2	15/19	78

Note. Numerator, number of persons with positive results; denominator, total number tested.

TABLE 97. Presence of Interferon and Survival Rate of
Influenza A2 Virus in Group B

Preparation administered	Number of subjects with interferon in nasal washings		Survival rate of influenza virus as shown by			
			isolation in chick embryos		increase in antibody titer	
	abs.	%	abs.	%	abs.	%
Interferon inducer	9/25	36	7/25	28	13/25	52
Normal allantoic fluid	10/29	34	8/24	33	11/24	45

Note. Numerator, number of persons with positive results: denominator, total number tested.

The results in Table 96 show that administration of UV-inactivated influenza A2 virus led to stimulation of interferon formation by the cells of the upper respiratory tract.

Administration of the interferon inducer had a well-marked prophylactic action. The mean values for the survival rate of the virus, as shown by its isolation in chick embryos, in the experimental and control groups showed statistically significant differences when analyzed by the Van der Waerden method (χ^2 = 2.14; n' = 38; p = 0.05).

The relative survival rate in the control group was 2.2 times higher than in the experimental group. The results for survival of the influenza virus determined on the basis of isolation in chick embryos and increase in antibody titer agreed almost completely.

Different results were obtained in group B. The first feature in Table 97 to attract attention is the frequent discovery of interferon in the nasal washings of subjects receiving normal allantoic fluid, and the frequency with which interferon was detected in the nasal washings was virtually identical (about 30%) in the control and experimental groups.

The results of a study of the survival rate of influenza vaccine virus were also in agreement with these findings. In this case no statistically significant difference could be found between the control and experimental groups. The survival rate was at

TABLE 98. Geometric Mean Titers of Antibodies and Indices of Their Increase

Group	Subgroup	Number of pairs of sera tested	Blood sample	Against influenza A virus				Against adenoviruses			
				M	multiplicity of increase in antibodies	χ^2	probability of correlation between indices	M	multiplicity of increase in antibodies	χ^2	probability of correlation between indices
A	Control	19	I	6.1	4	4.6	0.01	4.6	2.8	3	0.01
			II	24.2				13.0			
	Experiment	21	I	7.0	2.3	2.4	0.05	8.0	2.1	3	0.01
			II	16.0				17.1			
B	Control	24	I	7.5	2	3	0.01	2.7	8.9	9.7	0.01
			II	14.9				24.2			
	Experiment	25	I	6.1	2.7	2.4	0.01	2.6	10.0	6.6	0.01
			II	13.9				26.0			
	Patients	23	I	8.6	1.1	0.5	0.5	3.7	14.0	10	0.01
			II	9.8				52.0			

Legend: M) reciprocal of geometric mean titer; χ^2) statistical index of difference.

TABLE 99. Distribution of Multiplicities

Group	Subgroup	Number of pairs of sera tested	Against influenza		
			Change in antibody titer		
			no increase	twofold increase	fourfold increase
A	Control	19	4	8	7
	Experiment	21	14	3	4
B	Control	24	13	9	2
	Experiment	25	12	8	5

the level of the experimental subgroup of group A, i.e., it was reduced by 1.5-2 times compared with the control subgroup of group A.

The difference between the results obtained in experiments conducted by the same method can evidently be attributed to differences in the epidemic situation in the two groups at the time of the tests and in the preceding period.

As has already been mentioned, persons who had shown clinically identifiable forms of acute respiratory infection were excluded from the experimental and control subgroups. However, together with clinically manifest forms of acute respiratory infection, abortive cases also occurred among the groups, and the number of cases of latent infection in group B, in which the incidence of the disease was higher, was also 5-6 times greater than in group A.

It will be clear from Table 98 that in all subgroups except the patients the antibody titer was increased by 2-10 times in the two sera both against influenza A2 virus and against adenovirus. Determination of the statistical significance of the difference between the titers of the antibodies in sera I and II by calculation of the ratio between the difference of the mean titers and its mean error yielded values of χ^2 which point to a high level of significance of the immunological changes. However, these changes in the different subgroups differed quantitatively. These differences were revealed most clearly by statistical analysis of the ranks of distribution of the multiplicities of increase in the antibody titers.

of Increase in Antibody Titers

A2/M21/65 virus		Against adenoviruses				
Criterion of correlation (χ^2)	Probability of correlation (p)	Change in antibody titer			Criterion of correlation (χ^2)	Probability of correlation (p)
		no increase	twofold increase	fourfold increase		
10.4	0.01	9	7	3	0.47	0.7
		8	10	3		
		2	5	17		
1.93	0.8				1.16	0.3
		1	6	18		

Table 99 shows that the changes in titers of antibodies against influenza virus in the control subgroup of group A were observed more frequently than in the experimental subgroup. Statistical analysis of the significance of this difference in the distribution of multiplicities of increase in the antibody titer showed that it was very high (χ^2 = 10.4; n' = 2; p = 0.01). This indicates that the immunological reaction in the experimental subgroup of group A to administration of living influenza A2 virus was less marked not by chance but as the result of the prophylactic action of the interferon inducer.

7.6. Conclusion

The interferon-inducing activity of influenza virus, both infectious and when inactivated by various methods, was studied experimentally. The highest activity when administered intranasally to volunteers was exhibited by the vaccine virus, and this was followed by partially inactivated virus; inactivated viruses were least capable of inducing interferon formation. Of the last group, influenza A2 virus, inactivated by ultraviolet radiation, gave the greatest interferon-inducing effect. The ability of UV-inactivated influenza virus to induce interferon production in mice was demonstrated previously by Ermol'eva and co-workers [60]. Similar results were obtained by us in human studies. However, unlike in mice, interferon was found in the nasal washings of most volunteers for only 24 h, and it was present only rarely after 48 h. From this standpoint the results obtained by Sokolov and Kulikova [152], who studied the dynamics of immunogenesis during vaccination against influenza, are of considerable interest. After intranasal administration of killed influenza virus these workers found two phases in the development of immunity to influenza. The second phase, occurring on the 7th-10th day after immunization, was connected with antibody formation. At the same time, the animals were found to be resistant immediately after administration of the vaccine. This first phase of resistance is attributed by these workers to blocking of susceptible cells by influenza antigen. The results of our investigations suggest that these phenomena are due to stimulation of endogenous interferon.

The titers of the interferon induced by different stimulators were higher when the living virus was given. Under these circumstances interferon could also be detected for longer in the nasal washings. Considering that the survival rate of the vaccine virus depended on the interferon titers at the time of its administration, it can be concluded that the best results from intranasal administration of interferon inducers are given by active viruses, which reproduce for a long time and induce adequate quantities of interferon. At the same time, we suggest that prophylaxis of respiratory and other virus infections can be achieved by the administration of interferon inducers not only intranasally, but also by other routes. This is shown, in particular, by the results obtained with intramuscular injection of interferon inducers.

It must be remembered that the antivirus activity resulting from administration of an interferon inducer is of short duration; in order to obtain prolonged resistance to viruses it is therefore necessary to repeat the administration of the inducers. For this purpose, because of their antigenic activity, it is evident that the same interferon-inducing viruses whose action is due to their reproduction in the body must not be used repeatedly. An assortment of infectious, nonpathogenic interferon inducers, differing in their antigenic structure, is therefore required. Noninfectious, inactivated viruses can be used for these purposes, or preference may be given to nonviral agents such as statolon, helenine, or chemical compounds with adequate interferon-inducing activity. However, the use of interferon-inducing viruses which have already been studied for the prevention and treatment of generalized infections does not seem very promising at the present time because large doses of the inducer must be injected in order to stimulate a sufficiently high interferon concentration in the body. In order to obtain a clearly defined effect, about 10^{10} p.f.u. of Newcastle disease virus must be administered. The injection of such large doses of the virus must run the risk of harmful or dangerous effects [189]. Similar risks apply in the case of administration of bacteria and their lipopolysaccharides.

There is thus a strong case at the present time for the local administration of interferon inducers. In particular, results obtained by us and other workers with stimulators of endogenous interferon have shown that their use during an epidemic for the prevention of respiratory infections is promising. An urgent task at the present time is the search for highly active interferon inducers which, in our opinion, could prove to be an effective method of controlling virus infections.

PART III

Interferon Formation and Virus Infection

Interferon Formation in the Body during Virus Infections and Its Pathogenic Role

8.1. Interferon Formation in Virus Infections of Animals

The first important investigations to study interferon formation and the role of this process in experimental influenza were carried out by Isaacs and Hitchcock [37]. They studied the dynamics of formation of interferon and antibodies and its relationship to the character of reproduction of the virus. By infecting mice with a sublethal dose of influenza A virus these workers found that interferon appears in the lungs from the 2nd until the 5th day and that its maximal titer coincides with the beginning of a decrease in the concentration of virus in the tissues. Since antibodies appeared much later, Isaacs and Hitchcock postulated that inhibition of reproduction of the virus in the respiratory organs was due to the accumulation of interferon.

Subsequently a similar dynamics of virus reproduction and interferon formation in mice with influenza has been confirmed by many investigators [113, 215, 287, 290, 432, 495].

Baron and co-workers [215] compared interferon production with reproduction of influenza A virus (strain PR-8) in the lungs of mice during sublethal influenzal infection. They found that interferon appears in the lung immediately after reproduction of the virus, and that it can be detected until the 5th day but not later

despite the high titer of virus. In the discussion of their results
Baron and co-workers [215] postulated that in the late stage of
development of the infection many cells may produce small quantities of interferon which are, however, retained by the cells. They
suggested that interferon still participates in the late stage of
recovery even though no more of it is being produced, for antibody
formation was first prevented by immunodepression. The antiviral
action of the interferon adsorbed by the tissues may be observed
for several days, confirming the hypothesis put forward [376, 436,
483].

Link and co-workers [433] studied the relationship between
reproduction of the virus and interferon formation in the lungs of
mice after infection with adapted and nonadapted influenza A1
viruses. They found that the unadapted virus, which is less pathogeni
for mice, also induced smaller quantities of interferon. During
adaptation, however, it increased its pathogenicity and at the same
time induced larger amounts of interferon. They concluded from
these results that interferon can be used as an indicator of adaptation of a virus to the animal organism. Similar results were
obtained by Inglot and co-workers [361] with influenza A2 virus.
These workers also found that the adapted virus is more sensitive
to interferon than the unadapted virus. In all the investigations
cited above a direct correlation was observed between reproduction
of the virus and interferon formation. However, this correlation
was observed in the initial period of the disease until the 5th-6th
day after infection. Later no interferon could be found despite
further reproduction of the virus.

Ability to induce interferon formation during reproduction
in the animal body has also been demonstrated in the arboviruses.

The appropriate investigations have been carried out with
O'nyong-nyong [343], West Nile [553, 561], Semliki forest [284,
285], tick-borne encephalitis [5, 575], Sindbis [572], and Tahyna
[203] viruses.

Other evidence of interferon formation during reproduction
of viruses in the animal body has been obtained by experiments
in which animals were infected with other viruses: guinea pigs
with vaccinia virus [296], mice with lactic dehydrogenase virus [215],
chickens with Coxsackie B1 [518] and NDV [171], murine smallpox [553], mice [35], rabbit [292], and guinea pigs [557] with her-

pes, and mice with vesicular stomatitis [247]. Interferon has also
been found in the lungs of mice infected with parainfluenza viruses
of type 1 [526, 527] and type 3 [256]. A direct correlation was observed in adult animals between reproduction of the virus and interferon formation. A similar phenomenon has also been found in
hamsters [547] and mice [95] infected with fixed rabies virus.

Unsuccessful attempts to discover interferon in animals infected with several viruses also have been described. In particular,
no interferon was found in the organs of mice infected with the
viruses of Rauscher [487], Friend's leukemia [326], and cytomegaly
[477, 478], or in mice with chronic lymphocytic choriomeningitis
[587].

The results of the investigations carried out by these various
workers can be summed up in the statement that interferon formation usually proceeds parallel with reproduction of the virus.
In some cases, however, interferon production reaches its maximum
before [35] or a little after the maximum of virus reproduction in
selectively vulnerable tissues [343]. Meanwhile, in some virus infections interferon disappears from the body sooner than the virus
[35, 210, 296].

Interferon is produced in the body in response to administration of both avirulent and virulent strains of viruses regardless
of the character of the infection (lethal or sublethal) in animals
of different species [171, 361, 433, 553].

8.2. Interferon Formation in Human Virus Infections

Facts concerning interferon formation in human subjects
infected with attenuated vaccine strains and also with inactivated
viruses were described earlier in this book. At this stage only the
results obtained by the study of interferon formation in natural
human infections will be considered.

Gresser and Dull [324] investigated nasopharyngeal washings
of 13 patients with influenza. A virus was isolated from 9 of them
and in 12 cases the diagnosis was confirmed serologically. Interferon was found in the nasopharyngeal washings of 4 patients in
the first 2 days of the illness. Interferon was found in the cerebro-
spinal fluid (CSF) of 23 of 58 patients with aseptic virus meningitis.
It was also found in 3 of 25 patients with bacterial meningitis and

in 2 of 69 patients in whom a noninfectious disease of the central
nervous system was diagnosed. No direct correlation was found
between the presence of virus and the presence of inhibitor in the
CSF but the leukocyte count was found to be directly dependent on
the interferon concentration [327].

Wheelock [591] demonstrated the presence of interferon in
the scabs of the healing pustules of persons vaccinated against
smallpox. The inhibitor was found in 4 of 5 persons vaccinated.
Wheelock postulated that if the vaccination followed a severe
course interferon was absent. Vaccination with interferon formation in his opinion must give a mild reaction.

The interferon concentration in the CSF has also been
studied in children with diseases of the central nervous system
[414]. Interferon was found in 39 (13.6%) of 287 samples of CSF
tested. It was found in 26 of 51 children with aseptic meningitis.
The titers of the inhibitor in patients with meningitis as a com-
plication of mumps were 7-8 times higher than in patients with
meningitis of enterovirus etiology. The interferon level in both
groups was higher if the patient had a high fever. No correlation
was found between the presence of interferon and isolation of the
virus from the CSF. Other workers had previously reported the
discovery of interferon in the CSF of patients with aseptic meningitis caused by ECHO 9 virus [248, 498]. Workers studying the
interferon concentration in the CSF attempted to demonstrate a
correlation between the leukocyte count, the interferon concentration, and the frequency of isolation of the virus. However, no
definite correlation could be found between these indices.

Serum interferon was found in low titers in 4 of 17 children
with respiratory syncytial infection [594] and in the nasopharyngeal
washings of volunteers infected with Coxsackie A21 virus and
rhinovirus NIH 1734. No correlation was found between the interferon titer and the severity of the disease or the frequency of
isolation of the virus [594].

Attempts to find interferon in the serum of patients with
infectious hepatitis have also proved unsuccessful. No interferon
was found in any of the samples obtained from 34 patients in various
stages of acute and chronic forms of the disease over a period of
6 months [594]. The investigations of Lee and co-workers, who

studied the ability of the leukocytes of patients with leukemias to produce interferon, deserve special mention. In their initial studies [420] these workers found that suspensions of leukemic leukocytes gave a much lower yield of interferon than leukocytes from healthy donors. The mean titers of leukocytic interferon were 1:152.6 for healthy donors, 1:24.7 for patients with acute leukemia, and 1:37 for patients with chronic leukemia. Subsequently [418] they obtained further evidence that reduced ability to produce interferon is also a feature of patients with acute lymphatic and myeloid leukemia and with chronic lymphatic leukemia. In patients with recently diagnosed chronic lymphatic leukemia interferon production was normal, while in patients with chronic myeloid leukemia it was actually increased.

8.3. Effect of Various Factors on Interferon Production *in vivo*

Interferon production *in vivo* depends on the properties of the virus, its dose, and its mode of administration and also on the species and age of the animals. The relationship between the quantity of interferon produced and the above factors is seen particularly clearly after intravenous injection of the virus. The effect of factors modifying the course of a virus infection on interferon production will be examined below. These factors include the external environmental temperature, age, hormones, the virulence of the viruses, stress, and certain others.

Sawicki [526] found that newborn mice infected intranasally with Sendai virus produced much less interferon in the lungs than adult animals. The intensity of virus reproduction behaved in the opposite way and was greater in young mice. There are reports of the formation of much smaller quantities of interferon in newborn mice infected with Coxsackie B1 virus than in animals aged 6 weeks [332, 333, 518]. Newborn mice died by the 3rd day after infection without forming detectable quantities of interferon, whereas interferon formation in the adult mice reached a maximum on the 4th-5th day and the animals recovered.

Intravenous injection of a large dose of Powassan virus into chickens led to the formation of four times more interferon in birds aged 3 months than in birds aged 6 days [413]. Less interferon was found to be produced by young animals than by adults when Semliki forest virus also was used [45].

On the basis of results such as those described above it has been concluded that interferon is one of the principal factors accounting for the higher resistance of adult animals to virus infections. However, other workers have been unable to find any difference in the ability of animals of different ages to produce interferon [572, 575, 499, 256, 287].

Keeping animals at a low temperature considerably depresses their ability to produce interferon. This has been demonstrated for mice and Coxsackie B1 virus [518], for rabbits and NDV [500], and also for chick embryos [168].

Steroid hormones inhibit interferon production *in vivo*, as experiments on developing chick embryos [168, 395, 538] and on mice [168, 450, 501, 521] have shown. This applies to any inducer of interferon, whether of virus or nonvirus (endotoxin, helenine) nature. The only exception is one investigation [449] which showed that steroids stimulate interferon production by mouse peritoneal leukocytes *in vitro*.

Besides the factors mentioned above, interferon formation in animals is also inhibited by certain other factors which lower the resistance of the body. It has been shown [139], for example, that ionizing radiation depresses the ability of mice to form interferon in response to administration of influenza virus. This coincided with an increase in the titer of virus in the lung tissue of the mice and increased mortality among the infected animals. Reduced formation of serum and cutaneous interferons induced by herpes simplex virus in guinea pigs irradiated with x-rays has been observed [557]. Interesting results were obtained by Jullien and De Maeyer [386], who showed that different virus inducers react unequally to irradiation. If, for instance, Sindbis virus was used as the interferon inducer, the inhibitory action of irradiation was manifested after 24 h, but if NDV was used, the effect was delayed until 48 h. These workers found that the reduced ability to produce interferon in the case of Sindbis virus resembled the curve of disappearance of the circulating lymphocytes after irradiation, while in the case of NDV it resembled the curve of disappearance of the granulocytes. They accordingly postulate that the peripheral leukocytes play an important role in interferon production; depending on the character of the virus inducer, different types of leukocytes participate in this process.

Exposure of mice to noise stress for 3 h daily for 6–8 days led to a marked decrease in interferon production and to a more intensive and prolonged reproduction of the virus [247]. Prolonged exposure of mice to vibration had a similar effect [382].

The production of serum interferon is inhibited by the leukopenic agent methotrexate, by large doses of vitamin A, by various types of shock (histamine, endotoxin), and by alcohol poisoning. Interferon production in the skin of guinea pigs infected with herpes virus was also reduced in the Arthüs phenomenon [557].

Several investigations into the effect of antilymphocytic serum on interferon formation *in vivo* have recently been published.

For instance, Hirsch et al. [658] found no change in the intensity of interferon formation in mice treated with serum after intravenous infection with vaccinia virus. However, in the experiments of Barth et al. [630] antilymphocytic serum strongly inhibited the production of serum interferon induced by NDV and by synthetic double-stranded RNA (poly I : C). A decrease in serum interferon production has also been described in mice receiving antilymphocytic serum and infected with West Nile virus [651]. At the same time, according to Hirsch et al. [659], antilymphocytic serum had no effect on interferon formation in mice induced by injection of pyran. Similar results were obtained by Inglot et al. [661] in mice infected with Sindbis virus. At the same time, if instead of virus, the replicative form of the virus was injected into mice receiving a single injection of antilymphocytic serum, interferon formation was reduced by 4–10 times compared with the control.

A. M. Sorokin, working in our laboratory, also studied the effect of antilymphocytic serum on interferon and antibody production induced by intravenous injection of mice with NDV. The production of serum interferon was undisturbed if antilymphocytic serum was injected at the time of infection, but it was reduced by 8 times if the serum was injected 2 h before infection. Interferon production was inhibited to an even greater degree if the antilymphocytic serum was injected 3 days before infection. The production of interferon was largely restored if induced 3 days after a single injection of the serum.

Finally, it has been shown that in mice infected with Rous virus [562] and cytomegaly virus [477, 478] the quantity of interferon induced by intravenous injection of NDV is reduced.

In a series of investigations published recently [635a, 659a, 666a] evidence was obtained that cycloheximide increases the synthesis of interferon induced *in vivo* and *in vitro* by viruses and synthetic polyribonucleotides.

8.4. Interferon Production in the Immune Organism

Few attempts have been made to study interferon production in the immune organism. No interferon has been found in the lung tissues of immune mice infected with a sublethal dose of influenza virus. If a lethal dose of the virus was given, interferon appeared for a short time only. In the control group of animals interferon was found from the 2nd to the 5th day after infection [113, 407, 495]. Other results were obtained when interferon production by leukocytes of the immune animal was determined. Glasgow [311], for instance, found an increase in the production of interferon by the peritoneal leukocytes of immune mice vaccinated intraperitoneally with Chikungunya virus. One month after the last immunization, peritoneal leukocytes treated with homologous virus were tested. Interferon production varied from one experiment to another, but most frequently the immune leukocytes produced from 2 to 8 times more interferon than leukocytes of the control animals. Determination of interferon production by leukocytes with heterologous virus gave similar results with the immune and control animals. Consequently, stimulation of interferon production in the immune organism was specific in character.

Other work has not confirmed Glasgow's results. Grokhovskay [54] found no difference in the ability of leukocytes from mice vaccinated with tick-borne encephalitis virus and of control mice to produce interferon. Incidentally, Glasgow worked with freshly obtained leukocytes in which interferon was induced immediately, whereas in Grokhovskaya's investigation the cells were used after preliminary growth in tubes. During this period, a new population of cells presumably appeared, and as the work of Solov'ev and Alekseeva [154] has shown, immunity is not transmitted from an immune parent population to the progeny *in vitro*.

Meanwhile no increase in the production of serum and leukocytic interferons likewise was found in our experiments in mice immune to the viruses of Newcastle disease and Western equine encephalomyelitis. The quantity of interferon formed by the immune animals and by their leukocytes was always smaller than that formed by control (unvaccinated) mice.

8.5. The Role of Interferon in the Pathogenesis of Virus Infections

One of the most interesting aspects of the problem of interferon is its role in the pathogenesis of virus infection. However, the results so far obtained in this direction are contradictory.

The discovery of interferon in the organ most severely affected by a particular infection, the decrease in the concentration of virus after accumulation of interferon in its maximal concentration, and the fact that virus and interferon disappear simultaneously in experimental influenza all provided the basis on which Isaacs and Hitchcock [371] postulated that interferon is one of the most important factors of defense against primary virus infection. It is important to emphasize that in these experiments interferon appeared much earlier than antibodies. Antibodies did not appear until the 7th day, when the concentration of virus in the lungs was already considerably reduced. Consequently, a correlation was found between the beginning of recovery of the animals and the time of maximal interferon production. These results were confirmed by other investigations [343].

Friedman and co-workers [296] found that if antibody formation and hypersensitivity of delayed type were blocked by methotrexate or x-ray irradiation in guinea pigs infected with vaccinia virus, the process of recovery followed a normal course. In their opinion this result indicates that recovery is controlled by mechanisms other than antibodies. As a result of the discovery of interferon in the sites of skin lesions they consider that interferon formation must in fact play a role in the recovery process. This view is supported by evidence to show that persons with hypo- or agammaglobulinemia recover from virus infections despite their inability to produce antibodies, although they are still capable of producing interferon [319].

A number of factors reducing resistance of the body to virus infection are known but the mechanism of their action so far eludes discovery. Attempts have therefore been made to attribute it to interferon formation. Reference has previously been made to investigations which demonstrated a decrease in interferon production during exposure to cold, x-rays, noise stress, prolonged vibration, poisoning with alcohol, and histamine and endotoxin shock. In particular, as several workers have shown, the effect of temperature is mediated through interferon [438, 439, 500, 516, 518].

Lwoff [438] postulated that interferon is the most important nonspecific factor of immunity, for the other factors (temperature, partial oxygen pressure, etc.) act indirectly, only through their effect on interferon production.

The effects of hormones, which reduce interferon production and which aggravate the course of virus infections, must also be mentioned.

The important role of interferon in pathogenesis is also shown by the fact that young animals, which are more susceptible to virus infections, have been shown to produce less interferon and to be less sensitive to the antiviral action of interferon than mature animals.

Factors determining the virulence of viruses have received little study. In this connection some very interesting investigations have shown that there is a connection between virulence and interferon-producing activity and between virulence and sensitivity to interferon.

Investigations have shown that virulent strains of viruses are inferior inducers of interferon and are less sensitive to its action than avirulent strains. The vaccine strain of measles virus, for instance, is a more active interferon inducer than the virulent strain [260]. Attenuated strains of polioviruses induced interferon production in titers of $1:2$ to $1:4$, whereas more virulent strains (Brunhilde, MEF-1, Leon, and CHAT) induced no interferon whatever. Cultivation of virulent and attenuated strains of foot and mouth disease virus in tissue cultures showed that virulent viruses reproduce to higher titers. Meanwhile avirulent strains, reproducing less readily in these cells, induced larger quantities of interferon than virulent strains [533, 534].

A study of Semliki forest virus in calf kidney cells [517] showed
that more virulent strains are less sensitive to interferon and induce
the production of less interferon than avirulent strains. Other investigators have drawn attention to the lower sensitivity of more
virulent viruses to interferon [143, 147, 148, 259, 516-518]. Some
of them associate the interferon-inducing activity of the oncogenic
viruses with their oncogenic activity. In particular, Friedman [298]
and co-workers claim that interferon induced by the M-variant of
polyoma virus plays an important role in its low oncogenic activity.
A variant of the same virus possessing high oncogenic activity did
not induce interferon production, according to these workers'
observations, in tissue cultures. Similar relationships were subsequently found in experiments on mice [299].

The experiments of Solov'ev and co-workers [171] showed
that more virulent strains of NDV are less sensitive to interferon
than avirulent strains. According to Ho [346], since virulent viruses
actively inhibit biosynthesis in cells they cannot be good inducers
of interferon.

Some workers associate a long stay of the virus in the body
with weak induction of interferon by the virus and low sensitivity
to it. Hypotheses of this type have been expressed in relation to
the viruses of herpes [302] and cytomegaly [314, 477, 478]. Yet
it must be noted that in some virus infections the virulence of the
agents cannot be correlated sufficiently reliably with their interferon-inducing activity or with their sensitivity to interferon.

In particular, experiments on mice have shown that virulent
and avirulent variants of Sindbis virus possess similar interferon-
inducing activity. Despite identical quantities of interferon in
the brain of the mice, the outcome of the infection differed. It
was accordingly concluded that interferon evidently has no role
to play in the pathogenesis of virus diseases affecting the central
nervous system [502, 572, 575].

Mention has already been made of investigations with influenza virus [361, 433] and with Tahyna virus [203] in which
adaptation of the virus to mice and an increase in its virulence
for the animals were accompanied, not by a decrease but, on the
contrary, by an increase in interferon production.

In the experiments of Solov'ev and co-workers [170] no difference was found between the interferon-inducing activity of

strains of NDV of different virulence in chickens. In experiments on chick embryos with 8 strains of NDV differing in their virulence to chickens, Baron [206, 208] found no definite relationship between virulence and interferon-inducing activity.

It can accordingly be considered that the virulence of viruses can be associated only partially with their activity as interferon inducers and with their sensitivity to interferon.

Several investigations have been undertaken to determine the role of interferon in the species- and race-specific resistance of animals to certain viruses.

Vainio and co-workers [561], in order to study the mechanism of natural resistance of lines of inbred mice genetically resistant and sensitive to viruses, infected animals intracerebrally with West Nile virus. They found that less interferon is produced in the brain of mice resistant to this virus than in the brain of highly susceptible animals. They accordingly concluded that interferon does not play a role in the natural resistance of mice to West Nile virus. A similar conclusion was reached by Rusanova and Solov'ev [138], who studied the mechanisms of natural immunity in A2G mice to influenza virus. These workers consider that inborn immunity to influenza is due to genetic mechanisms other than the intensity of interferon formation.

Many of the results cited above demonstrate the important role of interferon in the pathogenesis of virus infections. At the same time, some experimental results cannot be explained on the ground of the effect of interferon. Correlation has not always been found between interferon formation and the outcome of the virus infection. Despite a high interferon concentration in the brain of animals, as a rule they die from certain virus infections causing encephalitis. For this reason interferon has not been ascribed a role in the pathogenesis of infections leading to involvement of the central nervous system. In our view, however, if consideration is paid to the natural pathways whereby arboviruses enter the body, and to the presence of a viremia in the pathogenesis of these infections, it does not seem possible to draw definite conclusions purely from the discovery of interferon in the mouse brain.

Baron and co-workers [205, 210, 211, 212] consider that endogenous interferon may not only play a role in the elimination

of virus from the body in an established infection, but also that
it may exhibit an antiviral action from the beginning of the infection,
both at the time of its passage through the portals of entry and
also during the viremia.

8.6. A Study of Interferon Formation *in vivo* and *in vitro* (by Leukocytes) in Experimental Virus Infections

To study the role of interferon in the pathogenesis of and immunity to virus infections, investigations of various types have
been carried out. Experiments were performed on animals infected with viruses differing in their tropism. Concurrently, interferon formation was studied in patients with known virus, presumptive virus, and nonvirus diseases. Most of the investigations were
connected with the study of the formation of leukocytic interferon
under normal and pathological conditions and with the possibility
of using this test as an indicator of the reactivity of the body.

Depending on the properties of the viruses, the animals
were infected intracerebrally (WEE), intranasally (influenza), or
intraperitoneally (ectromelia). In some special experiments the
viruses were injected by other routes. At various times (usually
at intervals of 24 h) after infection, the spleen, liver, kidneys, lungs,
brain, and blood were taken from 5-10 mice.

A 10% suspension was prepared from the organs in medium
199, centrifuged at 3000 rpm for 20 min, and the supernatant was
divided into two parts. One part was investigated for the presence
of the virus by infection of chick embryos (influenza) or mice (ectromelia, WEE), while the other part was immediately treated as
described previously to inactivate the virus. Blood was obtained
for estimation of the concentration of virus and interferon and
treated in the usual manner. Newcastle disease virus was used
at the rate of 10 TCD_{50} per cell as the interferon inducer for the
leukocytes *in vitro*. For determination of interferon, materials
from the mice were titrated on primary mouse fibroblasts or
transplanted L cells, and materials from the human subjects on
primary cultures or strains of diploid cells of human embryonic
myodermal tissue. Vesicular stomatitis virus was used as the
test virus.

In the study of interferon production in virus infections the
problem of how to judge the ability of the host to produce inter-

feron was encountered. Considering that leukocytes are active
interferon producers and that they can be obtained comparatively
easily, the correlation between production of serum interferon
by the organism *in vivo* and by its leukocytes *in vitro* was studied.
By determining this correlation it was possible to judge to what extent interferon production by leukocytes depends on the genotypical
properties of the individual and whether, by using leukocytes, the
ability of the organism to produce interferon can be assessed. In
order to study these problems inbred lines of mice were used.

Inbred lines of mice differ in their genotypical characters
and in their sensitivity to viruses. Eleven lines of mice were used
for the experiments. Interferon was determined in the serum 4 h
after intravenous injection of 10^8 TCD_{50} of NDV. The results of
the tests are given in Table 100. The experiments were carried
out jointly with N. R. Gutman and Yu. B. Fedorova.

Compared with mice of other lines and with noninbred mice,
those of lines A and CC57Br produced interferon in higher
intensity. Four hours after injection of the virus, interferon was
detected in their serum in dilutions of up to 1 : 128, while in the

TABLE 100. Discovery of Interferon in Serum of Various Lines
of Mice and Its Production
by Leukocytes

Line of mice	Interferon titer	
	serum	leukocytic
Noninbred	16	n.i.
C3H	16	4
C57BL/6	16	n.i.
CBA	32	n.i.
BaLB/c	32	n.i.
A2G	32	n.i.
C3HA	64	n.i.
AKR	б4	n.i.
DBA	64	n.i.
C3Hf/Pul	64	n.i.
A	128	32
CC57Br	>128	32

Note: n.i., not investigated

serum of the inbred animals and of certain other lines it was found in dilutions no greater than 1 : 16 to 1 : 32.

It can accordingly be concluded from this investigation that the level of interferon production *in vivo* depends to some extent on the genotypical characters of the animal.

Later lines of mice yielding the highest and lowest titers of serum interferon (CC57Br, A, and C3H) were used. Newcastle disease virus was injected intravenously into 10 animals of each line; leukocytes were obtained from the same number of animals and treated *in vitro* with the same virus. The concentration of interferon in the serum and in the culture fluid of the leukocyte suspension was then determined.

On the basis of the results of these experiments, which are also given in Table 100, it can be concluded that if leukocytes are removed from the body it is possible to determine whether the body is able or not to produce interferon. We later used the opportunity thus afforded to assess reactivity in experiments on animals and in clinical trials. Another reason why the ability of leukocytes to produce interferon was used as a test is that the leukocytes are the most important interferon-producing cells in the body.

8.6.1. Interferon Formation in Experimental Influenza

Noninbred mice weighing 7-8 g were infected intranasally under ether anesthesia with influenza A virus, strain PR-8, and the organs of the animals were investigated at different times after infection by the method described at the beginning of this section.

The dynamics of the interferon content in the various organs of mice and its correlation with reproduction of the virus in the lungs of animals infected with 100 LD_{50} of the virus were determined in the initial experiments. All the infected animals died by the 7th day after infection.

As Table 101 and Fig. 11 show, the concentration of virus in the lung tissues reached a maximum after 48 h and remained at a constant level until death of the animals. Until the 3rd or 4th day after infection there was a direct correlation between reproduction of the virus and the interferon concentration in the lung. Later, however, despite a high virus concentration, the interferon concentration fell. No interferon was found in the lung on the 6th-

TABLE 101. Dynamics of Interferon Formation and Reproduction of Virus in Lungs of Mice

Day of investigation	Titer of virus, $ID_{50}/0.1$ ml	Interferon titer
0	10^1	<20
1	10^5	640
2	10^7	640
4	10^7	640
5	10^7	320
6	10^7	<20
7	10^7	<20

7th day, when mortality among the animals was very high. Similar results were obtained by estimation of interferon in the plasma, spleen, and kidneys. The interferon concentration in these tissues also corresponded to its level in the lungs of the infected animals, but its concentration in the serum and spleen was lower. The interferon concentration in the kidneys and lungs was similar, which could be evidence of the excretion of interferon through the kidneys.

Having established the direct correlation between interferon production in healthy animals and by leukocytes *in vitro*, it was interesting to investigate the interferon levels in mice infected with influenza virus. A similar relationship was found in these experiments also. At the beginning of the infection the leukocytes formed the inhibitor equally with the control, but later, after the 4th day, their reactivity decreased and by the 6th–7th day, at the stage of development of lethal pneumonia, it was completely lost. Consequently, the ability of leukocytes to produce interferon *in vitro* was thus revealed as the mirror image of the progressive deterioration in the state of the experimental animal (Fig. 12).

The dynamics of antibody formation also was investigated by the neutralization, hemagglutination inhibition (HIT), and complement fixation (CFT) tests. The most interesting results were obtained by the study of animals from the 4th to the 7th day after infection, when the leukocytes had lost their ability to produce

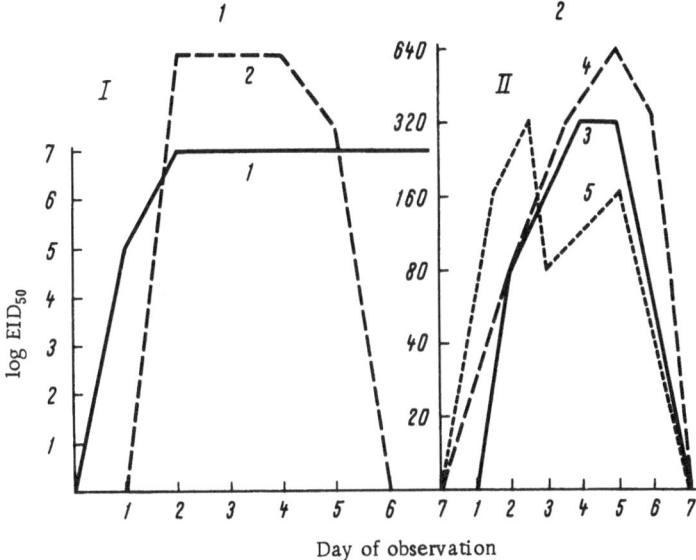

Fig. 11. Correlation between reproduction of virus and interferon formation in mice infected with influenza A virus in a
dose of 100 LD_{50}: I) concentration of virus (1) and interferon
(2) in lung; II) concentration of interferon in plasma (3),
spleen (4), and kidney (5).

interferon and before virus-neutralizing antibodies or antihemag-
glutinins had appeared in the blood stream. Complement-fixing
antibodies in a titer of 1:20 were not found in the surviving animals
until the 7th day (Table 102).

In the subsequent experiments interferon formation was
studied in mice and in their leukocytes *in vitro* after infection with
sublethal doses of virus (about 1 LD_{50}). In these experiments the
mice developed a nonlethal influenza and it was possible to investigate the leukocytic interferon in the course of the infectious
disease and during convalescence.

Organs and leukocytes were taken for investigation only from
those animals in which pneumonic foci had developed. The results
show that after infection with a sublethal dose of virus, just as
after infection with 100 LD_{50}, no interferon could be found in the
lungs even though the virus was present in them. Meanwhile, in
nonlethal influenza the leukocytes did not lose their ability to

TABLE 102. Results of Determination of Antibodies in Serum and Ability of Leukocytes to Produce Interferon in Mice Infected with
Influenza Virus

Day of observation	HIT	CFR	Neutralization test	Titer of leukocytic interferon
1	0	0	0	64
2	0	0	0	64
3	0	0	0	8
4	0	0	0	0
7	0	20	0	0

Note: 0 means that no antibodies were found in a dilution of
1:10 or higher.

produce interferon at any time during the period of observation
(Fig. 12).

8.6.2. Interferon Formation in Experimental Ectromelia

Experiments were carried out on noninbred mice weighing
7-8 g which were infected intraperitoneally with 1000 LD$_{50}$ of the

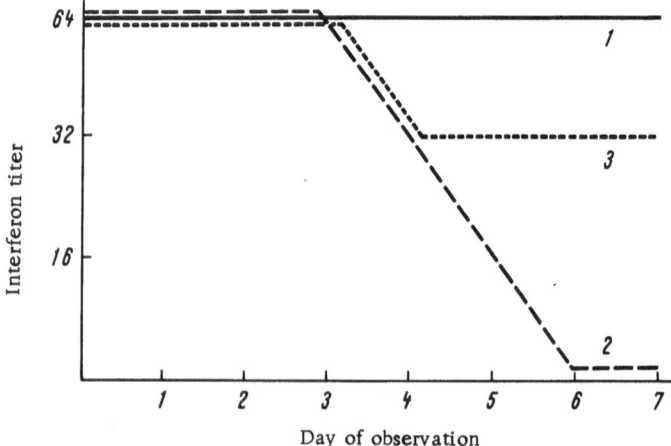

Fig. 12. Ability of mouse leukocytes to produce interferon
during lethal and sublethal influenza: 1) healthy mice; 2)
lethal infection; 3) sublethal infection.

TABLE 103. Dynamics of Reproduction of Virus and Interferon Formation in Organs of Mice Infected with Ectromelia Virus

| Organ or tissue | Day of observation | | | | | |
| | 1st | | 2nd | | 3rd | |
	virus	interferon	virus	interferon	virus	interferon
Liver	$10^{3.0}$	640	$10^{6.0}$	640	$10^{6.0}$	320
Spleen	$10^{3.0}$	640	$10^{6.0}$	640	$10^{6.0}$	320
Kidney	n.i.	320	n.i.	640	n.i.	160
Lung	n.i.	80	n.i.	320	n.i.	80
Blood	10^1	8	10^5	16	10^3	32

| Organ or tissue | Day of observation | | | | | |
| | 4th | | 5th | | 6th | |
	virus	interferon	virus	interferon	virus	interferon
Liver	$10^{7.0}$	80	$10^{7.0}$	40	$10^{7.0}$	20
Spleen	$10^{7.0}$	80	$10^{7.0}$	40	$10^{7.0}$	20
Kidney	n.i.	80	n.i.	80	n.i.	40
Lung	n.i.	20	n.i.	<20	n.i.	<20
Blood	10^3	16	10^3	4	10^3	2

Note: n.i., not investigated.

virus (strain T). Organs and blood were taken at various times after infection and the ability of the leukocytes to produce interferon was tested. The interferon and virus concentrations were determined in the organs and serum. As a rule the animals died by the 5th-6th day after infection. The results are given in Table 103.

As Table 103 shows the concentration of virus reached a maximum in the liver and spleen 48 h after infection and remained at that level until the animals died. The interferon concentration in the other organs also reached a maximum after 48 h, but by the 5th-6th day either interferon could no longer be found in them or its titers were extremely low.

The study of the ability of leukocytes to produce interferon *in vitro* during the development of experimental ectromelia in mice showed that in this diesase, just as in experimental influenza, at the time of death of the mice the ability of their leukocytes to produce interferon had fallen sharply in the absence of virus-neutralizing antibodies.

TABLE 104. Detection of Interferon and Virus in the Brain of Mice Infected Intracerebrally with WEE Virus

Day of observation	Virus titer	Interferon titer
1st	10^6	320
2nd	10^6	320
3rd	10^7	640
4th	10^7	640

TABLE 105. Interferon Production by Leukocytes of Mice of Different Ages

Age or weight	Interferon produced by leukocytes
25-30 g	16
7-8 g	8-16
Newborn, aged 1-2 days	<2-4

8.6.3. Interferon Formation in Experimental Western Equine Encephalomyelitis (WEE)

Mice were infected intracerebrally or intramuscularly with WEE virus. The subsequent tests were carried out as in influenza.

A direct correlation was observed in the animals' brain between reproduction of the virus and interferon formation (Table 104), and titers of both virus and interferon reached almost their maximum levels 24 h after infection, remaining at these levels until death of the animals. Most animals died on the 4th day after infection. Interferon also was found in the serum of the animals in a titer of 1:8 to 1:64. No interferon was found in the spleen, liver, and lungs. WEE virus evidently induced interferon formation only in the brain tissue, and the serum interferon was the result of its formation in the brain and subsequent passage into the blood stream or it might possibly have been the result of the viremia.

The ability of the leukocytes to produce interferon also was studied in mice infected with WEE virus. The intensity of production of leukocytic interferon fell during observations over a period of 4 days. Consequently, a state of areactivity of the leukocytes as regards interferon production also developed at the time of death of the mice, thus demonstrating the essential similarity between interferon production in experimental WEE and in influenza and ectromelia.

8.6.4. Interferon Formation *in vivo* in Animals of Different Ages

Considering the conflicting nature of data in the literature on the intensity of interferon production in animals of different ages, comparative studies were carried out jointly with A. E. Gumennik and M. S. Bektemirova with influenza and WEE viruses. Newborn mice aged 1-2 days and mice aged 4-5 weeks (weighing 7-8 g) were used in the experiments. The animals were infected intranasally with influenza virus and intracerebrally with WEE virus. The content of virus and interferon was determined in the affected organ in four animals of each age group at various times after infection with 100 LD_{50}. The virus was detected by titration in chick embryos (influenza) and in cultures of chick fibroblasts (WEE). Interferon was titrated in L cells with vesicular stomatitis virus.

As Table 105 shows, interferon production was weaker in the newborn mice than in mice weighing 7-8 g.

Considering the great importance of cells of the reticulo-endothelial system, the ability of the leukocytes of newborn mice weighing 7-8 and 25-30 g to produce interferon also was determined. The interferon inducer was NDV in a dose of 10 TCD_{50} per leukocyte.

The results given in Table 106 show that leukocytes of newborn mice produce 4-16 times less interferon than the leukocytes of adult mice.

Besides studying the interferon-synthesizing activity of leukocytes *in vitro*, together with A. E. Parushina we investigated age differences in serum interferon production in animals of different species. Experiments were carried out on albino mice, rabbits, and guinea pigs, animals which differ in their postembryonic state. In mice, because of the sharp changes in their sensitivity to viruses (arboviruses, Coxsackie viruses) during the first week of life, serum interferon production was determined at the ages of 1-2 days, 4 days, 7 days, and 4-5 weeks. The dose of inducer (NDV) injected depended on the animals' body weight.

As Table 107 shows, mice aged 1-2 days produced the least quantities of interferon. However, their ability to synthesize interferon increased rapidly, so that mice aged 4 days produced 2.6 times more, those aged 7 days nearly 3 times more, and those aged 4 days produced 8 times more interferon than the mice aged 1-2 days. The mice aged 4-5 weeks produced 32 times more interferon than the newborn mice.

TABLE 106. Dynamics of Reproduction of Virus and Interferon Formation in Animals of Different Ages

Infecting virus	Age or weight	Organ tested	Titration of	Day of observation						
				1st	2nd	3rd	4th	5th	6th	7th
Influenza PR-8	7-8 g	Lung	Virus	$10^{2.0}$	$10^{6.0}$	$10^{7.0}$	$10^{7.0}$	$10^{7.0}$	$10^{7.0}$	$10^{7.0}$
			Interferon	80	80	160	160	20	<20	<20
	Newborn, aged 1-2 days	Lung	Virus	$10^{2.0}$	$10^{7.0}$	$10^{8.0}$	$10^{8.0}$	$10^{8.0}$	$10^{8.0}$	$10^{8.0}$
			Interferon	40	40	40	80	20	<20	
	7-8 g	Brain	Virus	$10^{6.0}$	$10^{6.0}$	$10^{7.0}$	$10^{7.0}$	Animals died		
			Interferon	320	320	320	640			
WEE	Newborn, aged 1-2 days	Brain	Virus	$10^{7.0}$	$10^{7.0}$	$10^{8.0}$	$10^{8.0}$	Animals died		
			Interferon	40	40	20	20			

It will be clear from Table 108 that the production of serum interferon in the groups of rabbits tested differed significantly. Animals aged 6 months produced almost 20 times more interferon than newborn rabbits. However, by contrast with the rabbits, newborn guinea pigs produced serum interferon just as actively as the adult animals.

In this connection it must be mentioned that guinea pigs are distinguished by being born in a highly developed state; they can see, they are covered with hair, and they have the typical movements of adults. The high level of immunoreactivity of newborn guinea pigs by comparison with rabbits is also known from the observations of Khalyapina (1949) and others. Consequently, the reticuloendothelial cells of newborn mice and rabbits are much less capable of producing interferon, and this reflects the imperfect development of this protective mechanism in these species.

8.6.5. Individual Differences in Interferon Formation

The role of the factor of individuality in the onset and development of virus diseases is now established beyond all doubt and

TABLE 107. Production of Serum
Interferon by Mice of Different Ages

Age, days	Geometric mean interferon titer	P
1-2	64 ± 1.9	
4	177 ± 1.4	0.001
7	512 ± 1.0	
28-35	2048 ± 1.0	

TABLE 108. Results of Determination of Serum
Interferon Formation in Rabbits and Guinea Pigs

Species	Age	Number tested	Geometric mean interferon titer
Rabbit	3 days	25	1,780 ± 1.3
	6 months	12	32,768 ± 1.6
Guinea pig	1-2 days	29	1,910 ± 1.2
	2-3 months	15	1,910 ± 1.5

is confirmed by everyday clinical and epidemiological observation. This can be clearly illustrated by experiments in which animals are infected with minimal lethal doses of virus. The differences in sensitivity under these conditions may vary from complete immunity to the same infecting dose in some animals and development of the disease followed by death in others.

In immunology the factor of individuality is linked with extraordinary variability of the complex system of protective reactions. In this system the individual differences in the quantity of interferon produced and in the mechanism of its production have received the least study. Nevertheless, we and other workers have shown that the level of resistance conferred on cells by interferon is directly proportional to its concentration. Consequently, the individual intensity of endogenous interferon production may have a significant effect on the onset and course of virus infections.

In conjunction with M. S. Bektemirova and A. E. Parushina we studied individual differences in interferon production in man and animals. The results obtained by animal experiments are given below.

8.6.5.1. Individual Differences in Serum Interferon Production in Noninbred and Inbred Mice

The results of determination of serum interferon in noninbred and inbred mice are given in Table 109. Mice received 1 ml NDV (titer 10^8 TCD_{50}/ml) by injection into the caudal vein. After an interval of 4 h, 0.02 ml blood was taken from the same caudal vein, diluted in medium 199, treated with HCl, and then tested for its interferon concentration in fourfold dilutions starting with 1:400. Interferon-synthesizing activity was detected in 102 noninbred and 272 inbred mice (Table 109).

The individual ability to produce interferon varied within wide limits among noninbred mice. While in some animals (12.7%) no interferon was found in the serum, others possessed high interferon-synthesizing activity. The most numerous group (45%) consist ed of mice producing interferon in titers of 1:6400, 26.5% of animals synthesized interferon in titers of 1:400 to 1:1600, and 14.7% in a titer of 1:25,600.

The lines of mice which were tested were not absolutely uniform as regards their ability to produce interferon after injection of NDV. However, most animals of the same strain formed interferon with the same intensity. For instance, after receiving injections of NDV, the interferon titers in mice of line BALB/C did not exceed 1 : 1600 in 95% of cases, in 80% of line A mice the serum interferon titers were between 1 : 400 and 1 : 6400, and in 85% of the CC57Br mice the titers were between 1 : 6400 and 1 : 25,600.

Consequently, among the strains of mice tested, those which produced interferon most actively belonged to strain CC57Br, and those which were least active to strain BALB/C.

8.6.5.2. Individual Interferon Production in Mice Infected with WEE Virus

Albino mice aged 1-2 and 7 days and 4-5 weeks were infected intracerebrally. On the appearance of signs of the disease in the animals the brain was removed and tested individually for its interferon content. The results, given in Table 110, show that individual interferon production varies with the general age pattern of interferon formation: with an increase in age the individual indices are shifted toward higher titers although they still retain their wide variation.

For instance, among mice aged 1-2 days the most numerous group consisted of animals which produced interferon in a titer below 1 : 80; the corresponding titer for 7-day mice was 1 : 5120 and for mice aged 4-5 weeks it was 1 : 20,480.

8.6.5.3. Individual Differences in Serum Interferon Production in Rabbits and Guinea Pigs

Experiments were carried out on rabbits aged 3 days and 6 months and on guinea pigs immediately after birth and at the

TABLE 109. Individual Differences in Serum Interferon Production in Mice

Strain of animals	Total number tested	Number with interferon titer of							
		below 400		400-1600		6400		25,600	
		abs.	%	abs.	%	abs.	%	abs.	%
Noninbred	102	13	12.7	27	26.5	46	45.0	15	14.7
BALB/C	105	10	9.5	90	85.7	5	4.8	0	0
A	57	11	19.2	21	36.8	25	43.9	0	0
CC57Br	60	0	0	9	15.0	18	30.0	33	55.0

TABLE 110. Individual Interferon Production in Brain of Mice
Infected with WEE Virus

Age, days	Number of animals tested	Animals (%) with interferon titer of						
		below 80	80	320	1,280	5,120	20,480	81,920
1-2	32	40.62	31.22	15.62	9.37	3.12	0	0
7	26	3.84	7.69	19.23	19.23	38.46	0	7.69
28-35	14	0	0	7.14	7.14	35.71	42.57	0

age of 2-3 months. The rabbits received injections of 0.5 and
5 ml NDV, and the guinea pigs 0.2 and 5 ml NDV, respectively,
intraperitoneally.

The results given in Table 111 indicate wide individual differences in the ability of the animals to synthesize serum interferon. The interferon titers in rabbits varied from 1:1024 to
1:262,144 in adults and from 1:64 to 1:16,384 in the newborn
animals. The range of variation of newborn and adult guinea pigs
was from 1:64 to 1:16,384.

Different species of animals thus showed wide individual
variations in their ability to form interferon, and the deviations
from the mean level of interferon production by different individuals
were statistically significant.

8.6.6. Effect of Cooling, Internal Irradiation, and ACTH on
Production of Serum Interferon in Mice

We have also studied the effect of the environmental temperature of animals, ACTH, and internal irradiation on the

TABLE 111. Individual Serum Interferon Production by Rabbits and
Guinea Pigs

Species	Age	No. of animals tested	Number with interferon titer of						
			64	256	1,024	4,096	16,384	65,536	26,214
Rabbit	3 days	25	1	3	9	8	4	0	0
	6 mon.	12	0	0	1	2	2	4	3
Guinea	1-2 days	29	3	3	5	14	4	0	0
pig	2-3 mon.	24	1	3	3	17	0	0	0

formation of serum interferon in mice induced by intravenous injection of NDV.

Animals weighing 18-20 g were used in the experiment. To determine the effect of the environmental temperature of the animals on interferon formation the mice were divided into 3 groups and kept for 18-20 h before injection of NDV and for 4 h thereafter at 4°, 18-20°, and 37°C, respectively. The mice were then exsanguinated and their serum interferon concentration determined in a primary culture of mouse fibroblasts.

The results confirmed that the environmental temperature of animals exerts a marked effect on interferon production *in vivo.* Interferon production reached its highest intensity at 37°C, while mice kept at 4°C produced no interferon (Table 112).

In joint experiments with Yu. B. Fedorova the effect of ACTH on interferon production was studied. Injection of 50 units 24 h before the virus completely inhibited interferon formation. Meanwhile, interferon was detected in the serum of control animals not receiving ACTH in dilutions of up to 1 : 16. ACTH, which stimulates corticoid synthesis *in vivo,* evidently inhibits interferon formation.

In experiments to study the effect of internal irradiation mice received P^{32} in a dose of 2 μCi/g body weight (specific activity 89 mCi/ml). One week after injection of 35 μCi P^{32} the animals received an intravenous injection of 10^7 TCD_{50}/ml NDV and they were exsanguinated 4 h later. Control animals were injected with virus only. The results showed that internal irradiation

TABLE 112. Effect of Temperature of Keeping Animals on Production of Serum Interferon

Temperature	Interferon
4°	<4
18-20°	16
37°	32

TABLE 113. Effect of Internal Irradiation on Interferon Formation

Group of animals	Interferon titer
Irradiated	256
Control	>4096

of the animals sharply inhibited interferon production *in vivo*. The titers of serum interferon in the irradiated animals were more than 16 times lower than in the unirradiated controls (Table 113).

The experiments thus confirmed that lowering the environmental temperature of animals and administration of ACTH reduce the production of serum interferon. It was also shown for the first time that interferon production is significantly inhibited after internal irradiation with P^{32}. We [26] and others have previously shown that internal irradiation aggravates the course of virus infections. It can be concluded from the results now described that this effect is partly due to a decrease in interferon production.

8.7. Relationship between Interferon Formation and Sensitivity of Animals to Some Virus Infections

8.7.1. Relationship between Interferon Formation and Reproduction of Viruses in Chick Embryos of Different Ages

The relationship between interferon formation and the reproduction of Sindbis and WEE viruses was studied in chick embryos aged 6 and 13 days.

The chick embryos were infected in the allantoic cavity and the fluid obtained from it 48 h after infection was used as the test material. The dose given for infection was 10 TCD_{50} of virus per embryo. The results are given in Table 114.

As Table 114 shows, 6-day embryos produce less interferon than 13-day embryos. At the same time, significant differences were observed in the intensity of reproduction of the virus, which was almost 100 times higher in the younger chick embryos.

These results suggest that the lower interferon-synthesizing activity of 6-day than of 13-day chick embryos is responsible for the more rapid reproduction of Sindbis and WEE viruses in the former.

8.7.2. Relationship between the Reproduction of WEE Virus and Interferon Formation in the Mouse Brain

The relationship between interferon production and reproduction of WEE virus was investigated in mice aged 1-2 and 7 days,

TABLE 114. Relationship between Interferon Production and Reproduction of Sindbis and WEE Viruses in Chick Embryos

Virus	6-day embryos			13-day embryos			
	Number of observations	Geometric mean titer, M ± n		Number of observations	Geometric mean titer, M ± n		
		of virus, TCD_{50}	of interferon		of virus, TCD_{50}	of interferon	P
Sindbis	29	7.5 ± 0.43	2.4 ± 2.2	29	5.6 ± 0.48	14.8 ± 1.1	<0.01
WEE	14	7.5 ± 0.46	1.2 ± 1.1	16	5.0 ± 0.38	7.8 ± 0.8	<0.01

TABLE 115. Relationship between Course of WEE and Interferon Formation in Mice

Age	Number in group	Geometric mean titers, M ± m		Number of mice dying after					
		virus, TCD_{50}	interferon	1 day	2 days	3 days	4 days	5 days	6 days
1-2 days	32	8.0 ± 0.3	23.98 ± 1.6	26/81.2	6/18.8	0	0	0	0
7 days	26	8.2 ± 0.4	1,349 ± 1.5	0	24/92.3	2/7.7	0	0	0
4-5 weeks	28	8.0 ± 0.6	6,166 ± 1.4	0	20/71.3	8/28.7	0	0	0
1 year	28	n.i.	22,910 ± 1.1	0	0	16/57.1	7/25.0	5/17.0	0

Note: Numerator represents absolute number of mice dying, denominator shows number dying as a percentage of the total.

4-5 weeks, and 1 year. The mice of the first two age groups received 10 LD_{50} of the virus, and those aged 4-5 weeks and 1 year received 30 LD_{50} of the virus intracerebrally.

The duration of the incubation period and the mortality (in %) were subsequently recorded. The brain was taken from the mice just before death and tested individually for its content of virus and interferon. The results are given in Table 115.

It is clear from Table 115 that in all age groups the animals began to die when reproduction of the virus reached approximately 10^8 TCD_{50}/ml, at which time the intensity of interferon formation varied very considerably. At first glance the intensity of interferon production did not affect the level of reproduction of the virus. However, it must be remembered that the results given in this table were obtained by investigation of the brain only during the period of development of paralysis, which took place at different times in mice of different age groups. The lower the intensity of interferon production in the mice, the shorter the incubation period of the disease and the more rapidly the virus accumulated up to the critical lethal level.

8.7.3. Relationship between Individual Interferon Formation and Susceptibility of Animals to WEE Virus and to Fixed Rabies Virus

The results given in Table 116 were obtained jointly with M. S. Bektemirova after determination of individual differences in interferon production by rabbits and their relationship to sus-

TABLE 116. Relationship between Interferon-Inducing Activity and Susceptibility of Rabbits to Fixed Rabies Virus

Interferon titers	Distribution of animals			
	interferon titers		susceptibility to virus	
	abs.	%	abs.	%
4,096-16,384	18	26.46	17[*]	94.44
32,788-65,576	14	20.58	4	28.57
131,152-262,304	21	30.88	1	4.75
524,608-4,196,864	15	22.05	0	0

[*]Number of rabbits developing disease of the total number infected.

ceptibility to fixed rabies virus (the animals were infected intramuscularly 30 days after determination of their individual interferon production).

Table 116 shows that the individual interferon-synthesizing
activity of animals varied inversely with their susceptibility to
fixed rabies virus. For instance, of 18 animals with a low titer
of serum interferon (4096-16,384) 17 developed disease, while
among 15 rabbits with the highest titer, not one developed rabies.

The correlation between the intensity of interferon formation by inbred mice and their susceptibility to WEE was next
investigated. Susceptibility of the animals was estimated by determination of LD_{50} of the same virus-containing material for different strains of animals. The results are given in Table 117.

The results given in Table 117 clearly indicate the important
role of interferon in the pathogenesis of WEE. Mice of strain
CC57Br produce interferon more actively than BALB/C mice and
were more resistant than the latter to WEE virus.

8.7.4. Relationship between Individual Interferon Formation and
Skin Reaction of Rabbits to Vaccinia Virus.

In a joint investigation with A. E. Parushina the intensity
of the skin reaction of rabbits infected with vaccinia virus was
compared with individual differences in interferon formation.

Chinchilla rabbits weighing 2.5-3 kg were used. On the day
before the experiment an area of skin measuring 10 × 5 cm on
the lateral surface of the animals' trunk was shaved. The rabbits

TABLE 117. Relationship
between Production of Serum Interferon in Mice and Their Susceptibility to WEE Virus

Strain of animals	Most typical interferon titer	LD_{50} of material
BALB/C	400-1,600	$10^{4.5}$
A	6,400	$10^{3.0}$
CC57Br	25,600	$10^{2.0}$

were infected by intradermal injection of material from tenfold
dilutions of vaccinia virus, strain Tashkent. The skin reaction
was assessed on the 4th-5th day after infection by Groth's test.

Later, 1 month after infection, the concentration of hemagglutinins against vaccinia virus in the animals' blood was determined and the ability of the rabbits to produce serum interferon
investigated. For this purpose the rabbits were injected intravenously with 5 ml NDV (titer 10^8 TCD_{50}/ml) and blood samples
were taken after 1, 2, 4, and 6 h for determination of the interferon
concentration.

Experiments were carried out on 51 rabbits. The results
showing individual interferon production are given in Table 118.

As Table 118 shows, 1 h after injection of the interferon
inducer no interferon could be found in the blood serum, while
in the rest its titer varied from 1 : 16 to 1 : 1024. Later, in tests
carried out after 2 and 4 h, the interferon titer was much higher,
but after 6 h the concentration of the inhibitor showed a marked
decrease. It should be emphasized that in the overwhelming
majority of animals the maximal interferon concentration in the
serum was found 4 h after administration of the inducer, and only
in a few rabbits was the concentration at its highest after 6 h.

In most cases the sensitivity of the animals to vaccinia
virus and the intensity of the skin reaction (assessed by Groth's
test) were inversely proportional to the intensity of the interferon formation in the particular rabbit. The correlation between
the serum interferon titers and the arithmetic mean results of
assessment of the skin reaction by Groth's test is shown in Table
119.

The results given in Table 119 give some explanation of the
differences in susceptibility of rabbits to vaccinia virus. At the
same time, it should be noted that in individual animals the
interferon titers were not inversely proportional to the severity
of the skin reaction. In these animals, despite ability to produce
large quantities of the inhibitor, the skin reaction was actually
more marked than in weaker producers of interferon. The results
of one experiment illustrating this state of affairs are given in
Table 120.

TABLE 118. Individual Interferon Production Determined in Rabbits

Time of observation, h	Number of observations	Number of animals with an interferon titer of										
		below 16	16	64	256	1,024	4,096	16,384	65,576	262,304	1,049,216	4,196,864
1	47	23	8	4	11	1	*	—	—	—	—	—
2	50	—	—	2	3	6	15	17	5	1	1	—
4	51	—	—	—	—	4	7	10	14	10	4	2
6	27	—	—	—	2	3	9	3	7	2	1	—

* No animals with these interferon titers were found.

TABLE 119. Correlation between Intensity of Interferon Formation and Intensity of Skin Reaction in Rabbits

Serum interferon titer 4 h after injection of inducer	Number of rabbits	Arithmetic mean results of titration of vaccinia virus (by Groth's test)
1,024–4,096	11	$69/10^{4.72}$
16,394–65,576	24	$55/10^{3.75}$
262,304–4,196,864	16	$35/10^{2.2}$

TABLE 120. Individual Data on Correlation between Intensity on Skin Reaction to Vaccinia Virus in Rabbits and Serum Interferon and Antibody Titers

Rabbit No.	Interferon titer	Skin reaction (by Groth's test)	Titer of hemagglutinins*
51	4,096	$125/10^{5.0}$	320
49	16,384	$102/10^{4.0}$	640
47	65,536	$103/10^{4.0}$	80
48	65,536	$103/10^{4.0}$	320
45	262,144	$70/10^{4.0}$	160
50	262,144	$60/10^{3.0}$	320
46	1,048,576	$70/10^{4.0}$	640
52	1,048,576	$115/10^{5.0}$	320

*Hemagglutinins were titrated 2 weeks after infection with vaccinia virus.

It will be clear from Table 120 that in this experiment 7
of the 8 rabbits showed a definite inverse relationship between
the interferon titers and the intensity of the skin reaction. However, in rabbit No. 52, an active interferon producer, the intensity
of the skin reaction was the same as in the weakest interferon
producer (rabbit No. 51).

In connection with these results it was important to determine
whether the skin reaction depends on the character of antibody
formation. For this purpose, the blood serum of the animals was
tested in the passive hemagglutination test 2 weeks after infection
with vaccinia virus.

As the same table shows, rabbits Nos. 51 and 52, which differed sharply in their ability to produce interferon, formed identical
amounts of hemagglutinins. Moreover, the intensity of the skin
reaction, not only in these but also in the other animals, was neither
directly nor inversely related to the intensity of antibody formation.

These results thus demonstrate the important role of interferon in the skin reaction of rabbits to vaccinia virus. At the same
time, the intensity of the visible skin reaction may be influenced
by other factors which cannot yet be analyzed.

8.8. Relationship between the Pathogenicity and Interferon-Inducing Ability of Strains of Vaccinia Virus

To study this problem, in conjunction with L. S. Shenkman
we investigated the correlation between the pathogenicity of certain strains of vaccinia virus and their interferon-inducing activity.

In the initial experiments the interferon-inducing activity
of the various strains was compared in cell cultures *in vitro* and
in mice infected intravenously.

Infection of monolayer cultures of chick fibroblasts and of
transplanted mouse L cells in different multiplicities (from 0.001
to 1 TCD_{50}/cell) was not accompanied by the formation of detectable quantities of interferon.

In the comparative study of serum interferon production,
mice were injected intravenously with 10^7 p.f.u./ml of the cor-

responding virus. Blood was taken 4 h later, the serum separated and, after inactivation of the virus in it, titrated for its interferon content.

The results showed that when the inducer was administered in this way, the most highly pathogenic Tashkent strain induced the highest concentration of interferon, while the rest were similar in their activity and induced the formation of smaller quantities of interferon. The geometric mean titer of interferon induced by strains EM-63, L-IVP, and B-51 was 1:28.96, whereas for the Tashkent strain it was 1:77.5.

The next experiments were carried out on newborn mice which were infected intracerebrally, and the interferon concentration in the brain was determined at various times thereafter. None of the tested strains of vaccinia virus induced detectable quantities of interferon in the brain of mice aged 24-48 h.

Different results were obtained by the study of interferon formation in the brain of mice weighing 6-7 g, infected intracerebrally with these same strains of vaccinia virus. These tests revealed a definite relationship between the virulence of the strain to mice and its ability to induce interferon. Substantial differences were found in the dynamics of interferon formation. In particular, strains EM-63 and B-51 induced most interferon 48 h after infection, whereas strain Tashkent and also strain L-IVP induced most interferon after 96 h. It must also be emphasized that strains EM-63 and B-51, in a lower concentration of virus (10^3 p.f.u./ml), induced the formation of the same amount of interferon as could be induced by strains Tashkent and L-IVP only in a higher concentration of the virus (10^4 p.f.u./ml). It should be noted that the decrease in the concentration of virus in the mouse brain began only when the interferon concentration was maximal for that particular strain.

Differences in the interferon-inducing activity of the strains were seen particularly demonstratively when the virus and interferon concentrations were compared in the brain of animals 48 h after infection (Table 121). The results given in this table show that with an equal or lower concentration of virus in the animals' brain, strains EM-63 and B-51 induced much more interferon (titers 1:7235 to 1:5116) than strains L-IVP and Tashkent (titers 1:452 to 1:319.9).

TABLE 121. Correlation between Concentrations
of Virus and Interferon in Mouse Brain 48 h
after Infection

Strain	Pathogenicity for animals	Titer of virus, p.f.u./ml	Geometric mean interferon titer
EM-63	1/10	1.0×10^3	1:7235
B-51	1/10	1.8×10^3	1:5116
L-IVP	4/10	1.3×10^4	1:452.3
Tashkent	4/10	4.3×10^3	1:319.9

Legend: Numerator gives number of mice dying; denominator, total number of mice infected.

A similar pattern was found in the skin of rabbits infected
with different doses of these strains. The results of investigation
of the correlation between the concentrations of virus and interferon in the rabbit skin indicate that strains EM-63 and B-51 can
induce large quantities of interferon if the virus concentration is
smaller than or equal to the concentration of strains L-IVP and
Tashkent. Particularly demonstrative results were obtained by
determination of virus and interferon in the skin of rabbits 48 h
after infection (Table 122). For instance, when the rabbits' skin
contained 10^6 p.f.u./ml of virus of strains EM-63 and B-51, interferon was found in titers of 1:1809 to 1:1280, whereas strains
L-IVP and Tashkent in a higher concentration (10^7 p.f.u./ml)
induced the production of interferon in titers of 1:160 to 1:56.
It is important to emphasize that just as during the study of interferon formation in the mouse brain, the concentration of virus
in the rabbit skin began to decrease precisely when the interferon
concentration was maximal for that strain.

The sensitivity of the tested strains to interferon was also
determined in these experiments. For this purpose, 8 units of
interferon (determined by titration with vesicular stomatitis virus)
was added to one row of tubes containing chick fibroblasts, medium
199 was added to another row of tubes, and the virus was titrated
in the experimental and control cultures after 18-20 h. The sensitivity of the strain to interferon was estimated from the number
of TCD_{50} of virus inhibited by the interferon.

TABLE 122. Correlation between Concentrations
of Virus and Interferon in Rabbits' Skin
48 h after Infection

Strain	Maximal intensity of skin reaction in rabbit	Titer of virus, p.f.u./ml	Geometric mean interferon titer
EM-63	1.0 × 1.5 cm	4.6×10^6	1:1899
B-51	1.0 × 1.5 cm	3.4×10^6	1:1279
L-IVP	1.5 × 0.2 cm	1.4×10^7	1:56.25
Tashkent	2.0 × 2.5 cm, necrosis 0.2 × 0.2 cm	1.7×10^7	1:160.0

The results given in Table 123 show a marked difference
between the sensitivity of the strains to interferon. The virulent
Tashkent strain showed low sensitivity to interferon. The remaining strains were equally susceptible to the inhibitory action of
interferon.

8.9. Conclusion

Interferon production *in vivo* was studied in mice infected
with viruses differing in their tropism: influenza, ectromelia,
and WEE viruses. In every case a direct correlation was observed
in the mice between reproduction of the virus and interferon formation in the organs. However, this correlation was observed
only until a certain period, namely the 3rd-4th day after infection.
Later interferon production fell in influenza and ectromelia, but
remained unchanged in WEE. It was also noted that in the first
two infections interferon was found in virtually all organs, whereas in WEE it was found only in the brain and in the blood. These
results relating to the detection of interferon in the organs are
in general agreement with those of Subrahmanyan and Mims [553],
obtained with West Nile, ectromelia, and influenza viruses.

The results of these experiments also confirm observations
[215] that in the late stage of experimental influenza, despite
continuing reproduction of the virus, there is a marked decrease
in interferon production in the lung tissue. We also showed that
a similar decrease in the interferon concentration is observed

TABLE 123. Sensitivity of Strains of
Vaccinia Virus of Different Pathogenicity to Interferon

Strain	Pathogenicity	Number of TCD_{50} inhibited by 8 units interferon
EM-63	Low	10^4
B-51	Low	10^4
L-IVP	Moderate	10^4
Tashkent	High	10^2

not only in the lungs, but also in other tissues and, in particular,
in the spleen and kidneys.

These relationships were found to be characteristic not only
of experimental influenza, but also of ectromelia.

Investigations conducted with the leukocytes of mice infected
with influenza and ectromelia viruses are particularly interesting.
The results show that the ability of leukocytes to produce interferon may be used as an indicator of the general reactivity of the
body in certain infections. If interferon is regarded as one of the
factors determining resistance, presumably the loss of the ability
to produce interferon by cells of the corresponding organs and
migrating elements of the reticuloendothelial system is an essential element in the pathogenesis of lethal influenza and ectromelia
infection. Hence it follows that in the first stage of the infection
in mice with influenza and ectromelia interferon is an important
factor in protection against infection. Probably loss of the ability
to produce interferon and delay in the appearance of antibodies
at a time when the conflict between virus and host organism has
ended in favor of the former must be regarded as one of the causes
of death in experimental influenza and ectromelia. In lethal influenza and ectromelia, when interferon disappears and antibodies
have not yet appeared, there is evidently a negative phase of immunoreactivity during which the absolute majority of the infected
animals must die.

After infection with sublethal doses of influenza virus and
the development of a sublethal infection antibodies appear while
the leukocytes and other reticuloendothelial cells still remain

capable of producing interferon. In that case the negative phase
does not arise and the infection terminates in recovery. Similar
relationships are possibly observed also in sublethal ectromelia,
as other investigators have found [553]. In particular, when single
tests were carried out on the organs of mice infected with attenuated
ectromelia virus on the 6th day after infection, interferon was found
in the lymph glands, spleen, liver, and blood.

We obtained different results in experiments on animals infected intracerebrally with WEE virus: interferon was found only
in the brain tissue. The animals died at a time of reduced ability
of their leukocytes to produce interferon, the concentration of
which in the brain was adequate. On the basis of these results some
remarks can be made on the role of interferon in the pathogenesis
of WEE in mice. The first feature to be noted is the apparently
total absence of effect of endogenous interferon formed in the
brain tissue. Presumably the endogenous interferon formed in
the brain after intracerebral infection or, more precisely, after
penetration of virus into the brain has little or no power to restrict
reproduction of the virus in the brain. This conclusion is supported
by the findings of Karakuyumchan and Bektemirova [96], who showed
that "brain" interferon is relatively ineffective in experimental rabies
if the animals are infected intracerebrally. However, its action is
clearly revealed if infection is by a peripheral route. This may be
because antiviral protein, induced by interferon, is not formed or
is formed only in small amounts, whereas after extraneural infection its induction takes place in high intensity. It is thus difficult
to agree with those writers who deny a role of interferon in the
pathogenesis of neurovirus infections [54, 572]. Considering that
infection with neuroviruses takes place through the skin and that
viremia is one of the essential elements in its pathogenesis, the
role of interferon as a protective factor at the time of penetration
of the virus through the portal of entry of the infection and in its
viremic phase can be postulated. It therefore seems to us that
the role of interferon cannot be assessed purely on the basis of
the discovery of large quantities of it in the brain. It is known
that animals are much less sensitive to infection with neuroviruses
by the peripheral route and that they are almost absolutely resistant
to intracerebral infection with minimal doses. There are now sufficient grounds for attributing these differences in resistance to
the effect of endogenous interferon formed after infection through
peripheral channels.

Experiments on animals of different ages revealed clear differences in interferon production in selectively vulnerable organs in influenza and WEE. Much less interferon was formed in the body of newborn mice than in animals aged 4-5 weeks. However, variations in the degree of difference were noted. In newborn mice, for instance, the interferon titers in influenza were only 2-4 times lower than in adult mice, whereas in WEE they were 8-16 times lower.

In our opinion the results obtained by the study of the production of serum interferon and the production of interferon by leukocyt *in vitro* are particularly interesting. Young mice and newborn rabbits in our experiments produced little or no interferon. This indicates that cells of the reticuloendothelial system of newborn mice and rabbits are imperfect producers of interferon. Considering that the production of serum interferon is a function predominantly of the lymphoid tissue it can be concluded that perfection of the process of interferon formation is evidence of the maturation of the lymphoid tissue during growth of the animal. If, therefore, interferon is accepted as one of the factors determining resistance of the living organism, the agents of infections in whose pathogenesis viremia is an essential element must exhibit greater pathogenicity toward newborn animals in the case of infection through peripheral routes than toward adult mice. The available evidence confirms these results. For instance, whereas the lethal dose for adult animals infected intramuscularly with arboviruses is 1000-10,000 times greater than after intracerebral infection, in newborn animals these sharp differences between the lethal dose for different routes of infection are not found.

The results so far as interferon production by animals of different ages are concerned agree with those obtained by some investigators [45, 332, 333, 413, 518, 523, 526] but not by others [287, 499, 572, 575]. These differences can perhaps be attributed to the different viruses used in the experiments, giving rise to diseases with a different pathogenesis. For example, no differences were found in work with tick-borne encephalitis, Sindbis, and West Nile viruses. Other workers, however, found differences in the rate of interferon production in newborn and adult mice in experiments with Sendai, Coxsackie, Powassan, and Semliki forest viruses.

The equal ability of newborn and adult guinea pigs to sen-
sitize interferon, confirming data in the literature [614, 624] on
the high immunoreactivity of newborn guinea pigs, is interesting.

Our results obtained by animal experiments confirm the
role of endogenous interferon in the pathogenesis of virus infections. This conclusion is supported by the close correlation between the interferon-synthesizing activity of animals and their
susceptibility to virus infections studied.

At the same time these experiments also shed considerable
light on the mechanism of individual variation in resistance to
virus infection. They suggest that interferon is one of the most
important factors determining resistance of the host to viruses,
and the experiments with inbred mice demonstrate that the ability
of an individual to form interferon is dependent on the inborn
genetic constitution of that individual. Consequently, the phenotypic
resistance of animals to virus infections can be considered to be
based upon their interferon-forming ability.

In connection with the fact that interferon production by individual mice of the same strain is not absolutely uniform it is
interesting to remember the results described by Ipsen [662]. In
his experiments, after vaccinating inbred mice with tetanus toxoid
he found individual variations in antibody formation. He attributed his results to individual differences in the ease and rapidity
of maturation of the cells producing specific antibodies. Our own
results can evidently be explained by individual variations in the
number of interferon-component cells [227, 228] or by differences
in their ability to synthesize interferon.

In connection with these results it should be pointed out
that some workers [561] had previously concluded that interferon
does not play a role in the differences between the sensitivity of
inbred mice to virus infections. However, these conclusions were
drawn from the results of determination of interferon in an organ
selectively attacked by the particular infection concerned and in
the course of development of the virus disease. Our own results
indicate that the role of interferon must not be assessed on the
basis of how much of it was formed during the development of the
disease, but from the ability of the animal to produce interferon

before infection, since the action of interferon is exhibited in the earliest stages of infection.

Our experiments showed that the intensity of interferon formation and, consequently, its effect on the pathogenesis of infection depended not only on the properties of the host, but to a large extent they were also determined by the interferon-inducing activity and the sensitivity to interferon of the virus causing the disease. This was clearly revealed by experiments with different strains of vaccinia virus. An inverse relationship was clearly found between pathogenicity and interferon-inducing activity. Strains with low pathogenicity were found to induce interferon production more actively and also earlier than the pathogenic Tashkent and L-IVP strains.

Our observations show that the concentration of virus in the mouse brain and rabbit skin begins to decrease as soon as the interferon concentration reaches its maximum for that particular strain. It is this early accumulation of high concentrations of interferon and, consequently, the early inhibition of the virus which may explain the absence of necrosis in rabbits and of mortality in mice.

The results of these experiments thus suggest that interferon-inducing activity and sensitivity to interferon are among the important factors which determine the pathogenicity of the strains of a virus. It can also be concluded from these results that the choice of an adequate interferon-inducing system is vital to a correct interpretation of the role of interferon in the pathogenesis of infection. This system must be sensitive to the virus to be tested. Another conclusion which can be drawn from these results is that in order to evaluate the degree of correlation between the pathogenicity of strains and their interferon-inducing activity, of the three models tested only one (intravenous infection of mice) proved to be unsuitable, whereas the other two (intradermal infection of rabbits and intracerebral infection of mice) revealed clearly defined patterns.

We have confirmed that keeping animals at a low temperature or administration of ACTH reduces the production of serum interferon. We have also shown that interferon production is essentially inhibited by internal irradiation with P^{32}. Considering that internal irradiation with P^{32} aggravates the course of virus infections, it can be postulated that it does so by inhibiting interferon production.

Chapter 9

Interferon Formation in Man under Normal and Pathological Conditions

Our earlier experiments on animals showed that the ability of leukocytes to produce interferon *in vitro* reflects the reactivity of the animals. Besides determining interferon in various materials obtained from healthy and sick subjects, the interferon-producing ability of their leukocytes accordingly was investigated also. The basic assumption was that leukocytic interferon can be used as an indicator of the reactivity of the donor in certain virus infections. So that the results obtained by investigation of patients could be correctly evaluated, it was first necessary to investigate whether interferon may be present in the serum and urine of healthy persons and also to determine the mean levels of production of leukocytic interferon. With possible age variations in mind, tests were carried out with leukocytes from persons of different ages (the leukocytes of healthy and sick children were investigated jointly with N. V. Vorotyntseva, Z. N. Kleimenova, and M. P. Korzhenkova).

9.1. Interferon Production by Leukocytes of Healthy Persons of Different Ages. Detection of Interferon in the Urine and Serum

Blood was obtained from healthy persons and mixed with heparin. A suspension of leukocytes was diluted to a concentration of 500,000 cells/ml and the interferon-inducing virus (NDV) was added at the rate of $10 \, TCD_{50}$ per leukocyte. The interferon was titrated on primary cultures of human myodermal tissue with vesicular stomatitis virus. Leukocytes were obtained from adults aged 19-52 years and children aged from 1 month to 12 years.

TABLE 124. Interferon Production by Suspensions of Leukocytes from Healthy Adults and Children

Age of subjects	Number of subjects tested	Number with interferon in a titer of			
		below 1:4	1:4 to 1:8	1:16 and above	Geometric mean titer
1 month to 1 year	50	32	9	9	2.36
1-3 years	37	19	7	11	3.38
3-12 years	23	3	6	14	9.3
18-55 years	134	0	21	113	24.8
60-89 years	30	16	14	0	2.3

Altogether 134 adults were tested: 62 aged from 19 to 30
years, 34 aged from 31 to 40 years, and 38 aged 51 and 52 years.
The distribution of the children by age was as follows: 50 from
1 to 12 months, 37 from 1 to 3 years, and 23 from 3 to 12 years.
It is clear from Table 124 that the leukocytes of most adults (84.3%)
produced interferon in titers of 1:16 or above, in 15.6% the titers
were from 1:4 to 1:8, and in none of the volunteers was the titer
below 1:4. Different relationships were found in the group of
children and old people.

Whereas the leukocytes of none of the individual adults were
incapable of producing interferon, those of most of the children
under 1 year of age tested in these experiments were found to be
weak producers of interferon. With age the interferon-producing
ability of the leukocytes increased to reach a maximum at 12-18
years.

In old age, however, the ability of the leukocytes to produce
interferon declines sharply, to lower levels even than in the young-
est infants.

The immaturity of imperfection of this protective mechanism
is evidently one of the factors responsible for the increased susceptibility of children and old people to virus infection.

The serum and urine of healthy adults also were tested for
their interferon content. These materials were treated with
hydrochloric acid to pH 2.4-3.0 for 48 h and then with sodium hy-
droxide to pH 7.4 before titration. Altogether 47 samples of serum
and 29 samples of urine were tested. The inhibitor was found in

a titer of 1 : 4 in the serum of 3 persons and in the same titer in
the urine of 4 subjects. Inhibitors found in the serum and urine
were studied for species specificity and virus specificity. In particular, the inhibitors tested in chick fibroblasts showed no inhibitory action on vesicular stomatitis virus. In cultures of human
cells the inhibitor depressed the reproduction of vesicular stomatitis and smallpox viruses. The antiviral action of the inhibitor
also rendered the cells resistant if it was removed after preliminary
contact with the cells. Consequently, the inhibitor found in the
urine and serum was interferon. This is evidence that interferon
can sometimes be found in clinically healthy persons, although in
comparatively low titers.

9.2. Interferon Production by the Leukocytes of Newborn Infants

The blood of newborn infants possesses certain distinguishing
features: increased viscosity, an increased concentration of hemo-
globin and erythrocytes, and a marked increase in the number of
leukocytes.

The most interesting feature distinguishing the blood of
newborn infants in this case is that leukocyte count is more than
twice that of the adult and neutrophils are in a clear majority. An
attempt was accordingly made to determine the ability of the leukocytes in the blood of newborn infants to produce interferon.
Blood was taken from the umbilicus immediately after birth of
the child. In joint experiments with N. I. Barancheev and Yu. B.
Fedorova leukocytes were obtained from 67 newborn infants. In
18 of these 67 cases the mothers' leukocytes also were tested. Data
on interferon production by the leukocytes of infants aged 1-12
months are also shown for comparison.

TABLE 125. Interferon Production by Leukocytes of Newborn Infants

Group of infants tested	Total number tested	Number with interferon in a titer of			
		below 1 : 4	1 : 4 to 1 : 8	1 : 16 and above	geometric mean titer
Newborn	67	17	17	33	9.2
Aged 1-12 months	50	32	9	9	2.36

As Table 125 shows the leukocytes of newborn infants are
more active producers of interferon than leukocytes of infants
aged 1-12 months. The titers of leukocytic interferon in the newborn infants were similar to the interferon titers in adults. The
interferon concentration in most infants and in their mothers was
the same, but in 7 cases the leukocytes of the infant were more
active producers. Consequently, increased ability of the leukocytes
of newborn infants to form interferon is a distinguishing feature
of their blood.

9.3. Production of Leukocytic Interferon by Patients with Leukemia

The interferon-synthesizing ability of leukocytes from
patients with leukemia was studied jointly with V. T. Morozova
and Yu. B. Fedorova. Altogether 15 patients with myeloid and 10
with lymphatic leukemia were studied. The disease in all these
patients was of the chronic form and its duration ranged from 1 to
15 years.

It was shown previously that the titers of leukocytic interferon in most healthy adult persons were 1 : 16 or over. It was now
found that in most patients with leukemia the leukocytes were far
less capable of producing interferon. Comparison of the mean
interferon titers for healthy adults (1 : 24.8) and patients with leukemia (1 : 1.6 to 1 : 2.6) shows that the patients produced about 10
times less interferon than the healthy subjects. Differences in
interferon production by the leukocytes of patients with lymphatic
and myeloid leukemia also were found. The leukocytes of the
former produced slightly less interferon.

These results suggest that a possible explanation of the
severity of the course of virus infections in leukemic patients
is their decreased ability to produce interferon. Diseases such
as measles and chickenpox are known to run a severe course in
such patients and vaccination against smallpox is frequently at-
tended by serious complications.

9.4. Production of Leukocytic Interferon in Other Internal Diseases

Since the lymphoid tissue determines the reactivity of the
body in infectious diseases and is responsible for the formation

of antibodies and interferon, it is important to study the changes
which take place in it in various pathological states. So far, however, little work has been done to develop criteria for use in
defining the functional activity of lymphoid tissue. Essentially
the only test which can be used *in vitro* is the determination of
phagocytic activity. Since the intensity of interferon production
by leukocytes reflects the state of its production as a whole, this
test can evidently be used as a criterion or reactivity of the body
as a whole. Patients with chronic internal diseases are known
to be more prone to infectious (including virus) diseases. If
the interferon-synthesizing ability of the leukocytes to some extent
reflects the reactivity of the body, it can be assumed that this index
will be lowered in patients with internal diseases. On these grounds,
jointly with G. P. Shul'tsev, Yu. B. Fedorova, and G. V. Dibizheva
we investigated 88 patients, 23 of them repeatedly. The distribution of the patients by diagnosis and the results of the tests are
given in Table 126.

It will be clear from Table 126 that very low activity of the
leukocytes in producing interferon was found in patients with various diseases. Titers of 1:16 and above were observed in these
patients 10 times less frequently than in healthy subjects. In 23
patients the production of leukocytic interferon was tested repeatedly over a period of time and the intensity of the process was
compared with the course of the disease. It was found that in
most cases with an improvement in the patients' general condition,
the intensity of their interferon production also increased. Among
23 patients tested repeatedly at intervals of 10, 20, and 30 days,

TABLE 126. Leukocytic Interferon in Patients with Various Diseases

Diagnosis	Number of patients tested	Number with interferon titers of			
		below 1:4	1:4 to 1:8	1:16 and above	geometric mean titer
Bronchial asthma	24	11	9	4	3.0
Rheumatic fever	23	9	10	4	3.6
Tuberculosis, Boeck's sarcoid	14	10	3	1	2.0
Lymphogranulomatosis	9	1	6	2	6.7
Rheumatoid arthritis	7	3	1	3	4.7
Cirrhosis of the liver	6	4	1	1	2.5
Systemic lupus erythematosus	3	2	1	0	1.9

a marked improvement was observed in 11. The production of
leukocytic interferon also was increased in 9 of them (by 4 times or
more). In 12 patients there was no appreciable improvement in
health at the time of taking the second blood sample. In 9 of these
12 patients the leukocytic interferon production was unchanged,
while in 3 of them it was increased and these 3 were subsequently
discharged in a satisfactory condition.

These preliminary results suggest that this method of determining the functional activity of leukocytes in fact reflects changes
in the reactivity of the body as a whole during disease and that it
can be used to assess the functional state of the lymphoid tissue
in various pathological processes.

It is even possible that this method of the interferon reaction of the leukocytes (which can be abbreviated to IRL) may also
be used to evaluate the effects of treatment.

Interferon formation in 38 children under 3 years of age
after primary vaccination with smallpox vaccine was studied
jointly with A. F. Sokolova and Yu. B. Fedorova. The interferon
concentration in the serum was determined in children with a
typical vaccination reaction. The production of leukocytic interferon *in vitro* also was investigated. Blood was taken from the
children before vaccination and on the 8th and 21st-22nd days
thereafter. Consequently, three lots of material were obtained
from each vaccinated child. The blood and leukocytes were treated as described above; NDV was used to induce interferon production.

It will be clear from Table 127 that on the 8th day after
vaccination, at the height of the reaction, interferon could be
detected in the serum of more than two-thirds of the vaccinated
children in titers of 1 : 4 to 1 : 32, and that it had disappeared by
the end of the 3rd week.

The results of the investigation of the leukocytes show that
at the height of the vaccination reaction the production of leukocytic
interferon was reduced, and that it was increased again 2 weeks
later.

These results are in agreement with those of the investigation of other groups of sick children in whom a decrease in the
production of leukocytic interferon also was observed at the height

TABLE 127. Serum and Leukocytic Interferon in Children
Vaccinated against Smallpox

Time of testing	Serum interferon		Leukocytic interferon	
	number of tests	titer (geo-metric mean)	number of tests	titer (geo-metric mean)
Before vaccination	28	<1.0	28	3.0
8 days after vaccination	30	6.3	23	1.5
21-22 days after vaccination	33	<1.0	26	4.0

of the disease, followed by an increase in the period of convalescence.

9.6. Interferon Production in Adults with Influenza

As was pointed out above, the role of interferon in the
pathogenesis of influenza has been studied mainly in experimental
animals and the conclusion has been drawn that interferon undoubtedly plays a role in the development of the infectious process
and also, perhaps, in recovery from the infection. However, its
formation in the human influenza patient has so far received little
study. Together with L. I. Neklyudova, we investigated interferon
formation in influenza patients during an epidemic in January and
February, 1967.

Observations were made on 61 outpatients aged from 17 to
53 years with the typical picture of influenza. To isolate the virus
nasopharyngeal washings were collected and tested on chick embryos
by intra-amniotic injection. The clinical diagnosis was confirmed
by the HIT, carried out by the usual method on two successive samples of blood serum. Interferon was determined in the nasal washings, the blood, and urine of the patients.

Altogether 24 strains with similar properties were isolated
in chick embryos and 9 of them were identified as influenza A2
virus. Two samples of serum were tested from all patients: in
31 cases the titer of antibodies against influenza A2 virus and in
3 the titer against influenza B virus was increased by 4 times or
more.

These investigations were thus carried out on patients with a clinical and, in most cases, a virological and serological diagnosis of influenza. In 44 cases the tests were carried out on the 1st-2nd day of the disease, in 14 on the 3rd-4th day, and in 1 patient on the 5th, 6th, and 9th days after the beginning of the disease. It was interesting to determine the frequency with which interferon was found in the patients in the early periods of the illness. The results are given in Table 128.

As Table 128 shows, interferon was found in all material studied from most patients during the first days of the disease. On the first 2 days of the disease it was found more frequently in the serum and urine than in the nasal washings. The mean interferon titers also were determined in the washings, serum, and urine on different days of the illness.

The results given in Table 129 show that the interferon titers of the first 3-4 days of the disease remained at almost the same level in the materials tested; only in the washings was there a tendency for the titer to fall on the second day of the illness and to rise again on the 3rd-4th day. This probably led to inhibition of reproduction of the virus in the epithelial cells of the respiratory tract, thus promoting recovery. The high titers of interferon in the urine will be noted, for they were 1.5-2 times higher than the titers in the serum and 4-4.5 times higher than

TABLE 128. Frequency of Detection of Interferon in Influenza Patients at Various Times after the Beginning of the Illness

Day of illness	Material investigated	Total number tested	Number in which interferon was found	
			abs.	%
1-2	Nasal washings	44	27	61.3
	Serum	39	37	94.8
	Urine	37	36	97.2
3-4	Nasal washings	14	13	92.8
	Serum	14	13	92.8
	Urine	14	13	92.8

those in the nasal washings. However, there is an important reservation to be made here, which applies when the interferon concentration is judged in these materials. It must be remembered
that serum and urine were used in the untreated form for titration
whereas the nasal washings were diluted with medium 199 approximately 5 times when they were obtained. It was calculated
that each gauze swab introduced into the nasal passages absorbed
0.1-0.2 ml of secretion and was then immersed in 2 ml of medium
The results are thus inaccurate and must be regarded as purely
relative. Moreover, when the sites of the highest interferon concentration in the body are estimated, its titer in the washings
should be increased by 5-10 times. These titers are accordingly
shown in parenthesis in Table 129. In the subsequent tables interferon titers in the washings are given as a rule multiplied by 5.

With this reservation in mind it can be deduced that the
interferon concentrations in the nasal washings and in the urine
were approximately equal and were higher than its concentration
in the blood serum.

The interferon levels in groups of patients with serologically
confirmed and unconfirmed influenza were compared and the intensity of interferon formation was studied in relation to the blood
antibody titer at the beginning of the disease.

It was found that the interferon titer in the nasal washings
and blood serum was higher in patients with serologically confirmed influenza. Possibly in patients with no increase in antibody titer the clinical symptoms similar to those of influenza
could have been due to other viruses or to bacteria with weak interferon-inducing properties.

It was also found that the initial antibody titer has an appreciable effect on the intensity of interferon production. The difference
in the interferon concentration in the nasal washings was particularly marked. In patients with an antibody titer of 1:40 or more the
interferon concentration was almost 2.5 times less than in patients
with a low antibody titer or with absence of antibodies. These
results agree with those obtained previously in experiments on
animals [113, 495], which revealed a lower intensity of interferon
formation in the respiratory organs of immune animals infected
with influenza virus.

The interferon level was studied in relation to the intensity of the fever in the patients. To obtain comparable results, tests carried out on the first day of the disease were compared (Table 130).

As the results in Table 130 show, the concentration of interferon in the nasal secretion and urine was higher in patients with a higher temperature.

The ability of the leukocytes to produce interferon and its connection with the body temperature and duration of the illness also were determined in patients with influenza.

The results in Table 131 show that the height of the fever has a marked influence on interferon production by leukocytes, and that there is a direct correlation between the increased interferon production by the leukocytes at a higher body temperature and the interferon concentration in the nasal secretion and urine. A raised body temperature, regarded as a beneficial factor in the pathogenesis of virus infections [440], can be regarded in the same light as a factor affecting interferon production in the human body.

The results of the investigation of the relationship between the duration of the illness and the intensity of interferon production by the leukocytes are of great interest (Table 132). Earlier work in experiments on animals showed that interferon production in the animal body may be one of the criteria of its reactivity. The results of the investigation just described are confirmation of this view.

TABLE 129. Mean Titers of Interferon in Material from Patients on Various Days of the Disease

Day of illness	Number tested	Interferon titers (geometric mean) in		
		nasopharyngeal washings	serum	urine
1	35	3.5(17.5)*	11.1	17.2
2	9	2.2(11.0)	10.8	12.5
3-4	17	4.3(21.5)	8.7	17.6

*Explanation in text.

TABLE 130. Interferon Concentration in Relation to
Height of Fever

Body temperature	Number of patients	Interferon titers in		
		nasopharyngeal washings	serum	urine
Below 37.9°C	19	15.0	10.2	14.1
38°C and above	16	19.0	10.1	21.6

9.7. Interferon Production in Children with Acute Respiratory Virus Infections and Its Correlation with the Production of Leukocytic Interferon

These investigations were carried out on children admitted for treatment to the Institute of Pediatrics, Academy of Medical Sciences of the USSR. To confirm the diagnosis, two samples of serum from the patients were tested for the presence of antiviral antibodies in the CFT and HIT; the immunofluorescence method of Coons in Ketiladze's modification [99] and the method of rhinocytoscopy for the detection of DNA and RNA inclusions in the epithelium of the nasal mucous membrane also were used. Altogether 108 patients with acute respiratory virus infections aged from 3 months to 12 years were investigated. Their distribution by diagnosis is given in Table 133.

Considering that no appreciable difference in interferon production was found in the different groups of patients, the results described subsequently are pooled, without differentiation by diagnosis.

The tests showed (Table 134) that in the acute period of the illness interferon was found in low titers in the children's serum, especially in those under 1 year of age. Concentrations of 1 : 16 or more were never found in this group. This titer was found in about 10% of cases of children over 1 year old. The geometric mean titer of interferon in the children was 4 times lower than in adults.

A similar pattern was found in the different groups of patients when the leukocytic interferon was determined. Whereas the mean level of this parameter in children in the acute period

TABLE 131. Interferon Production by Blood Leukocytes in Relation to Patient's Body Temperature

Body temperature	Number of patients	Interferon titer
Below 37.9°C	21	17.0
38°C and above	18	23.5

TABLE 132. Relationship between Duration of Illness and Titer of Leukocytic Interferon

Duration of illness, days	Number of observations	Interferon titer
Under 5	28	31.0
Over 5	23	19.3

TABLE 133. Distribution of Patients by Diagnosis

Diagnosis	Number investigated
Influenza	42
Parainfluenza	8
RS infection	24
Adenovirus infection	13
Mixed (virus) infection	21

of the illness was of the order of 1 : 2.1 to 1 : 2.6, in the adults it was about 8 times higher.

The interferon concentration in the urine was determined in the acute period in 12 children aged under 1 year, in 32 children aged over 1 year, and in 51 adults. In the period of repair this parameter was determined in 12 children under 1 year old and in 20 over 1 year old. Since no significant differences were found in

TABLE 134. Comparison of Serum Interferon Concentration and Production of Leukocytic Interferon in the Acute Period of the Illness

Age of patients	Number tested	Interferon titer									
		in serum					leukocytic				
		below 1:4	1:4	1:8	1:16 and above	geometric mean	below 1:4	1:4	1:8	1:16 and above	geometric mean
Under 1 year	38	30	6	2	0	1.3	24	4	6	4	2.1
1-12 years	62	32	12	9	7	2.3	30	13	11	8	2.6
17-53 years	51	4	6	21	20	1:8.3	0	3	12	36	1:23.9

TABLE 135. Interferon Concentration in the Urine Compared with Production of Leukocytic Interferon

Age of patients	Period of illness	Number tested	Interferon titer									
			in urine					leukocytic				
			below 1:4	1:4	1:8	1:16 and above	geometric mean	below 1:4	1:4	1:8	1:16 and above	geometric mean
3 months to 12 years	Acute	44	17	8	10	9	3.6	27	9	5	3	2.0
	Repair	32	20	3	4	5	2.3	19	3	8	2	2.4
17-53 years	Acute	51	2	7	13	29	11.7	0	3	12	36	23.9

the results of the tests on the children of the different age groups, the combined data for the interferon concentration in the urine compared with the production of leukocytic interferon are given (Table 135).

The results given in Table 135 show a direct relationship between the production of leukocytic interferon and its concentration in the urine. In the adults, to correspond with the higher interferon production by the leukocytes, a higher interferon concentration was found in the urine. In most cases, it must be emphasized, correlation was found between these indices not only with respect to the mean results, but also when they were compared in individual patients.

Comparison of interferon production in the cells of the upper respiratory tract and by the leukocytes showed a definite correlation in this case. Admittedly, the differences in the interferon concentration in the nasal secretion in the various age groups were not so marked as in the serum and urine of the children and adults (Table 136).

Previous observations on adult patients with influenza showed that interferon production is stimulated by a high body temperature. In children with acute respiratory infections higher concentrations of interferon in the urine and serum also were found in the presence of a high fever (Table 137).

Interferon production *in vitro* by the leukocytes of sick children was studied in more detail. Besides patients with acute respiratory infections, 11 children with presumptive enterovirus infections also were tested.

The results of a study of leukocytic interferon in relation to the period of the illness are given in Table 138. For comparison, the geometric mean index of leukocytic interferon for healthy children of the corresponding age groups are given in the same table.

The results in Table 139 show that the ability of the leukocytes to produce interferon is clearly dependent on the period of the illness. On the first day of the disease the activity of the leukocytes was much higher than normal in children. On the 2nd-3rd day of the illness a marked fall in the ability of the blood

TABLE 136. Interferon Concentration in Nasal Washings and Its Correlation with Leukocytic Interferon Production

Age of patients	Number tested	Interferon titer									
		in nasal washings					leukocytic				
		below 1:2	1:2	1:4	1:8	1:16	geometric mean	below 1:4	1:4	1:8	1:16	geometric mean
Under 1 year	13	7	1	2	1	2	2.3	5	5	2	1	3.0
1–12 years	19	6	5	3	2	3	2.8	4	4	4	7	4.3
17–53 years	58	16	17	9	8	8	3.5	0	6	14	38	18.6

TABLE 137. Interferon in Urine and Serum of Sick Children in Relation to Body Temperature

Material tested	Body temperature	Number tested	Interferon titer (geometric mean)
Serum	Below 38.5°C	35	2.7
	Above 38.5°C	44	3.3
Urine	Below 38.5°C	26	4.3
	Above 38.5°C	18	6.3

TABLE 138. Intensity of Leukocytic Interferon Formation at Different Periods of Illness

Day and period of illness	Number tested	Interferon titer (geometric mean)
1st	15	6.7
2nd–3rd	62	2.3
Repair	75	4.14
Convalescence	84	5.76
Healthy children	110	3.2

leukocytes to produce interferon was observed. At the end of the
acute period of the illness the ability of the leukocytes to produce
interferon began to reappear and this coincided with the onset of
the recovery period. These relationships were particularly clear
when interferon-negative children, i.e., those constantly giving
negative results when tested for the production of leukocytic interferon, were excluded from the total number tested at the different
periods (Table 139).

During convalescence the titer of leukocytic interferon was
almost 3 times higher than during the acute period. Consequently,
the level of production of leukocytic interferon reflects the reactivity of the body in the various periods of the disease.

It must be emphasized that the indices of interferon production by the leukocytes in a period of the disease also depended
on the children's previous medical history. In children whose
previous medical history was suspect (early artificial feeding with
signs of malnutrition, frequent respiratory virus and bacterial infections, a predisposition toward chronic illnesses) the indices of
leukocytic interferon in all periods of the illness were lower than
in children with a satisfactory medical history (Table 140).

The next step was to determine how the production of leukocytic interferon depends on the severity and duration of the
disease. No definite correlation was found between the production
of leukocytic interferon and the acuteness of the initial period.
Meanwhile, in children over 1 year of age with a well-defined ability
to produce leukocytic interferon, there was a clear relationship
between the speed at which all the manifestations of the illness
cleared up and the intensity of interferon production by the leu-

TABLE 139. Titers of Leukocytic
Interferon with Exclusion of Interferon-Negative Children

Period of illness	Number tested	Interferon titer (geometric mean)
Height	78	3.8
Repair	47	5.6
Convales- cence	62	9.1

kocytes. In patients in whom the disease followed an abortive
course the geometric mean titer of interferon was 1:5.1, in
those with a subacute course it was 1.35, and in those with a
chronic course 1:2.2.

The difference between the indices in children under 1 year
of age in whom the disease followed an acute and subacute course
was not significant, evidently because these children were interferon-negative.

9.8. Conclusion

The purpose of the investigation described above was to
study the ability of the leukocytes of healthy adults and children
to produce interferon. There is little information on this question
in the literature. Our experiments represent the first comparative
investigation of human leukocytic interferon production at different
ages. Having regard to the correlation between interferon production *in vivo* and its production by leukocytes *in vitro* , it can be
concluded from the results obtained that the intensity of interferon
production depends on age. The much lower interferon production in small children is evidence of the immaturity or incomplete
development of this protective mechanism in infants, and this is
regarded as an explanation of the increased susceptibility of young
children to virus infections. It can also be considered that the activity of interferon production by different persons is reflected in

TABLE 140. Effect of Previous Medical
History on Production of Leukocytic Interferon in Sick Children

| Period of illness | Geometric mean interferon titers in children with | | | |
| | satisfactory med- ical history | | suspect medical history | |
	number of tests	inter- feron	number of tests	inter- feron
2nd–3rd day	25	2.23	23	2.06
End of acute period	10	3.02	12	2.11
Repair	34	4.24	40	3.35
Convalescence	15	5.78	24	3.26

their individual susceptibility. We mentioned above that cell cultures *in vitro* from different individuals also vary in their interferon-producing activity and in their sensitivity to interferon, and this is further confirmation of this conclusion.

The results of estimation of interferon formation by the leukocytes of newborn infants, which were found to be active producers of interferon, are interesting. In this respect infants in the first days of life differ from older children; the observations described in this chapter further show that interferon formation *in vivo* is increased in newborn infants.

The results of investigations of the serum and urine of healthy persons also deserve attention. Since the inhibitor discovered in these fluids was evidently interferon it can be assumed that viruses and bacteria permanently present in the body act as interferon inducers.

The results show that interferon can be found in children and adults with acute respiratory virus infections both at the site of reproduction of the virus (the respiratory tract) and in the blood serum and urine. It is interesting to note that on the first 2 days of the disease interferon is found more often in the serum and urine than in the nasal washings. This may indicate that interferon is produced in the influenza patient not only by the cells of the upper respiratory tract, but also by other tissues. No strict correlation is observed between the interferon concentrations in the nasal washings and serum or in the nasal washings and urine. Since interferon is found more often in the washings on the 3rd-4th day than during the first 2 days of the disease, we consider that this factor must play a role in the pathogenesis of infection with influenza virus, having regard to the short duration of the acute period of the illness.

The results obtained show that in influenza the initial antibody level has an appreciable influence on the intensity of interferon production: in patients with an antibody titer of 1:40 or above the interferon concentration was almost 2.5 times lower than in patients with a low titer or absence of antibodies.

From the standpoint of the study of the physiology and pathology of children the figures for the intensity of interferon production at different ages broaden our knowledge of immunity against respiratory virus infections. The correlation between the interferon concentration in the nasal washings, serum, and urine, on the one hand, and the levels of leukocytic interferon production, on the other hand, is interesting. It is clear from these results that the intensity of interferon formation in children (excluding the newborn) is much lower than in adults and this is evidently one reason for the more severe course of respiratory virus infections in children.

The fact that the leukocytes of sick children on the first day of the illness are more capable than those of healthy children of producing interferon must be noted. This may reflect the first reaction of the lymphoid system to dissemination of the virus and it may be associated with the activation of the whole range of immunological responses in the body.

The question of the origin of the interferon found in the urine requires special examination. Circulation through the kidney evidently explains the mechanism of its elimination from the body, which takes place at the same rate as the disappearance of interferon from the blood serum. It should be noted that substances with a molecular weight less than 70,000 are excreted freely via the kidneys, and human interferon has less than half this molecular weight (18,000-25,000).

The results of repeated investigation of the leukocytes at different periods of the disease and the marked dependence of the duration of the disease on the ability of the leukocytes to synthesize interferon are particularly interesting. In our observations recovery began to take place at the same time as the increase in the ability of the leukocytes to produce interferon, and greater ability to produce interferon corresponded to shortening of the course of the disease. Consequently, interferon production by the leukocytes reflected the reactivity of the organism and this corresponds to some degree with the results obtained in studies of experimental influenza in mice.

So far as the role of interferon in the pathogenesis of influenza is concerned, the results of these observations confirm and extend the existing views that this role is an important one. Proof of this is given by the increase in the interferon concentration and its more frequent detection at the time of disappearance of the acute manifestations in the clinical picture of the disease, the shorter duration of the illness in persons with a higher titer of leukocytic interferon, and the increased interferon production in patients with a higher fever.

At the same time, we consider that determination of the intensity of interferon production by the leukocytes is of importance not only in connection with the pathology of virus infections. Our investigations with the leukocytes of patients with internal diseases indicate that this test can be used both to determine the functional activity of lymphoid tissue in general and also the reactivity of the body as a whole. Determination of the intensity of leukocytic interferon production can be expected to find a useful role in many different fields of clinical medicine.

Mechanism of Formation
and Action of Interferon

To conclude this description of the results of investigations into the various aspects of the problem of interferon, a brief look must be taken at the mechanism of its formation and action.

The conditions of interferon formation have not yet been fully explained. What is known, however, is that the information required for its synthesis is coded in the cell DNA. This is confirmed by the fact that the interferon induced in the same cells by different RNA- or DNA-containing viruses possess common properties [410, 411, 451, 461]. It is further confirmed by the species and tissue specificity of interferon, and by the wide variation in the nature and chemical composition of the interferon inducers. The cistron which codes interferon synthesis is evidently in a repressed state in the cell genome. Under the influence of the inducer it is derepressed and initiates interferon synthesis; this process does not require the synthesis of new cell DNA but it does require the synthesis of messenger RNA and protein.

The fact that the synthesis of new cell DNA is not necessary is proved by experiments using 5-fluorodeoxyuridine and aminopterin, which block DNA synthesis but have no effect on interferon formation. However, interferon production takes place only if the cells remain capable of synthesizing cell RNA. This state of affairs has been confirmed by many investigations with actinomycin D, which inhibits DNA-dependent RNA synthesis.

Despite the fact that the formation of virus-induced interferon has been studied for over 10 years it is still impossible to

identify with confidence which components of the virus act as its
inducers.

Burke [233] considers that virus nucleic acid is the inducer.
A group of workers under Hilleman's direction has shown that
double-stranded RNA (including the replicative form) is the interferon inducer. However, the results obtained by these same workers showed that DNA does not possess interferon-inducing properties. The problem has thus been narrowed down in relation to
the induction of interferon in cells infected by RNA-containing
viruses and it is highly probable that replication of virus RNA is
an essential factor in the induction of interferon formation. At
the same time, it is not clear what determines interferon formation in the case of infection by DNA-containing viruses or when
inactivated viruses act upon the cell. In the last case it has to be
assumed that the inactivated virus can initiate a limited process of
nucleic acid replication which is insufficient for the formation of
the complete virus but which is capable of inducing interferon
formation. However, experiments with chick fibroblasts infected
with Semliki forest virus showed that interferon was formed in
the absence of synthesis of the mature virus and also in the absence of synthesis of its nucleic acid. It was concluded from
this observation that contact between virus and cell can lead to
interferon synthesis even in the absence of reproduction of the
virus. Furthermore, even virus-induced synthesis of its nucleic
acid is not necessary for interferon synthesis.

When analyzing the results obtained by a study of the mechanisms of interferon formation, Burke [233] compares it with induced synthesis of enzymes. Neither the induced enzyme nor
interferon is present under normal conditions but they appear in
the cell under the influence of appropriate stimulators and their
synthesis is controlled by cell mRNA. Burke suggests that the
process of interferon formation can be subdivided conventionally
into three phases: 1) that arising immediately after introduction
of the interferon-inducing virus; 2) the phase of interaction between the stimulator and the cell genome, resembling derepression
in its course; 3) synthesis of the messenger RNA controlling interferon synthesis.

On the basis of published data Agol [2] postulated the
following scheme of interferon formation. The structural cistron,

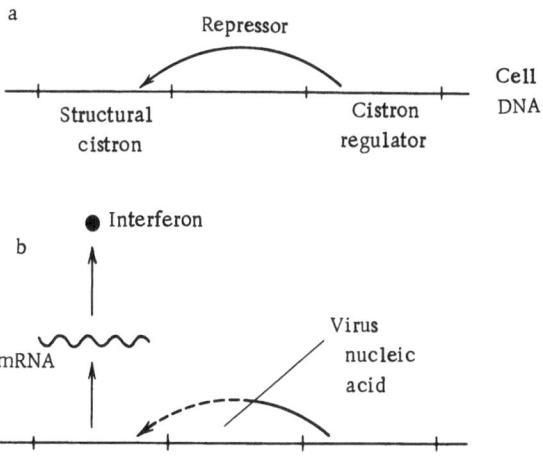

Fig. 13. Scheme of interferon formation
(after V. I. Agol). Explanation in text.

responsible for interferon formation, of the cell DNA is in a
repressed state in the cell so that the corresponding mRNA is not
formed. The action of the interferon inducer leads either to bind-
ing of the repressor or to the termination of its formation, as a
result of which the structural cistron begins to form interferon-
specific mRNA. Interferon is then synthesized in the cell ribosomes
(Fig. 13).

The mechanism of interferon formation under the influence
of inducers of nonviral nature has received little study. It has
been suggested [353, 606] that the interferon induced by bacterial
endotoxins is not synthesized *de novo* but is simply liberated under
the influence of the corresponding inducer. Evidence in support
of this view is given by the rapidity of interferon formation in
animals after administration of bacterial endotoxins. True, the
hypothesis of the preexistence of interferon in the body is silent
on the sources of its origin. There is likewise no definite opinion
on the location of the preexisting interferon in the body. It can be
postulated from the facts so far published that the preexisting
interferon can accumulate only in the cells of lymphoid tissue and,
in particular, in leukocytes. The reason for this is that bacteria
and their endotoxins which can induce interferon formation *in vivo*
are unable to induce its formation *in vitro* in cells other than leukocytes. Moreover, macrophages evidently secrete a certain

amount of interferon *in vitro* even if not stimulated by virus or lipopolysaccharide inducers.

Ho and Kono [353], who experimented on rabbits, showed that actinomycin D suppresses interferon synthesis induced by Sindbis virus but has no effect on interferon formation induced by bacterial endotoxin.

Youngner and co-workers [606] observed inhibition of interferon formation in mice *in vivo* under the influence of cycloheximide, an inhibitor of protein synthesis. Doses completely inhibiting protein synthesis in the liver also inhibited interferon formation under the influence of Brucella abortus but did not inhibit interferon formation induced by bacterial endotoxins. Puromycin, another inhibitor of protein synthesis, acted in the same way. Consequently, inhibition of protein synthesis *in vivo* also inhibited interferon formation induced by viruses and by Brucella abortus but did not affect interferon production induced by bacterial endotoxins.

In the discussion on the mechanism of action it must be remembered that interferon does not directly inactivate viruses or their nucleic acids but exerts its action on the intracellular stage of virus reproduction. Interferon does not prevent adsorption and penetration of the virus into the cell or its deproteinization. The intensity of inhibition of reproduction of a particular virus varies from partial to complete. For the antiviral action of interferon to be manifested, the cells must remain capable of synthesizing RNA and proteins, and this is evidence in support of its indirect action through an antiviral protein induced by interferon in the cells. This protein has been called translational inhibitory protein (TIP) or antiviral protein (AVP).

All the hypotheses which have so far been put forward in this field can be subdivided into two main groups:

1. TIP inhibits the synthesis of virus RNA or of mRNA by its direct inhibitory action [270].
2. TIP induces a specific block of the reading of information either by inhibiting the formation of polysomes [245, 246, 384] or by blocking translation of virus mRNA but not of cell mRNA [443, 479].

Regardless of which mechanism is the correct one, ultimately the formation of virus-specific enzymes [315, 524] and of replicative forms of virus RNAs [300, 317, 476, 524] is suppressed.

The hypothesis of interferon action according to which TIP disturbs the translation process is attractive [443]. Marcus and Salb, working with a cell-free system, used RNA of Sindbis virus and ribosomes from the cells of normal and interferon-treated chick embryos. Tritium-labeled virus RNA, by aggregating with 74S ribosomes from normal cells, formed polysomes with a sedimentation constant of 250S which functioned in protein synthesis. Ribosomes from interferon-treated cells formed only one-third as many polysomes and these did not function in protein synthesis. However, the ribosomes functioned normally if the cells were treated with actinomycin D together with interferon. In the analysis of their results these workers suggest that the mechanism of action of interferon is as follows. One or more interferon molecules penetrate into the cell and depress the host cistron coding mRNA synthesis for the formation of TIP in the cytoplasm. Contact between TIP and ribosomes renders the ribosomes incapable of synthesizing virus-specific proteins, but not cell proteins. Presumably union of TIP with the ribosomes specifically blocks the reading of proteins from the mRNA through a change in the three-dimensional configuration of the ribosomes. At the same time the translation of information from cell mRNA is undisturbed, and during the action of interferon on the cell synthesis of cell proteins, but not of virus proteins, can therefore take place in it. The results of this investigation have later been confirmed by other workers [479].

There is as yet no general agreement regarding the fate of exogenous interferon acting on the cell. Some workers have found that during the period of action of interferon on the cell there is a significant loss of interferon from the surrounding medium although it is still unknown whether this loss is the result of specific processes or whether it is due to nonspecific breakdown of the interferon. Other workers, however, have not found any decrease in the interferon concentration during the development of an antiviral state in the cells.

The absence of definite absorption of interferon by cells suggests that there are two ways by which interferon could react with the cell to induce TIP formation:

1. Action of the catalyst type. In this case the interferon is not used up but stimulates changes in the cell which lead to the production of antiviral protein.

2. Undetectably small quantities of interferon enter into irreversible combination with cell components and thereby induce TIP production.

The information now available is insufficient to allow a definite choice to be made between these two possibilities or even to judge the intensity with which exogenous interferon penetrates into the cell. It must be stated that integrity of the cell receptors must evidently be preserved for the action of interferon to be manifested. Their destruction by phospholipase C reduced the effectiveness of added interferon.

The antiviral activity of interferon varies with time. It appears between 1 and 4 h after the beginning of action of the interferon, rises steadily, and reaches a maximum after 7 h. The character of development of this antiviral activity depends on the interferon concentration in the extracellular medium: the more interferon was used, the quicker its antiviral activity was exhibited, and the higher the level it reached and the longer it remained at that level (provided that interferon was present in the medium in unchanged concentration).

The constant level of antiviral activity is evidently due to one or two causes:

1. The cells reach the level of the maximum possible reaction to the given concentration of interferon.

2. The intracellular antiviral substance formed is broken down at a rate which balances the rate of its synthesis.

Removal of the extracellular interferon does not lead to any appreciable loss of antiviral activity over a period of several hours. However, the level of antiviral activity subsequently falls, although it does so much more slowly than the activity rose initially.

This decrease in antiviral activity after the removal of the interferon indicates that the presence of extracellular (intracellular) interferon is essential for the maintenance of TIP synthesis. Removal of interferon evidently leads to a decrease in the production of antiviral protein through a decrease in the induction of messenger RNA for its synthesis. Delay in the loss of the performed antiviral activity and its relatively slow decline after the removal of interferon may correspond to the time required for breakdown of the previously induced RNA. This last hypothesis has been fully confirmed in experiments using inhibitors of RNA synthesis (actinomycin D) and of protein synthesis (p-fluorophenylalanine).

When actinomycin D was used the interferon activity fell. The dynamics of this phenomenon, moreover, was similar to the dynamics of the loss of antiviral activity by cells after removal of interferon from the culture medium. The workers concerned explained this observation on the assumption that during the action of actinomycin D only the synthesis of new RNAs was arrested, with no accompanying disturbance of protein synthesis as a result of activity of mRNAs already synthesized.

The use of p-fluorophenylalanine, on the other hand, led to a more rapid loss of antiviral activity by the cells through a disturbance of protein synthesis and, in particular, of the synthesis of antiviral protein (TIP); in the presence of p-fluorophenylalanine the protein was formed but was nonfunctioning. It is interesting to note that RNA synthesis was undisturbed in this case.

The greatest effect as regards a decrease in activity was given by the simultaneous use of actinomycin D and p-fluorophenylalanine, for their combined administration led to inhibition of synthesis of both RNA and protein.

These experiments, in conjunction with the results of experiments with removal of interferon from the culture medium, show that the primary cause of the loss of the antiviral state by the cells is cessation of the stimulation of mRNA formation. Cessation of the synthesis of protein with antiviral activity in this case is a secondary process.

In the discussion of the cell structures participating in interferon or antiviral protein production mention must be made of work carried out in the Department of Virology of the N. F. Gamaleya Institute of Epidemiology and Microbiology. Ya. E. Khesin, F. V. Voronina, and A. M. Amchenkova found that acid phosphatase ac-

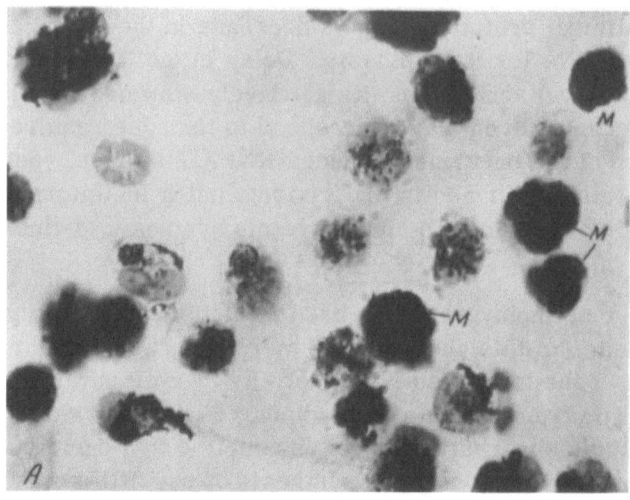

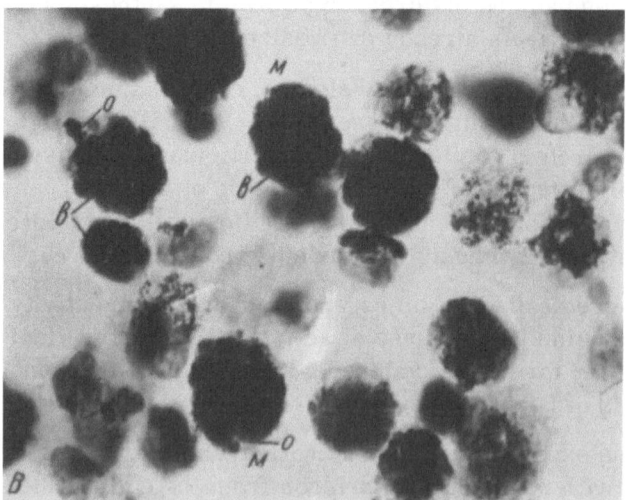

Fig. 14. Acid phosphatase activity in cells of 24-hour mouse peritoneal exudate. Gomori, 1100×. Photomicrographs show cells of exudate 1 h after addition of NDV (A, control; B, experiment). Enlargement of macrophages (M), vacuoles projecting above their surface (B), and rupture of vacuoles into medium (O) can be seen.

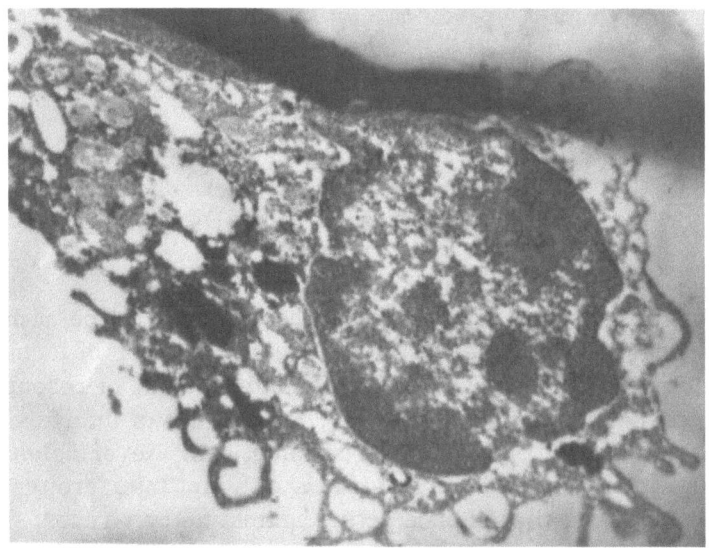

Fig. 15. Area of a macrophage with lysosome whose membranes
are partially ruptured after contact for 4 h with interferon-inducing
virus. Electron micrograph, 9000×.

tivity rises sharply in mouse peritoneal exudate cells under the
influence of interferon inducer, in this case NDV (Fig. 14).

This shows that lysosome activity was increased, and its
effects were seen particularly demonstratively in the macrophages,
in which the lysosomes swelled and formed large vacuoles. These
vacuoles were torn away from the cells and liberated their contents
into the culture medium. On the basis of these facts the hypothesis
of the direct (or indirect) participation of the lysosome system
of the cell in the production and liberation of interferon was put
forward.

Electron-microscopic investigations carried out at our Institute, in the laboratory directed by A. A. Avakyan, confirmed this
hypothesis. Specimens containing both control macrophages from
the peritoneal exudate and the corresponding cells after contact
for 4 h with an inducer virus were studied.

Examination of the specimens showed conclusively that
the membranes were ruptured under the influence of the interferon
inducer, leading to liberation of the contents of the lysosomes into
the cytoplasm. This process coincided with the time of intensive
interferon formation.

Conclusions and Prospects

As so frequently happens in the theory and practice of medicir the practical results of research into the mechanisms of formation and action of interferon have lagged far behind those of research in other directions and, in particular, into the use of interferon for the prevention and treatment of virus infections. Nevertheless the material which has now been obtained shows that interferon is a unique and universal substance acting against many viruses. Moreover it has been shown to be harmless both in its direct action on the body and in its freedom from late side effects of the allergic type.

The immediate future will show which of the methods of producing and using interferon are the most suitable, more especial ly since there are at least four directions in which its potential value can be exploited for practical purposes:

1. The use of homologous exogenous interferon in the most highly concentrated and purified form and in those pathological states which respond most successfully to its action.

2. The use of various stimulators of endogenous interferon, some of which must be substances harmless to the recipier and free from antigenic (sensitizing) side effects. Among the most active polynucleotides used as inducers of interferon under experimental conditions, investigators abroad have paid most attention to a complex of polyinosinic and polycytidylic acids.

3. The advantage of simultaneous administration of the final product and the inducer, thus resulting in the combined action of exogenous and endogenous interferons.

4. A combination of interferon with chemotherapeutic and other preparations.

Although the first two directions speak for themselves, the third requires an explanation. It is the prophylactic action of interferon which is least in doubt, or in other words the earlier interferon is used in an adequate concentration, the more marked its effect. Under experimental conditions this is nearly always attainable, but it is extremely difficult in practice because of the short duration of its action. For example, interferon prophylaxis of the respiratory infections is recommended in the presence of a source of infection, i.e., in an epidemic focus. Yet in such a focus there are healthy persons as well as those in the incubation period. It thus follows that interferon must be given within the shortest period of time and with maximum effectiveness.

One way in which this condition may perhaps be satisfied is by the combined administration of exogenous and endogenous interferons. The best procedure in this case is the preliminary administration of exogenous interferon. This is based on the results of experiments conducted in our laboratory by V. I. Marchenko and co-workers on cells of different origin: epithelial cells, fibroblasts, and leukocytes. Preliminary treatment with small doses of interferon (0.1-0.01 unit of interferon activity) followed by administration of the inducer virus 2 h later gave a level of interferon formation 4-10 times higher than in the control.

On the basis of existing experience of the use of interferon for influenza prophylaxis it can also be deduced that exogenous interferon does not only act alone. Its action is combined with that of endogenous interferon produced by the cells of the human respiratory tract. In other words, maximal prophylactic activity of artificially administered interferon arises when the individual concerned is infected, when he has developed a latent infectious process which is masked by the interferon, and the virus is reproducing without causing symptoms of the disease and is acting as an inducer of interferon formation by the epithelial cells of the respiratory tract. Special investigations have shown that the production of endogenous interferon varies both among animals and among man. Whereas minimal interferon production was found in 19.2% of pure-line mice receiving a large dose of interferon inducer intravenously, and under the same conditions in 26.4% of rabbits, the percentage of interferon-refractory human subjects receiving the interferon inducer intranasally was about 30. Different strains of influenza virus isolated during the 1969 epidemic differed in their ability to induce interferon. Of 46 strains of influenza A2 virus of the Hong Kong type tested from this point of view 7 were inactive as inducers of interferon in tests on mice, and this was subsequently confirmed by observations on volunteers.

The explanation of the fourth direction is based on the positive results of experiments in which interferon was combined with amantadin in experimental influenza.

Recent work has shown that the synthetic compound amantadin hydrochloride can prevent the development of influenza. Soviet investigators have shown that the combined administration of interferon and amantadin potentiates the synergic effect of inhibition of reproduction of influenza A/WSN virus in tissue culture [415]. Potentiation of the action of amantadin by interferon is interesting not only because these two substances have different mechanisms of action (amantadin changes the configuration of the cell membrane while interferon has an intracellular action), but also because amantadin is slightly toxic to man. Reducing the dose of amantadin by combining it with interferon thus increases its potential value in the prevention of influenza during epidemics.

This hypothesis was confirmed by observations on volunteers infected with influenza A2 vaccine virus. The volunteers were divided into four groups with 50 persons in each group; the first group received interferon and tablets of a placebo, the second received amantadin in medium 199, the third group amantadin and interferon, and the fourth group tablets of the placebo and medium 199. The preparations, which were identified by numbers, were given twice, 24 and 2 h before administration of the virus: interferon intranasally in a dose of 0.5 ml and amantadin in a dose of 150 mg by mouth. By recording the temperature reactions and by reisolation of the virus the following results were obtained from the groups (to save space the groups are identified by the name of the substances which they received) — general reactivity (pyrexia): interferon 8.5%, amantadin 7.1%, interferon + amantadin 2.4%, control 34.8%; reisolation of the virus: interferon 19.6%, amantadin 48.2%, interferon + amantadin 9.7%, control 46.6% [696].

These observations confirmed our previous results for the action of interferon during infection of volunteers with influenza virus and they justify the hope that combined prophylaxis of this type will be successful in practice.

The possibility of an association between exogenous interferon and specific antibodies can also be considered, since they act on extracellular virus.

Much, of course, depends on the development of research into the mechanism of action of interferon. If the theory or, more exactly, the hypothesis of the indirect action of interferon finds experimental confirmation and if the TIP is isolated, this will enable the potential therapeutic value of interferon to become a practical possibility very much sooner. So far as the prevention of virus infections is concerned, the use of interferon for this purpose already rests on a firm experimental basis. During the 1969 influenza epidemic controlled tests of interferon prophylaxis were carried out by the Central Institute of Epidemiology, Ministry of Health of the USSR, and the Department of Epidemiology of the N. F. Gamaleya Institute of Epidemiology of Microbiology, Academy of Medical Sciences of the USSR. They showed a decrease of between 40.5 and 73.8% in the incidence of influenza among 11,879 adults and children. As a result of this investigation to assess the effectiveness of interferon for the prevention of influenza and other virus respiratory infections, the Committee for Sera and Vaccines of the Ministry of Health of the USSR authorized the large-scale production of human leukocytic interferon and recommended the preparation for practical use.

If interferon is regarded from the standpoint of a protective reaction of immunity, it must be pointed out that the system forming the specific immunoreactivity of the organism is the lymphoid tissue. In particular, lymphocytes are ascribed the leading role as precursors of the antibody-forming cells and as carriers of the immunological memory. Unlike the antigen–antibody complex, the formation of interferon is one of the nonspecific reactions of the organism. In this case there is no definite antigen to which specific antibodies would be produced and with which they would need to combine. However, interferon formation in the organism is an activity of the same system of lymphoid organs and cells.

We consider that the process of immunoreactivity incorporates two stages: the immediate (primary) response of the organism to introduction of the virus, for which interferon is responsible, and the secondary response connected with antibodies. If antibodies are described as a humoral factor and interferon as a cellular factor, it is logical to regard them as links in the same chain of immunological reactions of the organism, both specific and nonspecific. According to this view it is not interferon but rather the antibodies which are the characteristic of recovery and which correspond to the development of postinfectious immunity. Interferon, on the other hand, determines the rate and intensity of the infectious process connected with the period of reproduction of viruses.

We have shown that in certain infections there is a negative phase of immunoreactivity, when the leukocytes become inert and do not produce interferon, and before antibodies can be found. This negative phase heralds a lethal outcome of the infectious process.

The use of interferon as a product of leukocytic metabolism, i.e., as an indicator of the functional state of the lymphoid organs maintaining the constancy of the internal environmental of the organism, is another promising development. Tests of lymphoid function have so far been restricted to the reaction of phagocytosis, which has a very low level of reproducibility and incorporates a number of changing components, so that it cannot be used in a standard and universal form. The IRL (interferon reaction of the leukocytes) test corresponds much more strictly to this purpose, as the writer has shown on several examples. Further and more extensive clinical trials are, of course, necessary in order to overcome all the technical problems, yet nevertheless the results so far obtained with this test when used to assess the functional state of the lymphoid organs in man, under both normal and pathological conditions, have proved very encouraging.

Bibliography

1. Abadzhyan, G. A., Vestn. Oftal'mol., 1:72 (1968).
2. Agol, V. I., in: Molecular Bases of the Biology of Viruses, Moscow (1966), p. 177.
3. Aksenov, O. A., Smorodintsev, A. A., Gvozdilova, D. A., et al., in: Influenza and Acute Respiratory Diseases, Leningrad (1967), p. 213.
4. Andzhaparidze, O. G., Bogomolova, N. N., and Grokhovskaya, A. A., Vopr. Virusol., 2:158 (1966).
5. Andzhaparidze, O. G., and Grokhovskaya, A. A., in: Inhibitors of Virus Activity, Riga (1967), p. 87.
6. Andzhaparidze, O. G., Grokhovskaya, A. A., and Bogomolova, N. N., Vopr. Virusol., 3:296 (1967).
7. Antonova, T. N., in: The Theory and Practice of Stomatology. Moscow Medical Stomatological Institute, No. 9 (1966), p. 214.
8. Ashmarin, Yu. Ya., and Vil'ner, L. M , in: Current Problems in Virus Infections, Moscow (1965), p. 389.
9. Ashmarin, Yu. Ya., Vil'ner, L. M., Zeitlenok, N. A., et al., in: Interferon and Interferon Inducers, Vol. 10, Moscow (1967), p. 69.
10. Babushkin, V. S., in: Interferon and Interferon Inducers, Moscow (1967), p. 103.
11. Balezina, T. I., Borisov, Yu. V., Ermol'eva, Z. V., et al., Vopr. Virusol., 2:235 (1966).
12. Balezina, T. I., Korable'nikova, N. I., Bostandzhyan, M. G., and Vilenchik, M. M., in: Problems in General Virology, Moscow (1966), p. 232.
13. Balezina, T. I., Korabel'nikova, N. I., Krupchatnikova, G. E., and Fadeeva, L. L., in: Acute Respiratory Virus Infections, Sverdlovsk (1966), p. 169.
14. Balezina, T. I., Korabel'nikova, N. I., Pyrikova, A. P., et al., Proceedings of the 5th Conference of Tallin IEMG, Tallin (1964), p. 23.
15. Balezina, T. I., Korabel'nikova, N. I., and Sklyanskaya, E. I., in: Relations between Virus and Cell, Riga (1965), p. 33.
16. Balezina, T. I., Korabel'nikova, N. I., Pyrikova, A. P., et al., Antibiotiki, 13(2):176 (1968).
17. Bektemirov, T. A., Med. Radiol., 10:62 (1961).
18. Bektemirov, T. A., in: Textbook of Epidemiology, Clinical Picture, and Microbiology of Infectious Diseases, Vol. 4, Moscow (1965), p. 273.
19. Bektemirov, T. A., in: The Epidemiology and Prophylaxis of Infectious Diseases, Moscow (1965), p. 102.

20. Bektemirov, T. A., in: The Epidemiology and Prophylaxis of Infectious Diseases, Moscow (1965), p. 73.
21. Bektemirov, T. A., Acta Virol., 9:546 (1965).
22. Bektemirov, T. A., Vopr. Virusol., 5:626 (1965).
23. Bektemirov, T. A., and Gumennik, A. E., Vopr. Virusol., 6:689 (1965).
24. Bektemirov, T. A., and Gumennik, A. E., Vopr. Virusol., 1:18 (1967).
25. Bektemirov, T. A., and Gumennik, A. E., Acta Virol., 11:165 (1967).
26. Bektemirov, T. A., and Mastyukova, Yu. N., Vopr. Virusol., 2:221 (1960).
27. Bektemirov, T. A., and Sokkar, I. M., Vopr. Virusol., 3:330 (1963).
28. Borecky, L., and Blaskovic, D., Uspekhi Sovr. Biol., 63:261 (1967).
29. Bostandzhyan, M. G., in: The Microbiology, Immunology, Epidemiology, and Natural Nidality of Human Diseases, Moscow (1966), p. 10
30. Bostandzhyan, M. G., The Production and Comparative Study of Purified Interferons of Different Origin. Author's Abstract of Candidate's Dissertation, Moscow (1966).
31. Bostandzhyan, M. G., in: Inhibitors of Virus Activity, Riga (1967), p. 112.
32. Bostandzhyan, M. G., Vopr. Virusol., 2:161 (1967).
33. Bostandzhyan, M. G., in: Influenza and Acute Respiratory Diseases, Leningrad (1967), p. 129.
34. Bostandzhyan, M. G., and Balezina, T I., in: Problems in General Virology, Moscow (1966), p. 228.
35. Bostandzhyan, M. G., and Bikbulatov, R. M., Acta Virol., 2:159 (1967).
36. Budnitskaya, P. Z., The Isolation, Chemical Characteristics, and Some Biological Properties of a Pyrogenal Preparation. Candidate's Dissertation, Moscow (1963).
37. Veselkin, P. N., in: Pyrogenal, Moscow (1965), p. 7.
38. Vil'ner, L. M., Zeitlenok, N. A., Rodin, I. M., Brodskaya, L. M., Gnuni, G. M., and Finogenova, E. V., in: Relations between Virus and Cell, Riga (1965), p. 35.
39. Vil'ner, L. M., Zeitlenok, N. A., Chumakov, M. P., Brodskaya, L. M., Rodin I. M., and Reizin, F. M., in: Interferon and Interferon Inducers, Moscow (1967), p. 37.
40. Vil'ner, L. M., Chumakov, P. M., Gol'dfarb, M. M., Mustafina, A. D., Brodskaya, L. M., and Mironova, L. L., in: Current Problems in Virus Infections, Moscow (1965), p. 382.
41. Vil'ner, L. M., Chumakov, M. P., and Zeitlenok, N. A., in: Poliomyelitis and Virus Encephalitis. Proceedings of a Committee of Inquiry, Academy of Medical Sciences of the USSR, Moscow (1967), p. 135.
42. Vil'ner, L. M., Chumakov, M. P., and Zeitlenok, N. A., Antibiotiki, 12:1093 (1967).
43. Vil'ner, L. M., Chumakov, M. P., Zeitlenok, A. N., and Brodskaya, L. M., Antibiotiki, 12:908 (1967).
44. Vil'ner, L. M., Chumakov, M. P., Zeitlenok, N. A., et al., in: Proceedings of the 9th International Congress of Microbiology, Moscow (1966), p. 560.
45. Vil'ner, L. M., Chumakov, M. P., Zeitlenok, N. A., et al., in: Interferon and Interferon Inducers, Moscow (1967), p. 123.
46. Vorob'eva, M. S., Selimov, M. A., and Safarov, R. K., in: Proceedings of the

13th Session of the Institute of Poliomyelitis and Virus Encephalitis, Moscow (1967), p. 70.

47. Vorotyntseva, N. V., Solov'ev, V. D., Bektemirov, T. A., et al., in: Problems in the Pathology of Children's Infectious Diseases, Leningrad (1967), p. 68

48. Gendon, Yu. Z., in: Relations between Virus and Cell, Riga (1965), p. 24.

49. Gendon, Yu. Z., Acta Virol., 2:186 (1965).

50. Gendon, Yu. Z., in: Virus and Cell, Riga (1966), p. 87.

51. Gendon, Yu. Z., Balandin, I. G., and Babushkina, L. M., Acta Virol., 10:268 (1966).

52. Globa, L. I., Production of Interferon with Inactivated Influenza Virus and Some Properties of the Preparation. Candidate's Dissertation, Kiev (1967).

53. Grokhovskaya, A. A., Vopr. Virusol., 2:163 (1966).

54. Grokhovskaya, A. A., A Study of the Phenomenon of Interference and of Interferon Formation in Experimental Arbovirus Infection. Candidate's Dissertation, Moscow (1968).

55. Demidova, S. A., and Smirnova, G. A., in: Inhibitors of Virus Activity, Riga (1967), p. 102.

56. Dubova, A. V., in: Current Problems in Virus Infections, Moscow (1965), p. 385.

57. Duisalieva, R. G., Gutman, N. R., and Marchenko, V. I., in: Inhibitors of Virus Activity, Riga (1967), p. 77.

58. Ermol'eva, Z. V., Antibiotics. Interferon. Bacterial Polysaccharides, Moscow, Meditsina (1968).

59. Ermol'eva, Z. V., Vaisberg, G. E., and Afanas'eva, T. I., Byull. Eksperim. Biol. i Med., No. 8, 77 (1961).

60. Ermol'eva, Z. V., Fadeeva, L. L., Balezina, T. I., et al., Vopr. Virusol., No. 2, 221 (1965).

61. Ermol'eva, Z. V., Furer, N. M., Balezina, T. I., et al., in: The Problem of Influenza, Leningrad (1961), p. 175.

62. Ermol'eva, Z. V., Furer, N. M., Balezina, T. I., et al., Antibiotiki, 3:196 (1961).

63. Ermol'eva, Z. V., Furer, N. M., Balezina, T. I., et al., Khim. Med., No. 10, 3 (1963).

64. Ermol'eva, Z. V., Furer, N. M., Bezdenezhnykh, I. S., et al., in: Influenza, Moscow (1966), p. 139.

65. Ermol'eva, Z. V., Furer, N. M., Vaisberg, G. E., et al., in: Abstracts of Proceedings of the Prague Congress on Virus and Rickettsial Diseases of the Respiratory Tract, Prague (1961), p. 11.

66. Ermol'eva, Z. V., Furer, N. M., Vaisberg, G. E., et al., in: Collected Transactions of the Central Postgraduate Medical Institute, Moscow (1963), p. 145.

67. Ermol'eva, Z. V., Furer, N. M., Nemirovskaya, B. M., et al., in: Virus and Cell, Riga (1966).

68. Ermol'eva, Z. V., Furer, N. M., Nemirovskaya, B. M., et al., in: Proceedings of the 17th Session of the D. I. Ivanovskii Institute of Virology, Part 1, Moscow (1964), p. 65.

69. Ermol'eva, Z. V., Furer, N. M., Pokidova, N. V., et al., in: Proceedings of the 13th Session of the Institute of Poliomyelitis and Virus Encephalitis, Moscow (1967), p. 268.

70. Ermol'eva, Z. V., Furer, N. M., Pokidova, N. V., et al., Antibiotiki, 12:1034 (1967).

71. Ermol'eva, Z. V., Furer, N. M., Fadeeva, L. L., et al., in: Problems in Medical Virology, Vol. 8, Moscow (1963), p. 127.

72. Ermol'eva, Z. V., Furer, N. M., Fainshtein, S. L., et al., in: Problems in General Virology, Moscow (1966), p. 222.

73. Ershov, F. I., in: General Virology, Moscow (1967), p. 164.

74. Ershov, F. I., and Zhdanov, V. M., Dokl. Akad. Nauk SSSR, 164:1165 (1964).

75. Ershov, F. I., and Zhdanov, V. M., in: Virus and Cell, Riga (1966), p. 103.

76. Ershov, F. I., Tazulakhova, E. B., and Ermol'eva, Z. V., Antibiotiki, No. 1, 32 (1966).

77. Zhdanov, V. M., Ermol'eva, Z. V., Fadeeva, L. L., et al., in: Proceedings of the 17th Scientific Session of the D. I. Ivanovskii Institute of Virology, Academy of Medical Sciences of the USSR, Part 1, Moscow (1964), p. 67.

78. Zhdanov, V. M., Ershov, F. I., Tazulakhova, E. B., et al., in: Relations between Virus and Cell, Riga (1965), p. 14.

79. Zhdanov, V. M., Yakovleva, L. S., Pyrikova, A. P., et al., Vopr. Virusol., No. 4, 496 (1965).

80. Zalmanzon, E. S., Balezina, T. I., Korabel'nikova, N. I., et al., in: Virus and Cell, Riga (1966), p. 17.

81. Zalmanzon, E. S., Balezina, T. I , Korabel'nikova, N. I., et al., in: Proceedings of the 9th International Congress of Microbiologists, Moscow (1966), p. 562.

82. Zalmanzon, E. S., Korabel'nikova, N. I., Balezina, T. I., et al., in: Relations Between Virus and Cell, Riga (1965), p. 6.

83. Zalmanzon, E. S., Korabel'nikova, N. I., Balezina, T. I., et al., in: Influenza and Acute Respiratory Diseases, Part 1, Leningrad (1967), p. 147.

84. Zeitlenok, N. A., in: Interferon and Interferon Inducers, Moscow (1967), p. 7.

85. Zeitlenok, N. A., Vil'ner, L. M., Brodskaya, L. M., and Roikhel', V. M., in: Relations between Virus and Cell, Riga (1965), p. 10.

86. Zeitlenok, N. A., Vil'ner, L. M., and Kasparov, A. A., Vestn. Oftal'mol., No. 6, 80 (1966).

87. Zeitlenok, N. A., Vil'ner, L. M., Rodin, I. M., et al., in: Inhibitors of Virus Activity, Riga (1967), p. 16.

88. Zeitlenok, N. A., Vil'ner, L. M., Chumakov, M. P., Rodin, I. M., and Solovei, É. A., in: Interferon and Interferon Inducers, Moscow (1967), p. 115.

89. Zlatkovskaya, N. M., Ulanovskaya, T. I., Furer, N. M., et al., in: Problems in the Pathology of Childrens' Infectious Diseases, Leningrad (1967), p. 67.

90. Ivanova, N. A., Principles Governing the Conditions of Interferon Formation and Manifestation of Its Biological Activity. Candidate's Dissertation, Leningrad (1965).

91. Ivanova, N. A., Byull. Éksperim. Biol. i Med., 61(12):75 (1966).

92. Ivanova, N. A., in: Virus and Cell, Riga (1966), p. 31.

93. Ivanova, N. A., and Polyak, R. Ya., in: Virus and Cell, Riga (1966), p. 95.

94. Ivanova, N. A., and Polyak, R. Ya., Vopr. Virusol., No. 1, 25 (1966).

95. Karakuyumchan, M. K., Bektemirova, M. S., and Vagabov, R. A., in: Current Problems in Veterinary Virology, Vol. 1, Moscow (1967), p. 166.

96. Karakuyumchan, M. K., and Bektemirova, M. S., Vopr. Virusol., No. 5, 596 (1968).
97. Kasparov, A. A., Vil'ner, L. M., and Zeitlenok, N. A., in: Interferon and Interferon Inducers, Moscow, (1967), p. 75.
98. Kasparov, A. A., Kunicheva, G. S., Kulikova, L. A., et al., in: Interferon and Interferon Inducers, Moscow (1967), p. 85.
99. Ketiladze, E. S., in: Virus Diseases of Man, Moscow (1967), p. 54.
100. Klemparskaya, N. N., Antibacterial Immunity and Radioresistance, Moscow (1963).
101. Korabel'nikova, N. I., Pyrikova, A. P., Balezina, T. I., et al., in: Problems in General Virology, Moscow (1966), p. 235.
102. Korsantiya, B. M., Conditions of Formation and Detection of Biological Activity of Interferon in Cell Cultures. Candidate's Dissertation, Leningrad (1967).
103. Korsantiya, B. M., and Smorodintsev, A. A., in: The Microbiology, Immunology, Epidemiology, and Natural Nidality of Human Diseases, Moscow (1966), p. 71.
104. Kunicheva, G. S., Kasparov, A. A., Vil'ner, L. M., and Zeitlenok, N. A., Vestn. Oftal'mol, No. 6, 17 (1966).
105. Lipkind, M. A., in: Inhibitors of Virus Activity, Riga (1967), p. 114.
106. Litvinov, A. N., in: Current Problems in Veterinary Virology, Part 1, Moscow (1965), p. 34.
107. Litvinov, A. N., in: Virus and Cell, Riga (1966), p. 123.
108. Litvinov, A. N , Conditions of Formation and Study of Some Biological Properties of Interferon. Author's Abstract of Candidate's Dissertation, Moscow (1967).
109. Litvinov, A. N., in: Current Problems in Veterinary Virology, Moscow (1967), p. 161.
110. L'vovskii, É. A., Effect of Ionizing Radiation on Interferon Formation in Irradiated Tissues. Candidate's Dissertation, Leningrad (1967).
111. Maichuk, Yu. F., Vil'ner, L. M., Andzhelov, V. O., Gushchina, A. V., and Rzhechitskaya, O. V., in: Interferon and Interferon Inducers, Moscow (1967), p. 95.
112. Martynov, L. A., in: Pyrogenal, Moscow (1965), p. 84.
113. Mentkevich, L. M., Vopr. Virusol., No. 4, 420 (1967).
114. Mentkevich, L. M., Virus Interference, Doctoral Dissertation, Moscow (1967).
115. Mentkevich, L. M., and Orlova, T. G., Acta Virol., 10:226 (1966).
116. Mentkevich, L. M., Orlova, T. G., and Eremkina, E. I., in: Interferon and Interferon Inducers, Moscow (1967), p. 173.
117. Ovsyannikova, N. V., and Zeitlenok, N. A., in: Interferon and Interferon Inducers, Moscow (1967), p. 165.
118. Peterson, O. P., and Li Yü, Vopr. Virusol., No. 3, 279 (1963).
119. Peterson, O. P., and Li Yü, Vopr. Virusol., No. 6, 719 (1963).
120. Peterson, O. P., Kozlova, I. A., Mel'nikova, L. A., and Bostandzhyan, M. G., in: Proceedings of the 19th Scientific Session of the D. I. Ivanovskii Institute of Virology, Moscow (1966), p. 231.
121. Peterson, O. P., Mel'nikova, L. A., Kozlova, I. A., and Balezina, T. I., Vopr. Virusol., No. 6, 662 (1966).
122. Pokidova, N. V., Furer, N. M., Sapozhnikova, G. A., et al., in: Virus and Cell, Riga (1966), p. 57.

123. Potekaev, N. S., Konstantinov, A. V., and Vil'ner, L. M., in: Current Problems in Virus Infections, Moscow (1965), p. 390.
124. Priimyagi, L. S., Vopr. Virusol., No. 6, 694 (1965).
125. Priimyagi, L. S., Production of Tissue Interferons and Determination of Their Spectrum of Action on Viruses. Author's Abstract of Candidate's Dissertation, Moscow (1965).
126. Priimyagi, L. S., Grinshpun, L. E., Oleinik, I. P., et al., in: Problems in General Virology, Moscow (1966), p. 236.
127. Priimyagi, L. S., Grinshpun, L. E., Raevskii, D. I., et al., in: Influenza and Acute Respiratory Diseases, Leningrad (1967), p. 196.
128. Priimyagi, L. S., Grinshpun, L. E., Raevskii, D. I., et al., in: Inhibitors of Virus Activity, Riga (1967), p. 98.
129. Priimyagi, L. S., and Iyks, S. R., in: Inhibitors of Virus Activity, Riga (1967), p. 105.
130. Priimyagi, L. S., and Fadeeva, L. L., in: Proceedings of a Scientific and Practical Conference of the Leningrad Pasteur Research Institute of Epidemiology and Microbiology, Leningrad (1965), p. 136.
131. Priimyagi, L. S., and Fadeeva, L. L., in: Proceedings of the 5th Scientific Conference in 1964, Tallin (1965), p. 66.
132. Priimyagi, L. S., and Fadeeva, L. L., in: Virus and Cell, Riga (1966), p. 23.
133. Pyrikova, A. P., Korabel'nikova, N. I., Balezina, T. I., et al., in: Inhibitors of Virus Activity, Riga (1967), p. 92.
134. Rakhmanov, V. A., Potekaev, N. S., Konstantinov, A. V., et al., in: Interferon and Interferon Inducers, Moscow (1967), p. 63.
135. Revazova, E. S., in: Inhibitors of Virus Activity, Riga (1967), p. 71.
136. Rodin, I. M., Vil'ner, L. M., Zeitlenok, N. A., et al., in: Current'Problems in Veterinary Virology, Vol. 1, Moscow (1967), p. 172.
137. Rostoka, A. A., and Églite, I. É., in: Inhibitors of Virus Activity, Riga (1967), p. 73.
138. Rusanova, N. A., and Solov'ev, V. D., Vopr. Virusol., No. 4, 398 (1966).
139. Sklyanskaya, E. I., Peterson, O. P., Balezina, T. I., and Korabel'nikova, N. I., in: Virus and Cell, Riga (1966), p. 135.
140. Smirnova, G. A., in: Virus and Cell, Riga (1966), p. 73.
141. Smirnova, G. A., Fadeeva, L. L., Korabel'nikova, N. I., et al., in: Respiratory Virus Infections, Moscow (1963), p. 56.
142. Smorodintsev, A. A., Vopr. Virusol., No. 5, 587 (1964).
143. Smorodintsev, A. A., Uspekhi Sovr. Biol., 62(3):398 (1966).
144. Smorodintsev, A. A., Aksenov, O. A., Burov, S. A., et al., in: Influenza and Acute Respiratory Diseases, Leningrad (1967), p. 215.
145. Smorodintsev, A. A., and Gvozdilova, D. A., in: The Microbiology, Immunology Epidemiology, and Natural Nidality of Human Diseases, Moscow (1966), p. 128.
146. Smorodintsev, A. A., Gvozdilova, D. A., Korsantiya, B. M., et al., in: Advances in the Diagnosis and Treatment of Virus Diseases, Leningrad (1967), p. 217.
147. Smorodintsev, A. A., Gvozdilova, D. A., and Aksenov, O. A., in: Problems in the Pathology of Children's Infectious Diseases, Leningrad (1967), p. 70
148. Smorodintsev, A. A., Gvozdilova, D. A., and Aksenov, O. A., in: Inhibitors of Virus Activity, Riga (1967), p. 90.

149. Smorodintsev, A. A., Korsantiya, B. M., and Gvozdilova, D A., in: Interferon and Interferon Inducers, Moscow (1967), p. 145.
150. Smorodintsev, A. A., in: Virus and Cell, Riga (1966), p. 39.
151. Smorodintsev, A. A., Kotenko, T. V., Gvozdilova, D. A., and Korshunova, V. A., in: Transactions of the Institute of Experimental Medicine, Academy of Medical Sciences of the USSR, Vol. 9, Moscow (1967), No. 5, p. 18.
152. Sokolov, M. I., and Kulikova, K. S., Annotations of Publications of the Institute of Virology, Academy of Medical Sciences of the USSR, for 1949, Moscow (1950), p. 16.
153. Solov'ev, V. D., Vestn. Akad. Med. Nauk SSSR, No. 5, 27 (1963).
154. Solov'ev, V. D., and Alekseeva, A. K., Acta Virol., 4(3):129 (1960).
155. Solov'ev, V. D., and Bektemirov, T. A., Tissue Cultures in Virology, Moscow (1963).
156. Solov'ev, V. D., Bektemirov, T. A., and Gumennik, A. E., Vopr. Virusol., No. 4, 420 (1965).
157. Solov'ev, V. D., and Bektemirov, T. A., in: Problems in General Virology, Moscow (1966), p. 226.
158. Solov'ev, V. D., Bektemirov, T. A., Gutman, N. R., and Fedorova, Yu. B., Vopr. Virusol., No 4, 418 (1966).
159. Solov'ev, V. D., Bektemirov, T. A., Vorotyntseva, N. V., et al., Vopr. Virusol., No. 1, 21 (1967).
160. Solov'ev, V. D., Bektemirov, T. A., Neklyudova, L. I., and Gumennik, A. E., in: General Virology, Moscow (1967), p. 89.
161. Solov'ev, V. D., Bektemirov, T. A., Neklyudova, L. I., et al., in: Proceedings of a Scientific Session of the Central Postgraduate Medical Institute, Moscow (1967), p. 24.
162 Solov'ev, V. D., Bektemirov, T. A., Porubel', L. A., and Rapoport, R. I., Vopr. Virusol., No. 3, 311 (1966).
163. Solov'ev, V. D., Bektemirov, T. A., Porubel', L. A., and Churkin, G. S., in: Interferon and Interferon Inducers, Moscow (1967), p. 55.
164. Solov'ev, V. D., Bektemirov, T. A., and Fedorova, Yu. B., in: Inhibitors of Virus Activity, Riga (1967), p. 66.
165. Solov'ev, V. D., Bektemirov, T. A., and Fedorova, Yu. B., Vopr. Virusol., No. 4, 415 (1967).
166. Solov'ev, V. D., Duisalieva, R. G., Gutman, N. R., and Marchenko, V. I., in: Interferon and Interferon Inducers, Moscow (1967), p. 111.
167. Solov'ev, V. D, and Mentkevich, L. M., Acta Virol., 9:308 (1965).
168. Solov'ev, V. D., and Mentkevich, L. M., Vopr. Virusol., No. 2, 154 (1966).
169. Solov'ev, V. D., Mentkevich, L. M., Orlova, T. G., and Eremkina, E. I., in: Proceedings of the 13th Session of the Institute of Poliomyelitis and Virus Encephalitis, Moscow (1967), p. 266.
170. Solov'ev, V. D., et al., Acta Virol., 10:104 (1966).
171. Solov'ev, V. D., Orlova, T. G., Mentkevich, L. M., and Tatarinova, Yu. N., in: Current Problems in Veterinary Virology, Vol. 1, Moscow (1967), p. 167.
172. Stepanyuk, T. I., and Goncharov, A. I., in: Inhibitors of Virus Activity, Riga (1967), p. 95.
173. Tikhonenko, T. I., Shatkin, A. A., Irlin, I. S., and Sinyakova, R. N., Vopr. Virusol., No. 4, 480 (1963).

174. Trubina, L. M., Yakovenko, Z. F., and Stratienko, L. M., in: Current Problems in the Virology and Specific Prophylaxis of Virus Diseases, Moscow (1967), p. 180.

175. Tyufanov, A. V., and Vil'ner, L. M., in: Current Problems in Virus Infections, Moscow (1967), p. 387.

176. Fadeeva, L. L., Balezina, T. I., Korabel'nikova, N. I., et al., in: Problems in General Virology, Moscow (1966), .p. 221.

177. Fadeeva, L. L., Balezina, T. I., and Korabel'nikova, N. I., in: General Virology, Moscow (1967), p. 161.

178. Fadeeva, L.L., Balezina, T. I., Korabel'nikova, N. I., Yakovleva, L. S., and Pyrikova, A. P., Proceedings of the 11th Scientific Conference of the Institute of Poliomyelitis and Virus Encephalitis, Moscow (1964), p. 74.

179. Fadeeva, L. L., Balezina, T. I., Furer, N. M., and Nemirovskaya, B. M., Problems in Medical Virology, Vol. 8, Moscow (1963), p. 133.

180. Fel'dmane, G. Ya., Érele, G. E., Smilga, Ya. M., Lozha, V. P., and Plander, É. M., in: Relations between Virus and Cell, Riga (1965), p. 18.

181. Furer, N.M., Nemirovskaya,. B. M., Kalabukhova, N. F., et al., in: Problems in General Virology, Moscow (1966), p. 223.

182. Furer, N.M., Nemirovskaya, B. M., Tazulakhova, E. B., and Ermol'eva, Z. V., Antibiotiki, 1:25 (1966).

183. Furer, N. M., Nemirovskaya, B. M., Khanina, L. A., and Ermol'eva, Z. V., in: The Epidemiology and Prophylaxis of Infectious Diseases, Moscow (1965), pp. 80 and 96.

184. Khesin, Ya. E., and Mentkevich, L. M., Acta Virol., 9:190 (1965).

185. Chernetsov, Yu. E., in: General Virology, Moscow (1967), p. 169.

186. Chumakov, M. P., Vil'ner, L. M., Gagarina, A. V., and Gol'dfarb, M. M., in: Problems in Neurovirus Infections, Kiev (1965), p. 47.

187. Chumakov, M. P., Vil'ner, L. M., Zeitlenok, N. A., et al., in: Relations between Virus and Cell, Riga (1965), p. 4.

188. Chumakov, M. P., Zeitlenok, N. A., Vil'ner, L. M., Rodin, I. M., and Ashmarin, Yu. Ya., in: Current Problems in Virus Infections, Moscow (1965), p. 380.

189. Chumakov, M. P., Zeitlenok, N. A., and Vil'ner, L. M., in: Interferon and Interferon Inducers, Moscow (1967), p. 15.

190. Yurov, K. N., Acta Virol., 11:494 (1967).

191. Action, J. B., and Myrvik, Q. N., J. Bact., 91:2300 (1966).

192. Alford, R. H., Kasel, J. A., Loda, F., and Knight, V., Ann. Intern. Med., 62:1312 (1965).

193. Allison, A. C., Virology, 15:47 (1961).

194. Anderson, S. G., Austr. J. Exp. Biol. Med. Sci., 43:345 (1965).

195. Anderson, C. D., and Atherton, J. G., Nature, 203:671 (1964).

196. Andrews, K. D., Brit. Med. J., 1:1728 (1961).

197. Asch, R. J., and Bubel, H. C., J. Infect. Dis., 111:1 (1966).

198. Atanasiu, P., and Chany, C., C. R. Acad. Sci., 251:1687 (1960).

199. Aurelian, L., and Roizman, B., Virology, 22:452 (1964).

200. Aurelian, L., and Roizman, B., J. Mol. Biol., 11:539 (1965).

201. Bader, J. P., Virology, 16:436 (1962).

202. Baltimore, D., Franklin, R., and Callender, J., Biochim. Biophys. Acta, 76:425 (1963).

203. Bardos, V., and Seeficova, L., Acta Virol., 10:80 (1966).
204. Baron, S., Adv. Virus Res., 10:39 (1963).
205. Baron, S., in: International Symposium on Nonspecific Resistance to Virus Infection, Interferon and Viral Chemotherapy, Smolenica, Sept. 8-11, 1964.
206. Baron, S., Inform. Exch. Gr., Vol. 6 (1964).
207. Baron, S., Barban, S., and Buckler, C. E., Science, 145:814 (1964).
208. Baron, S., and Buckler, C. E., Bact. Proc. Abstr., 63:142 (1964).
209. Baron, S., and Buckler, C. E., Science, 141:1061 (1963).
210. Baron, S., and Buckler, C. E., Fed. Proc., 23:507 (1964).
211. Baron, S., Buckler, C. E., McCloskey, R. V., and Kirschstein, R. L.,·J. Immunol., 96:12 (1966).
212. Baron, S., Buckler, C. E., Friedman, R. M., and McCloskey, R. V., J. Immunol., 96:17 (1966).
213. Baron, S., Buckler, C. E., McCloskey, R. V., and Kirschstein, R. L., Inform. Exch. Gr., Vol. 6 (1965).
214. Baron, S., Buckler, C. E., Levy, H. B., et al., Proc. Soc. Exp. Biol. Med., 125:1320 (1967).
215. Baron, S., Du Buy, H. G., Buckler, C. E., and Johnson, M. L., Proc. Soc. Exp. Biol. Med., 117:338 (1964).
216. Baron, S., Buckler, C., and Levy, H. B., Ninth International Congress of Microbiology, Moscow (1966), p. 558.
217. Baron, S., and Isaacs, A., New Sci., 11:81 (1961).
218. Baron, S., and Isaacs, A., Nature, 191:97 (1961).
219. Baron, S., and Isaacs, A., Brit. Med. J., 1:18 (1962).
220. Baron, S., Merigan, T., and McKerlie, M. L., Proc. Soc. Èxp. Biol. Med., 121:50 (1966).
221. Barski, G., and Cornefert, F., J. Nat. Cancer Inst., 28:823 (1962).
222. Blackmore, R. V., and Morgan, H. P., Acta Virol., 11:1 (1967).
223. Bocci, V., Russi, M., and Rita, G., Inform. Exch. Gr., Vol. 6 (1967).
224. Bodian, D., Am. J. Hyg., 60:339 (1954).
225. Borecky, L., and Lackovic, V., Acta Virol., 10:271 (1966).
226. Borecky, L., and Lackovic, V., Simposio Internationale sugli Interferoni, Siena, 1967.
227. Borecky, L., and Lackovic, V., Acta Virol., 11:150 (1967).
228. Borecky, L., Lackovic, V., Blaskovic, D., Masler, L., and Sikl, D., Acta Viról., 11:264 (1967).
229. Boudreault, A., and Pavilanis, V., Rev. Canad, Biol., 23:277 (1964).
230. Brailowsky, C., and Chany, C., Comp. Rend. Acad. Sci., 260:2634 (1965).
231. Buckler, C. E., and Baron, S., J. Bact., 91:231 (1966).
232. Buckler, C. E., Baron, S., and Levy, H. B., Science, 152:80 (1966).
233. Burke, D. C., in: Interferons, Amsterdam (1966), p. 55.
234. Burke, D. C., and Buchan, A., Virology, 26:28 (1965).
235. Burke, D. C., and Isaacs, A., Brit. J. Exp. Path., 39:78 (1958).
236. Burke, D. S., and Isaacs, A., Brit. J. Exp. Path., 39:452 (1958).
237. Burke, D. C., and Isaacs, A., Acta Virol., 4:215 (1960).
238. Cantell, K., Arch. Ges. Virusforsch., 10:510 (1961).
239. Cantell, K., Lapinieimu, K., Penttinoz, K., Saukkonen, J., and Urome, E., Acta Path. Microb. Scand., Suppl. 154:348 (1962).

240. Cantell, K., and Paucker, K., Virology, 19:81 (1963).
241. Cantell, K., and Paucker, K., Virology, 21:11 (1963).
242. Cantell, K., and Tommi, V., Lancet, 2:682 (1960).
243. Cantell, K., and Valle, M., Ann. Med. Exp. Fenn., 43:61 (1965).
244. Cantell, K., Valle, M., Schakir, R., Saukkonen, J. J., and Uroma, E., Ann. Med. Exp. Fenn., 43:125 (1965).
245. Carter, W. A., and Levy, H. B., Fed. Proc., 25:491 (1966).
246. Carter, W. A., and Levy, H. B., Science, 124:1254 (1967).
247. Chang, S., and Rasmussen, A. F., Nature, 205:623 (1965).
248. Chang, T. W., and Weinstein, L., J. A. M. A., 182:1040 (1962).
249. Chany, C., Virology, 13:485 (1961).
250. Chany, C., and Brailowsky, C., C. R. Acad. Sci., 261:4282 (1965).
251. Chany, C., and Brailovsky, C., Proc. Nat. Acad. Sci., USA, 57:87 (1967).
252. Cohn, Z. A., and Benson, B., J. Exp. Med., 121:153 (1965).
253. Cotito, C., De Maeyer, E., and De Somer, P , Life Sci., 12:753 (1962).
254. Cocito, C., De Maeyer, E., and De Somer, P., Life Sci., 12:759 (1962).
255. Cogniaux-Le Clerk, J., Levy, A. H., and Wagner, R. R., Virology, 28:497 (1966).
256. Craighead, S. F., Brit. J. Exp. Path., 47:235 (1966).
257. Deinhardt, F., and Burnside, J., Inform. Exch. Gr., Vol. 6 (1966).
258. De Maeyer, E., and De Maeyer, J., Nature, 197:724 (1963).
259. De Maeyer, E., and Enders, J. R., Arch. Ges. Virusforsch., 16:151 (1965).
260. De Maeyer, E., and Enders, J. R., Proc. Soc. Exp. Biol. Med., 107:573 (1961).
261. De Maeyer, E., and De Maeyer-Guignard, J., Virology, 20:536 (1963).
262. De Maeyer-Guignard, J., and De Maeyer, E., J. Nat. Cancer Inst., 34:265 (1965).
263. De Maeyer-Guignard, J., and De Maeyer, E., Nature, 205:985 (1965).
264. De Maeyer, E., and De Maeyer-Guignard, J., J. Nat. Cancer Inst., 32:1317 (1964).
265. De Maeyer, E., and De Somer, P., Nature, 194:1252 (1962).
266. Denys, P., Lancet, 2:174 (1963).
267. Denys, P., De Somer, P., and Prinzie, A., Antonie van Leeuwenhoek J. Microbiol. Serol., 27:261 (1961).
268. De Somer, P., and Billian, A., Arch. Ges. Virusforsch., 19:112 (1966).
269. De Somer, P., De Clercq, E., Schone, E., and Billiau, A., Inform. Exch. Gr., Vol. 6 (1966).
270. De Somer, P., Prinzie, A., Denys, P. J., and Schone, E., Virology, 16:63 (1962).
271. Diderholm, H., Arch. Ges. Virusforsch., 14:39 (1963).
272. Diderholm, H., and Dinter, Z., Proc. Soc. Exp. Biol. Med., 121:976 (1966).
273. Dinter, Z., and Philipson, L., Proc. Soc. Exp. Biol. Med., 109:893 (1962).
274. Duc-Nguyen, H., and Henle, W., J. Bact., 92:258 (1966).
275. Ermolieva, Z. V., and Furer, N. M., Proc. Microb. Res. Group, Hung. Acad. Sci., 2:49 (1968).
276. Falcoff, E., Proc. Microb. Res. Group, Hung. Acad. Sci., 2:43 (1968).
277. Falcoff, E., Falcoff, R., Fournier, F., and Chany, C., Ann. Inst. Pasteur, 111:562 (1966).
278. Falcoff, E., and Fauconnier, B., Proc. Soc. Exp. Biol. Med., 118:609 (1965).
279. Falcoff, E., Fournier, F., and Chany, C., Ann. Inst. Pasteur, 111:241 (1966).
280. Falcoff, E., Gresser, J., and Chany, C., C. R. Acad. Sci., 258:1096 (1964).

281. Falcoff, E., Levy, H., Colin, J., and Chany, C., C. R. Acad. Sci., 260:5405 (1965).
282. Fantes, K. H., in: Interferons, North Holland, Amsterdam (1966), p. 119.
283. Finter, N. B., Virology, 24:589 (1964).
284. Finter, N. B., Brit. Med. J., 2:981 (1964).
285. Finter, N. B., Nature, 204:1114 (1964).
286. Finter, N. B., J. Hyg. (Camb.), 62:337 (1964).
287. Finter, N. B., Nature, 206:597 (1965).
288. Finter, N. B., Brit. J. Exp. Path., 47:361 (1966).
289. Finter, N. B., in: Interferons, Amsterdam (1966), p. 232.
290. Finter, N. B., in: Interferon. Ciba Foundation Symposium, London (1968), p. 204.
291. Fitzgerald, G. R., and Pollard, M., Proc. Soc. Exp. Biol. Med., 126:245 (1967).
292. Force, E. E., Stewart, R. C., and Haff, R. F., Virology, 25:322 (1965).
293. Freshman, M., Merigan, T., Remington, J., and Brownlee, J., Inform. Exch. Gr., Vol. 6 (1966).
294. Friedman, R. M., Nature, 201:848 (1964).
295. Friedman, R. M., J. Immunol., 96:872 (1966).
296. Friedman, R. M., Baron, S., Buckler, C. E., and Steinmuller, R. J., J. Exp. Med., 116:347 (1962).
297. Friedman, R. M., and Cooper, H. L., Proc. Soc. Exp. Biol. Med., 125:901 (1967).
298. Friedman, R. M., Rabson, A. S., and Kirkham, W. R., Proc. Soc. Exp. Biol. Med., 112:347 (1963).
299. Freidman, R. M., and Rabson, A. S., J. Exp. Med., 119:71 (1964).
300. Friedman, R. M., and Sonnabend, J. A., Nature, 206:532 (1965).
301. Fruitstone, M. J., Michaels, B. S., Rudloff, D., and Sigel, M.M., Proc. Soc. Exp. Biol. Med., 122:1008 (1966).
302. Fruitstone, M. J., Waddel, G. H., and Sigel, M. M., Proc. Soc. Exp. Biol. Med., 117:804 (1964).
303. Gifford, G. E., J. Gen. Microbiol., 33:437 (1963).
304. Gifford, G. E., Proc. Soc. Exp. Biol. Med., 114:644 (1963).
305. Gifford, G. E., Nature, 200:91 (1963).
306. Gifford, G. E., and Heller, E., Nature, 200:50 (1963).
307. Gifford, G. E., Mussett, M. V., and Heller, E., J. Gen. Microbiol., 34:475 (1964).
308. Glasgow, L. A., J. Exp. Med., 121:153 (1965).
309. Glasgow, L. A., J. Exp. Med., 121:1001 (1965).
310. Glasgow, L. A., J. Pediat., 67:104 (1965).
311. Glasgow, L. A., J. Bact., 91:2185 (1966).
312. Glasgow, L. A., and Habel, K., J. Exp. Med., 115:503 (1962).
313. Glasgow, L. A., and Habel, K., J. Exp. Med., 117:149 (1963).
314. Glasgow, L. A., Hanshaw, J. B., Merigan, T. C., and Petralli, J. K., Proc. Soc. Exp. Biol. Med., 125:843 (1967).
315. Glasky, A. J., Simon, L., and Holper, J. C., Science, 144:1581 (1964).
316. Gledhill, A. W., Brit. J. Exp. Path., 40:195 (1959).
317. Gordon, J., Chenault, S., Stevenson, D., and Acton, J., J. Bact., 91:1230 (1966).
318. Gotlieb-Stematsky, T., Rotem, Z., and Karby, S., J. Nat. Cancer Inst., 37:99 (1966).

319. Gresser, I., Proc. Soc. Exp. Biol. Med., 108:799 (1961).
320. Gresser, I., Proc. Soc. Exp. Biol. Med., 108:303 (1961).
321. Gresser, I., Proc. Nat. Acad. Sci., USA, 47:1817 (1961).
322. Gresser, I., and Chany, C., J. Immunol., 92:889 (1964).
323. Gresser, I., Coppey, J., Falcoff, E., and Fontaine, D., Proc. Soc. Exp. Biol., 124:84 (1967).
324. Gresser, I., and Dull, H. B., Proc. Soc. Exp. Biol. Med., 115:192 (1964).
325. Gresser, I., and Enders, J. F., Virology, 16:428 (1962).
326. Gresser, I., Fontaine, D., Coppey, J., Falcoff, R., and Falcoff, E., Proc. Soc. Exp. Biol. Med., 124:91 (1967).
327. Gresser, I., and Naficy, K., Proc. Soc. Exp. Biol. Med., 117:285 (1964).
328. Grossberg, S. E., and Scherer, W., Am. J. Path., 45:519 (1964).
329. Hallum, J. V., Younger, J. S., and Stinebring, W. R., Virology, 27:429 (1965).
330. Hanna, L., Merigan, T. C., and Jawetz, E., Proc. Soc. Exp. Biol. Med., 122:417 (1966).
331. Harsfall, F. L., and McCarthy, M., J. Exp. Med., 85:623 (1947).
332. Heineberg, H., J. Pediat., 63:728 (1963).
333. Heineberg, H., Gold, E., and Robbins, F. C., Proc. Soc. Exp. Biol. Med., 115:947 (1964).
334. Heller, E., Biochem. J., 87:456 (1963).
335. Henderson, J. R., and Taylor, R. M., Virology, 13:477 (1961).
336. Henle, W., Henle, G., Deinhardt, F., and Bergs, V. V., J. Exp. Med., 110:525 (1959).
337. Henslova, E., and Libikova, H., Acta Virol., 10:475 (1966).
338. Hermodsson, S., Virology, 20:333 (1963).
339. Hermodsson, S., Acta Path. Microbiol. Scand., 2:224 (1964).
340. Hermodsson, S., and Philipson, L., Proc. Soc. Exp. Biol. Med., 114:574 (1963).
341. Hilleman, M. R., Am. J. Med., 38:751 (1965).
342. Hitchcock, G., and Isaacs, A., Brit. Med. J., 2:1268 (1960).
343. Hitchcock, G., and Porterfield, J. S., Virology, 13:363 (1961).
344. Ho, M., Virology, 17:262 (1962).
345. Ho, M., Proc. Soc. Exp. Biol. Med., 112:511 (1963).
346. Ho, M., Bact. Rev., 28:367 (1964).
347. Ho, M., Science, 146:1472 (1964).
348. Ho, M., Jap. J. Exp. Med., 37:169 (1967).
349. Ho, M., and Breinig, M. K., J. Immunol., 89:177 (1962).
350. Ho, M., and Breinig, M. K., Virology, 25:331 (1965).
351. Ho, M., and Enders, J. F., Proc. Nat. Acad. Sci., USA, 45:385 (1959).
352. Ho, M., and Enders, J. F., Virology, 3:446 (1959).
353. Ho, M., and Kono, J., Proc. Nat. Acad. Sci., USA, 53:220 (1965).
354. Ho, M., and Kono, J., J. Clin. Invest., 44:1059 (1965).
355. Ho, M., and Köhler, K., Arch. Ges. Virusforsch., 22:69 (1967).
356. Ho, M., Kono, J., and Breinig, M. K., Proc. Soc. Exp. Biol. Med., 119:1227 (1965).
357. Ho, M., and Postic, B., Nature, 214:1230 (1967).
358. Ho, M., Postic, B., and Ke, J. H., in: Interferon, Ciba Foundation Symposium, London (1968), p. 19.

359. Hopps, H. E., Kohno, S., Kohno, M., and Smadel, J. E., Bact. Proc. (1964), p. 115.
360. Hook, E., and Wogner, R., J. Immunol., 83:310 (1959).
361. Inglot, A. D., Lobadzinska, M., Biernacka, J., and Niedzwiedska, E., Arch. Immun. Ther. Exp., 14:333 (1966).
362. Isaacs, A., Virology, 9:56 (1959).
363. Isaacs, A., New Scientist, 14:213 (1962).
364. Isaacs, A., Bull. Schweiz. Akad. Med. Wiss., 17:477 (1962).
365. Isaacs, A., Cold Spring Harbor Symp. Quant. Biol.
366. Isaacs, A., Advances in Virus Res., 10:1 (1963).
367. Isaacs, A., Proc. Roy: Soc. Med 55:725 (1962).
368. Isaacs, A., and Baron, S., Lancet, 2:946 (1960).
369. Isaacs, A., and Burke, D. C., Nature, 182:1073 (1958).
370. Isaacs, A., Cox, H. R., and Rotem, Z., Lancet, 2:113 (1963).
371. Isaacs, A., and Hitchcock, G., Lancet, 2:69 (1960).
372. Isaacs, A., and Lindenmann, J., Proc. Roy. Soc. B, 147:258 (1957).
373. Isaacs, A., Lindenmann, J., and Valentine, P., Proc. Roy, Soc. B., 147:268 (1957).
374. Isaacs, A., Klemperer, H. G., and Hitchcock, G., Virology, 13:191 (1961).
375. Isaacs, A., Rotem, Z., and Fantes, K. H., Virology, 29:248 (1966).
376. Isaacs, A., and Westwood, M. A., Nature, 184:1232 (1959).
377. Isaacs, A., and Westwood, M. A., Lancet, 2:324 (1959).
378. Ianowska, I., Biul. Inst. Weteryn., Putawash., 9:7 (1965).
379. Jao, R. L., Wheelock, E. F., and Jackson, G. G., J. Clin. Invest., 44:1062 (1965).
380. Jenkin, A., and Lin, J., in: Proceedings of the 66th Annual Meeting of the American Society of Microbiologists, May (1966).
381. Jensen, K. E., Neal, A. L., Owens, R. E., and Warren, J., Nature, 200:433 (1963).
382. Jensen, M. M., and Rasmussen, A. F., J. Immunol., 90:31 (1963).
383. Johnson, T., and McLaren, L., J. Bact., 90:565 (1965).
384. Joklick, W. K., and Merigan, T. C., Proc. Nat. Acad. Sci., USA, 56:558 (1966).
385. Jones, B. R., Galbraith, J. E., and Al-Hussaini, M. R., Lancet, 1:875 (1962).
386. Jullien, P., and De Maeyer, E., Int. J. Rad. Biol., 11:567 (1966).
387. Kato, N., Okada, A., and Ota, F., Virology, 26:630 (1965).
388. Kato, N., Okada, A., and Ota, F., Arch. Ges. Virusforsch., 17:731 (1965).
389. Kato, N., and Ota, F., Arch. Ges. Virusforsch., 18:116 (1966).
390. Kato, N., Ota, F., and Okada, A., Virology, 28:785 (1966).
391. Kazar, J., Acta Virol., 10:277 (1966).
392. Ke, Y. H., Ho, M., and Merigan, T., Nature, 211:541 (1966).
393. Ke, Y. H., Singer, S. H., Postic, B., and Ho, M., Proc. Soc. Exp. Biol. Med., 121:181 (1966).
394. Kilbourne, E. D., Smart, K. M., and Pokorny, B., Nature, 190:650 (1961).
395. Kishida, T., Kalmata, J., Miyamoto, H., and Kato, S., Biken, J., 8:55 (1965).
396. Kishida, T., Kato, S., and Nagano, G., C. R. Soc. Biol., 159:782 (1965).
397. Kishida, T., Kawamata, J., Miyamoto, H., and Kato, S., C. R. Soc. Biol., 160:1765 (1966).
398. Kleinschmidt, W. J., Cline, J. C., and Murphy, E. B., Fed. Proc., 23:507 (1964).
399. Kleinschmidt, W. J., Cline, J. C., and Murphy, E. B., Proc. Nat. Acad. Sci., USA, 52:741 (1964).

400. Kleinschmidt, W. J., and Ellis, L. F., in: Interferon, Ciba Foundation Symposium, London (1968), p. 39.
401. Kleinschmidt, W. J., and Murphy, E. B., Virology, 27:484 (1965).
402. Kleinschmidt, W. J., and Murphy, E. B., Bact. Rev., 31:132 (1967).
403. Kono, Y., Proc. Soc. Exp. Biol. Med., 124:155 (1967).
404. Kono, Y., Arch. Ges. Virusforsch., 21:276 (1967).
405. Kono, Y., and Ho, M., Virology, 25:162 (1965).
406. Kreuz, L. E., and Levy, A. H., J. Bact., 89:462 (1965).
407. Lackovic, V., and Borecky, L., Arch. Ges. Virusforsch., 17:619 (1965).
408. Lackovic, V., and Borecky, L., Acta Virol., 10:365 (1966).
409. Lackovic, V., Borecky, L., Sikl, D., Masler, L., and Bauer, S., Acta Virol., 11:500 (1967).
410. Lampson, G. P., Tytell, A. A., Nemes, M. M., and Hilleman, M. R., Proc. Soc. Exp. Biol. Med., 112:468 (1963).
411. Lampson, G. P., Tytell, A. A., Nemes, M. M., and Hilleman, M. R., Proc. Soc. Exp. Biol. Med., 118:441 (1965).
412. Lampson, G. P., Tytell, A. A., Nemes, M. M., and Hilleman, M. R., Proc. Soc. Exp. Biol. Med., 121:377 (1966).
413. Larke, R. P. B., Proc. Soc. Exp. Biol. Med., 119:1234 (1965).
414. Larke, R. P. B., Canad. Med. Ass. J., 96:21 (1967).
415. Lavrov, S. V., Eremkina, E. J., Orlova, T. G., Gaiegow, G. A., Soloviev, V. D., and Zhdanov, V. M., Nature, 217:856 (1968).
416. Le Clerc, J., L., Cogniaux-Le Clerc, J., Acta Virol., 9:18 (1965).
417. Ledinko, L., Virology, 20:29 (1963).
418. Lee, S. H., Lewis, R. V., and van Rooyen, C. E., Interferon Sci. (1967).
419. Lee, S. H. S., and Ozere, R. L., Proc. Soc. Exp. Biol. Med., 118:190 (1965).
420. Lee, S. H. S., Ozere, R. L., and van Rooyen, C. E., Proc. Soc. Exp. Biol. Med., 122:32 (1966).
421. Levine, S., Proc. Soc. Exp. Biol. Med., 121:1041 (1966).
422. Levy, H., and Carter, W., Inform. Exch. Gr., Vol. 6 (1966).
423. Levy, H. B., and Merigan, T. C., Proc. Soc. Exp. Biol. Med., 121:53 (1966).
424. Levy, H. B., Shnellbaker, L. F., and Baron, S., Virology, 21:48 (1963).
425. Levy, H. B., Shnellbaker, L. F., and Baron, S., Life Sci., 3:204 (1963).
426. Levy, H. B., Shnellbaker, L., and Baron, S., Proc. Soc. Exp. Biol. Med., 121:630 (1966).
427. Libikova, H., Acta Virol., 9:279 (1965).
428. Lindemann, J., Z. Mittschr. Hyg., 146:287 (1960).
429. Lindemann, J., Burke, D. C., and Isaacs, A., Brit. J. Exp. Path., 38:551 (1957).
430. Lindemann, J., and Gifford, G. E., Virology, 19:283 (1963).
431. Lindemann, J., and Gifford, G. E., Virology, 19:302 (1963).
432. Link, F., Blaskovic, D., and Raus, J., Nature, 197:821 (1963).
433. Link, F., Blaskovic, D., and Raus, J., Acta Virol., 9:95 (1965).
434. Lockart, R. Z., J. Bact., 85:556 (1963).
435. Lockart, R. Z., J. Bact., 89:117 (1965).
436. Lockart, R. Z., and Horn, B., J. Bact., 85:996 (1963).
437. Lucas, B., and Hruskova, J., Acta Virol., 12:257 (1968).

438. Lwoff, A., Proceedings of the 9th International Congress of Microbiologists, Moscow (1966).
439. Lwoff, A., and Lwoff, M., Ann. Inst. Pasteur, 98:173 (1960).
440. Lwoff, A., Tournier, P., Lwoff, M., and Cathale, P., C. R. Acad. Sci., 250:2644 (1960).
441. Mahdy, S., and Ho, M., Proc. Soc. Exp. Biol. Med., 116:174 (1964).
442. Mao Chieng-shen and Huang Chen-hsiung, Acta Microbiol. Sinica, 11:326 (1965).
443. Marcus, P. J., and Salb, J. M., Virology, 30:502 (1966).
444. Mayer, V., Acta Virol., 6:92 (1962).
445. Mayer, V., Sokol, F., and Vilcek, J., Acta Virol., 5:264 (1961).
446. Mayer, V., Sokol, F., and Vilcek, J., Virology, 16:359 (1962).
447. Mayer, V., Zemla, J., and Vilcek, J., Acta Virol., 5:130 (1961).
448. Mecs, E., Acta Virol., 8:475 (1964).
448a. Melnick, J. L., and McCombs, R. M., Progr. Med. Virol., 8:400 (1966).
449. Mendelson, J., and Finland, M., Proc. Soc. Exp. Biol. Med., 123:98 (1966).
450. Mendelson, J., and Glasgow, L., J. Immunol., 96:345 (1966).
451. Merigan, T. C., Science, 145:811 (1964).
452. Merigan, T. C., Bact. Proc., (1966), p. 119.
453. Merigan, T. C., Clin. Res., 14:144 (1966).
454. Merigan, T. C., Nature, 1:416 (1967).
455. Merigan, T. C., in: Interferon, Ciba Foundation Symposium, London (1968), p. 50.
456. Merigan, T. C., Bact. Rev., 31:138 (1967).
457. Merigan, T. C., Gregory, D. F., and Petralli, J. K., Virology, 29:515 (1966).
458. Merigan, T. C., and Hanna, L., Proc. Soc. Exp. Biol. Med., 122:421 (1966).
459. Merigan, T. C., and Kleinschmidt, W. J., Nature, 208:667 (1965).
460. Merigan, T. C., and Regelson, W., Clin. Res., 15:3 (1967).
461. Merigan, T. C., Winget, C. A., and Dixon, C. B., J. Mol. Biol., 13:679 (1965).
462. Michaels, R. H., Weinberger, M. M., and Ho, M., New Eng. J. Med., 272:1148 (1965).
463. Nagano, Y., Jap. J. Exp. Med., 37:183 (1967).
464. Nagano, Y., and Kojima, Y., Compt. Rend. Soc. Biol., 162:1627 (1958).
465. Nagano, Y., Kojima, Y., and Suraki, T., Compt. Rend. Soc. Biol., 154:2166 (1960).
466. Nagano, Y., and Kojima, Y., Compt. Rend. Soc. Biol., 154:2172 (1960).
467. Nagano, Y., and Kojima, Y., Compt. Rend. Soc. Biol., 155:1183 (1961).
468. Nagano, Y., Kojima, Y., Arakawa, J., and Kanashiro, R., Jap. J. Exp. Med., 36:481 (1966).
469. Nagano, Y., Kojima, Y., Oda, M., Kim, T., Shirasaka, M., and Haneshi, T., Compt. Rend. Soc. Biol., 159:280 (1965).
470. Nagata, J., Kunii, A., and Ono, S., Inform. Exch. Gr., Vol. 6 (1967).
471. Neal, A. L., Jensen, K. E., and Warren, J., Fed. Proc., 23:507 (1964).
472. Nava, F. A., and Weller, T., J. Immunol., 93:466 (1964).
473. Miner, N., Ray, J., Jr., and Simon, E. H., Biochem. Biophys. Res. Commun., 24:204 (1966).
474. Oh, J. O., Proc. Soc. Exp. Biol. Med., 123:493 (1966).
475. Oh, J. O., and Gill, E. J., J. Bact., 91:251 (1966).

476. Ohno, S., and Nozima, T., Acta Virol., 10:310 (1966).
477. Osborn, J. E., and Medearis, D. N., Proc. Soc. Exp. Biol. Med., 121:819 (1966).
478. Osborn, J., and Medearis, D., Proc. Soc. Exp. Biol. Med., 124:347 (1967).
479. Oxman, M., Baron, S., Black, P., Takemoto, K., Habel, K., and Rowe, W., Virology, 32:122 (1967).
480. Paucker, K., J. Immunol., 94:371 (1965).
481. Paucker, K., and Boxaca, M., Ann. Med. Exp. Fenn., 44:274 (1966).
482. Paucker, K., and Cantell, K., Virology, 18:145 (1962).
483. Paucker, K., and Cantell, K., Virology, 21:22 (1963).
484. Paucker, K., Cantell, K., and Henle, W., Virology, 17:324 (1962).
485. Paucker, K., Skurska, L., and Henle, W., Virology, 17:301 (1962).
486. Pereira, J. G., Virology, 11:590 (1960).
487. Peries, J., Boiron, M., and Canivet, M., Ann. Inst. Pasteur, 109:595 (1965).
488. Petralli, J. K., Merigan, T. C., and Wilbur, J. K., New Engl. J. Med.,273:198 (1965
489. Petralli, J. K., Merigan, T. C., and Wilbur, J. K., Lancet, 2:401 (1965).
490. Phillips, A. W., and Wood, R. D., Nature, 201:319 (1964).
491. Phillipson, L., and Dinter, Z., J. Gen. Microbiol., 32:277 (1963).
492. Pollikoff, R., Inform. Exch. Gr., Vol. 6 (1967).
493. Pollikoff, R., Donikian, M. A., Paaron, A., and Lin, O. C., Proc. Soc. Exp. Biol. Med., 110:232 (1962).
494. Pollikoff, R., Donikian, M. A., and Lin, O. C., Bact. Proc. (1961), p. 158.
495. Pollikoff, R., Lieberman, M., and Lem, N. E., Proc. Soc. Exp. Biol. Med., 119:790 (1965).
496. Porterfield, J. S., Lancet, 2:326 (1959).
497. Porterfield, J. S., Burke, D. C., and Allison, A. C., Virology, 12:197 (1960).
498. Portnoy, B., et al., Am. J Med. Sci., 248:521 (1964).
499. Postic, B., Doctoral Dissertation, Univ. Pittsburgh (1965), pp. 1-123.
500. Postic, B., De Angelis, C., Breinig, M. K., and Ho, M., J. Bact., 91:1277 (1966).
501. Postic, B., De Angelis, C., Breinig, M. K., and Ho, M., Proc. Soc. Exp. Biol. Med., 125:89 (1967).
502. Postic, B., Singer, S. H., and Ho, M., Fed. Proc., 23:193 (1964).
503. Powell, H. M., Culbertson, C. G., McGuire, J. M., Hoehn, M. M., and Baker, L. A., Antibiot. Chemother., 2:432 (1952).
503a. Provisional Committee for Nomenclature of Viruses. Ann. Inst. Pasteur, 109:625 (1965).
504. Regelson, W., Proc. Intern. Symp. Atheros. Retic. Endoh. System, Italy, Sept. 1966.
505. Ray, C. C., Gravelle, C. R., and Chin, T. D. J., Bact. Proc. (1966), p. 124.
506. Ray, C. G., Gravelle, C. R., and Chin, T. D. J., J. Pediat., 71:27 (1967).
507. Reinicke, V., Acta Path. Microbiol. Scand., 60:528 (1964).
508. Reinicke, V., Acta Path. Microbiol. Scand., 64:339 (1965).
509. Reinicke, V., Acta Path. Microbiol. Scand., 64:543 (1965).
510. Reinicke, V., Acta Path. Microbiol. Scand., 64:553 (1965).
511. Riley, B., and Gifford, G., Inform. Exch. Gr., Vol. 6 (1966).
512. Riley, B., Toy, S., and Gifford, G., Proc. Soc. Exp. Biol. Med., 122:1142 (1966).
513. Rossum, W. V., and De Somer, P., Life Sci., 5:105 (1966).
514. Rotem, Z., Beewald, G., and Sachs, L., Virology, 24:483 (1964).

515. Rotem, Z., Cox, R. A., and Isaacs, A., Nature, 197:564 (1963).
516. Ruiz-Gomez, J., and Isaacs, A., Virology, 19:1 (1963).
517. Ruiz-Gomez, J., and Isaacs, A., Virology, 19:8 (1963).
518. Ruiz-Gomez, J., and Sosa-Martinez, J., Arch. Ges. Virusforsch., 17:295 (1965).
519. Russell, P. K., Bellanti, J. A., Buescher, E. L., and McCown, J. M., Proc. Soc. Exp. Biol. Med., 122:557 (1966).
520. Rytel, M., and Jones, T. C., Proc. Soc. Exp. Biol. Med., 123:859 (1966).
521. Rytel, M. W., and Kilbourne, E. D., J. Exp. Med., 123:767 (1966).
522. Rytel, M. W., Shope, R. E., and Kilbourne, E. D., J. Exp. Med., 123:577 (1966).
523. Sadiskis, R. J., and Schultz, J., J. Infect. Dis., 116:455 (1966).
524. Salzman, N. P., Shatkin, A. J., and Schring, E. D., J. Mol. Biol., 8:405 (1964).
525. Sandelin, Karin, Acta Path. Microbiol. Scand., Suppl. 154:143 (1962).
526. Sawicki, L., Nature, 192:1258 (1961).
527. Sawicki, L., Acta Virol., 6:347 (1962).
528. Scientific Committee on Interferon, Lancet, 1:873 (1962).
529. Schonne, E., Biochem. Biophys. Acta, 115:429 (1966).
530. Schulman, J. L., and Kilbourne, E. D., Proc. Soc. Exp. Biol. Med., 113:431 (1963).
531. Scientific Committee on Interferon, Lancet, 1:505 (1965).
532. Seymour, L., Virology, 17:593 (1962).
533. Sellers, R. F., Nature, 198:1228 (1963).
534. Sellers, R. F., J. Immunol., 93:6 (1964).
535. Sellers, R. F., and Fitzpatrick, M., Brit. J. Exp. Path., 43:674 (1962).
536. Sellers, R. F., and Fitzpatrick, M., Res. Veterin. Sci., 4:151 (1963).
537. Shope, R. E., J. Exp. Med., 123:213 (1966).
538. Smart, K. M., and Kilbourne, E. D., J. Exp. Med., 23:309 (1966).
539. Smith, T., and Wagner, R., J. Exp. Med., 125:559 (1967).
540. Smith, T., and Wagner, R., J. Exp. Med., 125:579 (1967).
541. Sonnabend, J. A., Nature, 203:496 (1964).
542. Sonnabend, J., Martin, E., and Mecs, E., J. Gen. Virol., 1:41 (1967).
543. Stancek, D., Acta Virol., 9:298 (1965).
544. Stancek, D., Acta Virol., 10:406 (1966).
545. Stancek, D., and Vilcek, J., Acta Virol., 9:1 (1965).
546. Stancek, D., and Vilcek, J., Acta Virol., 9:9 (1965).
547. Stewart, W. E., and Sulkin, S. E., Proc. Soc. Exp. Biol. Med., 123:650 (1966).
548. Stinebring, W. R., and Youngner, J. S., Nature, 204:712 (1964).
549. Strander, H., and Cantell, K., Ann. Med. Exp. Biol. Fenn., 44:265 (1966).
550. Strander, H., and Cantell, K., Proceedings of the 9th International Congress of Microbiologists, Moscow (1966), p. 560.
551. Strander, H., and Cantell, K., Ann. Med. Exp. Biol. Fenn., 45:20 (1967).
552. Strandström, H., Sandelin, K., and Oker-Blom, N., Virology, 16:384 (1962).
553. Subrahmanyan, T. P., and Mims, C. A., Brit. J. Exp. Path., 47:168 (1966).
554. Sutton, R. N. P., and Tyrell, D. A. J., Brit. J. Exp. Path., 42:99 (1961).
555. Takano, K., Warren, J., and Jensen, K. E., Fed. Proc., 23:507 (1964).
556. Takano, K., Jensen, K. E., and Warren, J., Proc. Soc. Exp. Biol. Med., 114:472 (1963).
557. Tokumaru, T., Arch. Ges. Virusforsch., 21:61 (1967).

558. Tomilla, V., Acta Ophtalm., 41:478 (1963).

559. Tyrell, D. A. J., Nature, 184:452 (1959).

560. Vaczi, L., Horvath, E., and Hadhory, G., Acta Microbiol. Acad. Sci. Hung., 12:345 (1965-1966).

561. Vainio, T., Gwatkin, R., and Koprowski, H., Virology, 14:385 (1961).

562. Vandeputte, M., De Lafonteyne, J., Billiau, A., and De Somer, P., Arch. Ges. Virusforsch., 20:235 (1967).

563. Versteeg, J., Proc. Koninkl. Nederl. Acad., 67:49 (1964).

564. Versteeg, J., Proc. Kon. Ned. Akad. Wet. Ser. C, 70:3 (1967).

565. Valle, M., and Cantell, K., Ann. Med. Exp. Fenn., 43:57 (1965).

566. Vilček, J., Acta Virol., 5:278 (1961).

567. Vilček, J., Nature, 187:73 (1960).

568. Vilček, J., Acta Virol., 4:308 (1960).

569. Vilček, J., Acta Virol., 6:144 (1962).

570. Vilček, J., Acta Virol., 7:107 (1963).

571. Vilček, J., Uspekhi Sovr. Biol., 55:391 (1963).

572. Vilček, J., Virology, 22:651 (1964).

573. Vilček, J., Towisova, J., Sokol, F., and Hanna, L., Acta Virol., 8:76 (1964).

574. Vilček, J., and Rada, B., Acta Virol., 6:9 (1962).

575. Vilček, J., and Stancek, D., Acta Virol., 7:331 (1963).

576. Volkman, A., J. Exp. Med., 124:241 (1966).

577. Wagner, R. R., Bact. Rev., 24:151 (1960).

578. Wagner, R. R., Virology, 13:323 (1961).

579. Wagner, R. R., Virology, 19:215 (1963).

580. Wagner, R. R., Immunol., 91:112 (1963).

581. Wagner, R. R., Nature, 204:49 (1964).

582. Wagner, R. R., Postgrad. Med., 35:512 (1964).

583. Wagner, R. R., Am. J. Med., 38:726 (1965).

584. Wagner, R. R., and Huang, A. S., Virology, 28:1 (1966).

585. Wagner, R., and Huang, A. S., Proc. Nat. Acad. Sci., USA, 54:1112 (1965).

586. Wagner, R., and Levy, H., Ann. N. Y. Acad. Sci., 88:1308 (1960).

587. Wagner, R., and Snyder, S., Nature, 196:393 (1962).

588. Wagner, R. R., Snyder, R. M., Hook, E. W., and Luttrell, C. H., J. Immunol., 83:87 (1959).

589. Wagner, R., and Wood, W. B., Trans. Assoc. Am. Phys., 76:92 (1963).

590. Wei Wen-pin, An Ch'ing-on, and Ch'ing Lo-huai, Acta Microb. Sinica, 12:33 (1966).

591. Wheelock, E. F., Proc. Soc. Exp. Biol. Med., 117:650 (1964).

592. Wheelock, E. F., Science, 149:310 (1965).

593. Wheelock, E. F., Inform. Exch. Gr., Vol. 6 (1966).

594. Wheelock, E. F., Inform. Exch. Gr., Vol. 6 (1966).

595. Wheelock, E. F., Proc. Soc. Exp. Biol. Med., 124:855 (1967).

596. Wheelock, E. F., and Dingle, J. H., New Engl. J. Med., 271:645 (1964).

597. Wheelock, E. F., and Sibley, W. A., Lancet, 2:382 (1964).

598. Wheelock, E. F., and Sibley, W. A., New Engl. J. Med., 273:194 (1965).

599. Zemla, J., and Vilček, J., Acta Virol., 5:129 (1961).

600. Zemla, J., and Vilček, J., Acta Virol., 5:367 (1961).
601. Youngner, J. S., and Kelly, M. E., J. Bact., 90:443 (1965).
602. Youngner, J. S., Scoff, A. W., Hallum, J. V., and Stinebring, W. R., J. Bact., 92:862 (1966).
603. Youngner, J. S., and Stinebring, W. R., Science, 144:1022 (1964).
604. Youngner, J. S., and Stinebring, W. R., Nature, 208:456 (1965).
605. Youngner, J. S., and Stinebring, W. R., Virology, 29:310 (1966).
606. Youngner, J. S., Stinebring, W. R., and Taube, S. E., Virology, 27:541 (1965).
607. Aksenov, O. A., Golovin, B. P., and Smorodintsev, A. A., in: Interferon, Leningrad (1970), p. 69.
608. Bektemirova, M. S., The Study of the Formation and Action of Interferon in Experimental Rabies, Candidate's Dissertation, Moscow (1970).
609. Bektemirov, T. A., Gumennik, A. E., and Bektemirova, M. S., Vopr. Virusol., No. 6, 709 (1968).
610. Bektemirov, T. A., Shenkman, L. S., and Marennikova, S. S., Vopr. Virusol., No. 5, 555 (1971).
611. Vorob'eva, M. S., Selimov, M. A., and Safarov, R. K., in: Proceedings of the 13th Session of the Institute of Poliomyelitis and Virus Encephalitis, Moscow (1967), p. 70.
612. Gaidamovich, S. Ya., and Agrba, V. Z., Vopr. Virusol., No. 5, 569 (1970).
613. Germanov, A. B., Rudneva, P. A., and Sokolov, M. I., Vopr. Virusol., No. 2, 166 (1970).
614. Zdrodovskii, P. F., Problems in Infection and Immunity, Medgiz, Moscow (1961).
615. Zeitlenok, N. A., Bresler, S. E., Vil'ner, L. M., Tikhomirova-Sidorova, N. S., Brodskaya, I. M., and Alpatova, G. A., in: Current Problems in Virus Infections, Moscow (1968), p. 21.
615a. Kasparov, A. A., Vestn. Oftal'mol., No. 2, 63 (1972).
615b. Kursinova, L. A., Bukharina, E. A., Makarova, G. I., and Neklyudova, L. I., Vopr. Virusol., No. 2, 194 (1971).
616. Marennikova, S. S., Svet-Moldavskaya, I. A., and Mal'tseva, N. N., Vopr. Virusol., No. 5, 579 (1969).
617. Marennikova, S. S., and Tashpulatov, G. M., Vopr. Virusol., No. 3, 266 (1966).
618. Novokhatskii, A. S., in: Problems in General Virology, Part 1, Moscow (1971), p. 129.
619. Oganesyan, R. Kh., Tikhonenko, T. I., Nikol'skaya, I. I., and Fadeeva, L. I., in: General Virology, Moscow (1968), p. 58.
620. Smorodintsev, A. A., Jr., The Theory and Practice of Interferon Induction, Doctoral Dissertation, Leningrad (1970).
621. Solov'ev, V. D., Bektemirov, T. A., Karakuyumchan, M. K., and Bektemirova, M. S., Vopr. Virusol., No. 4, 419 (1970).
622. Solov'ev, V. D., Neklyudova, L. I., Bektemirov, T. A., and Fedorova, Yu. B., Vopr. Virusol., No. 5, 548 (1971).
623. Tazulakhova, E. B., and Ershov, F. I., in: Problems in General Virology, Part 1, Moscow (1971), p. 131.
624. Khalyapina, T. K., in: Problems in Infectious Pathology and Immunology, No. 1, 28 (1949).

625. Shubladze, A. K., and Maevskaya, T. M., Vopr. Virusol., No. 1, 73 (1966).

626. Armstrong, R. W., Gurwith, M. J., Waddel, D., and Merigan, T. C., New Engl. J. Med., 283:1182 (1970).

627. Banks, G. T., Buck, K. W., Chain, E. B., Himmelweit, F., Marks, J. E., Tyler, J. M., Hollings, M., Last, F. L., and Stone, O. M., Nature, 218:542 (1968).

628. Baron, S., Arch. Intern. Med., 126:184 (1970).

629. Baron, S., Bogomolova, N. N., Billiau, A., Levy, H. B., Buckler, C. E., Stern, R., and Naylor, R., Proc. Nat. Acad. Sci. (Washington), 64:67 (1969).

630. Barth, R. F., Friedman, M. R., and Malmgren, R. A., Lancet, 2:723 (1969).

631. Baugh, C. L., Tytell, A. A., and Hilleman, M. R., Interferon Sci. Memo., August (1971).

632. Belady, J., and Bakny, M., Acta Virol., 7:477 (1963).

633. Buckler, C., Billiau, E. A., Dianzani, F., Uhlendorf, C., and Baron, S., Fed. Proc., 28:503 (1969).

634. Catalano, L. W. J., Proc. Soc. Exp. Biol. (New York), 133:684 (1970).

635. Cathala, F., and Baron, S., J. Immunol., 104:1355 (1970).

635a. Chester, T. Y., De Clercq, E., Nuwer, M. R., and Merigan, T. C., Infect. and Immun., 5(3):383 (1972).

636. Colby, C., and Duesberg, P. H., Nature, 222:940 (1969).

637. De Clercq, E., Eckstein, F., and Merigan, T. C., Science, 165:1137 (1969).

638. De Clercq, E., and Merigan, T. C., Nature, 222:1148 (1969).

639. De Maeyer, E., and de Maeyer-Guignard, G., J. Gen. Virology, 2:445 (1968).

640. Depoux, R., C. R. Acad. Sci., 260:354 (1965).

641. Dianzani, F., Cantagalli, P., Gagnoni, S., and Rita, G., Personal communication (1968).

642. Falcoff, R., and Falcoff, E. T., Biochem. Biophys. Acta, 182:501 (1969).

643. Fenje, P., and Postic, B., Interferon Sci. Memo. 311/1 (1970).

644. Field, A. K., Tytell, A. A., Lampson, G. P., and Hilleman, M. R., Proc. Nat. Acad. Sci. (Washington), 61:340 (1968).

645. Field, A. K., Lampson, G. P., Tytell, A. A., Nemes, M. M., and Hilleman, M. R., Proc. Nat. Acad. Sci. (Washington), 58:2102 (1967).

646. Field, A. K., Tytell, A. A., Lampson, G. P., and Hilleman, M. R., Proc. Nat. Acad. Sci. (Washington), 58:1004 (1967).

647. Field, A. K., Young, C. W., Krakoff, J. H., Tytell, A. A., Lampson, G. P., Nemes, M. M., and Hilleman, M. R., Proc. Soc. Exp. Biol. (New York), 136:1180 (1971).

648. Finkelstein, M. S., Bausek, G. H., and Merigan, T. C., Science, 161:465 (1968).

649. Finter, N. B., Arch. Intern. Med., 126:147 (1970).

650. Glasgow, L. A., Arch. Intern. Med., 126:125 (1970).

651. Haahr, S., Acta Path. Microbiol. Scand., 77(1):167 (1969).

652. Henson, D., and Smith, R. D., Proc. Soc. Exp. Biol. (New York), 117:517 (1964).

653. Hill, D. A., Baron, S., Levy, H. B., Bellanti, J., Buckler, C. B., Cannelos, G., Carbone, P., Chanock, R. M., De Vita, Guggenheim, M. A., Homan, E., Kapikian, A. Z., Kirchstein, R. L., Mills, J., Perkins, J. C., Van Kirk, J. E., and Worthington, M., Interferon Sci. Memo., February (1970).

654. Hilleman, M. R., J. Cell. Physiol., 71:43 (1968).

655. Hilleman, M. R., "Prospects for the use of double-stranded RNA (poly I : C) inducers in man."

656. Hilleman, M. R., J. Infect. Dis., 121:196 (1970).

657. Hilleman, M. R., Lampson, G. P., Tytell, A. A., Field, A. K., Nemes, M. M.; Krakoff, J., and Young, C. W., in: Biological Effects of Polynucleotides, Springer Verlag, New York-Heidelberg-Berlin (1971), p. 27.

658. Hirsch, M. S., Murphy, F. A., Nahmias, A. J., and Kaye, H. S., Fed. Proc., 27(2):734 (1968).

659. Hirsch, M. S., Zisman, B., and Allison, A. C., J. Immunol., 104(5):1160 (1970).

659a. Ho, M., Tan, Y. H., and Armstrong, J. A., Proc. Soc. Exp. Biol. (New York), 139(1):259 (1972).

660. Hoffman, H., Radda, A., and Kunz, C., Arch. ges. Virusforsch., 28(2):197 (1969).

661. Inglot, A. D., Radzikowski, C., and Szkudlarek, J., Interferon Sci. Memo. 344/1 (1970).

662. Ipsen, J., J. Immunol., 83:4 (1959).

663. Janis, B., and Habel, K., Fed. Proc., 29:636 (1970).

664. Joshing, K., Taniguchi, S., and Arai, K., Proc. Soc. Exp. Biol. (New York), 123:387 (1966).

665. Kaplan, M. M., Weckler, E., Forsek, Z., and Koprowski, H., Nature, 186:821 (1960).

666. Kato, N., and Eggers, H., Virology, 37(4):545 (1969).

666a. Lab, M., and Koehren, F., Ann. Inst. Pasteur, 122(3):569 (1972).

667. Lampson, G. P., Field, A. K., Tytell, A. A., Nemes, M. M., and Hilleman, M. R., Proc. Soc. Exp. Biol. (New York) (1970).

668. Lampson, G. P., Field, A. K., Tytell, A. A., Nemes, M. M., and Hilleman, M. R., Proc. Nat. Acad. Sci. (Washington), 58:782 (1967).

669. Lampson, G. P., Field, A. K., Tytell, A. A., Nemes, M. M., and Hilleman, M. R., Proc. Soc. Exp. Biol. (New York), 132:212 (1969).

670. Larson, V. M., Clark, W. R., Dagle, G. E., and Hilleman, M. R., Proc. Soc. Exp. Biol. (New York), 132:602 (1969).

671. Larson, V. M., Clark, W. R., and Hilleman, M. R., Proc. Soc. Exp. Biol. (New York), 131:1002 (1969).

672. Larson, V. M., Panteleakis, P. N., and Hilleman, M. R., Proc. Soc. Exp. Biol. (New York), 133:14 (1970).

673. Levy, H. B., Law, L. W., and Rabson, A. S., Proc. Nat. Acad. Sci. (Washington), 62:357 (1969).

674. Maeno, K., Joshii, S., and Nagata, M., Virology, 29:255 (1966).

675. Matumoto, M., Jap. J. Microbiol., 12:505 (1968).

676. Merigan, T. C., Am. J. Med., 43:817 (1967).

677. Merigan, T. C., and Finkelstein, M. S., Virology, 35:363 (1968).

678. Merigan, T. C., and Regelson, W., New. Engl. J. Med., 272:1283 (1967).

678a. Morahan, P. S., Munson, A. E., Regelson, W., Commerford, S. L., and Hamilton, L. D., Proc. Nat. Acad. Sci. (Washington), 69:4842 (1972).

679. Nemes, M. M., Tytell, A. A., Lampson, G. P., Field, A. K., and Hilleman, M. R., Proc. Soc. Exp. Biol. (New York), 132:776 (1969).

680. Nemes, M. M., Tytell, A. A., Lampson, G. P., Field, A. K., and Hilleman, M. R., Proc. Soc. Exp. Biol. (New York), 132:784 (1969).

681. Niblack, J. F., Knirsch, A. K., and Vora, K. R. M., Interferon Sci. Memo., March (1970).

682. Oh, J. O., Interferon Sci. Memo., May (1971).

683. Park, M. J. H., and Baron, S., Science, 162:811 (1968).

684. Parkman, P. D., Phillips, P. E., and Kirschstein, R. L., J. Immunol., 95:743 (1965).

685. Pollikoff, R., Cannavale, P., Dixon, P., and Dipuppo, A., Bact. Proc. (1969).

686. Postic, B., and Fenje, P., Bact. Proc. (1970).

687. Sarma, M., Proc. Nat. Acad. Sci. (Washington), 62:1046 (1969).

688. Sheaff, E. T., and Stewart, R. B., Canad. J. Microbiol. 14(9):965 (1968).

689. Truden, J. L., and Siegel, M. M., Virology, 33:95 (1967).

690. Tytell, A. A., Lampson, G. P., Field, A. K., and Hilleman, M. R., Proc. Nat. Acad. Sci. (Washington), 58:1719 (1967).

691. Vaczi, L., Hadhazy, G. J., and Horvath, E., Inst. of Microbiol. University Med. School. Hung. (1967).

692. Vilček, J., Ng, M. H., Friedman-Kien, A. E., and Krawciw, T., J. Virology, 2:648 (1968).

693. Vilček, J. J., and Fermina, V., J. Gen. Virology, 13(1):185 (1971).

694. Wiktor, T. J., Fernandez, M. V., and Koprowski, H. J., Immunol., 93:353 (1964).

694a. Worthington, M., and Hasenclever, H. F., Infect. and Immun., 2:199 (1972).

695. Youngner, J. S., and Wertz, G., J. Virol., 2(11):1360 (1968).

696. Fedorova, G. I., Lavrov, S. V., Obrosova-Serova, N. P., Pushkarskaya, N. L., Slepushkin, A. N., Galegov, G. A., Shal'nov, M. I., Orlova, T. G., Rybakov, M. T., Zhdanov, V. M., and Solov'ev, V. D. General Virology. Proceedings of a Scientific Conference on the Study of Biosynthesis, Antimetabolites, and Chemotherapy of Viruses and Virus Infections, December 19-20, 1968. D. I. Ivanovskii Institute of Virology, Academy of Medical Sciences of the USSR, Moscow (1968), p. 80.

Index